AF841071

HERALDRY & STAINED GLASS AT APOTHECARIES' HALL

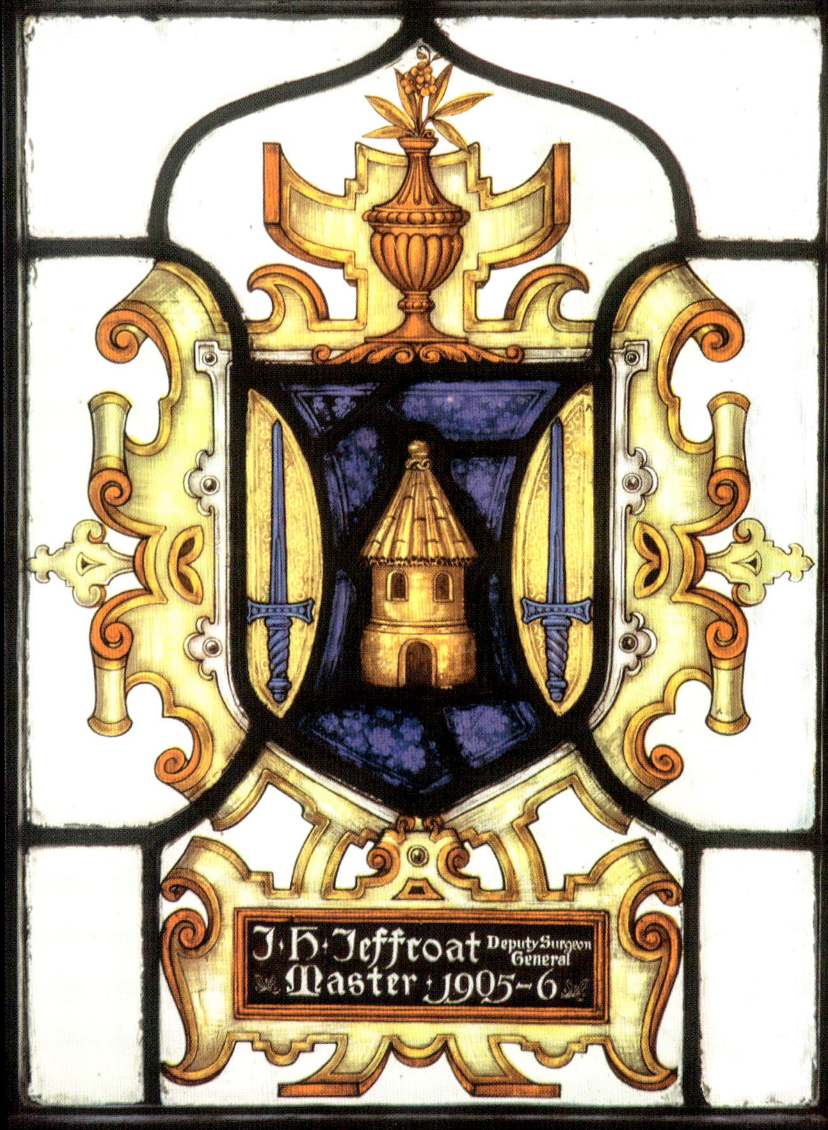
J·H·Jeffroat Deputy Surgeon General
Master 1905–6

HERALDRY & STAINED GLASS AT APOTHECARIES' HALL

WILLIAM SHAND &
ANDREW WALLINGTON-SMITH

PWP

PHILIP WILSON PUBLISHERS
Bloomsbury Publishing Plc
50 Bedford Square, London, WC1B 3DP, UK
1385 Broadway, 5th Floor, New York, NY 10018

BLOOMSBURY, PHILIP WILSON PUBLISHERS and the PHILIP WILSON logo are trademarks of Bloomsbury Publishing Plc

First published in Great Britain in 2020

Copyright © 2020 William Shand and Andrew Wallington-Smith

William Shand and Andrew Wallington-Smith have asserted their rights under the Copyright, Designs and Patents Act, 1988, to be identified as Authors of this work

All rights reserved. No part of this publication may be reproduced or transmitted in any form or by any means, electronic or mechanical, including photocopying, recording, or any information storage or retrieval system, without prior permission in writing from the publishers

Bloomsbury Publishing Plc does not have any control over, or responsibility for, any third-party websites referred to in this book. All internet addresses given in this book were correct at the time of going to press. The authors and publisher regret any inconvenience caused if addresses have changed or sites have ceased to exist, but can accept no responsibility for any such changes

A catalogue record for this book is available from the British Library

Library of Congress Cataloguing-in-Publication data has been applied for

ISBN: 978 1 78130 106 7

10 9 8 7 6 5 4 3 2 1

Designed and typeset in Adobe Jenson and Arno Pro by Christopher Bromley
Printed and bound in China by RR Donnelly Asia Printing Solutions Ltd

Bloomsbury Publishing Plc makes every effort to ensure that the papers used in the manufacture of our books are natural, recyclable products made from wood grown in well-managed forests. Our manufacturing processes conform to the environmental regulations of the country of origin

Frontispiece: The Arms of Dr James Henry Jeffcoat, Master 1905–06,
the probable initiator of the Great Hall glazing scheme in 1906

To find out more about our authors and books visit www.bloomsbury.com and sign up for our newsletters

CONTENTS

Acknowledgements

The authors wish to express their sincere gratitude to the many people who have given freely of their time to undertake research and engage in discussion, who have helped to provide the copious pictures necessary to illustrate the book and who have done much valuable work behind the scenes in order to bring this volume to fruition in printed form. The list which follows is long, but is not prioritised as the authors are equally grateful to all.

They do wish to begin by thanking all the members of staff at Apothecaries' Hall who have assisted in so many ways. In particular they are very grateful to Janet Payne, part-time Archivist to the Society, for much tireless research, wise counsel and admirable patience while dealing with their innumerable queries. Without her help this publication would not have been possible.

Dr John Ford, Liveryman of the Society, has provided immeasurable help with the more obscure areas of the Society's records and history, with the Wall Index and with apothecaries' biographies in general. Past Master Nicholas Wood, Curator of the Society's Archive, has given substantial advice and expertise, particularly with respect to the collection of drug jars. Briony Hudson, member of the British Society for the History of Pharmacy and President of the Society's Faculty of the History and Philosophy of Medicine and Pharmacy, has also given much guidance in dealing with the pharmacological aspects of subjects illustrated in some of the windows.

Dr Jasmine Allen, Curator of the Stained Glass Museum at Ely Cathedral gave her expert assessment of the seventeenth-century windows described in Chapter 5 and of the first-floor Landing panels described in Chapter 10. Christopher Parkinson contributed an insightful assessment of the older glass in the Hall.

Mr Geoffrey Lane, Librarian to the British Society of Master Glass Painters, has contributed a very scholarly assessment of the likely artist who painted the seventeenth-century panels described in Chapter 5.

Caroline Benyon supplied detailed information about her father's time at Apothecaries' Hall when he and his studio were tenants of the Society. She identified a number of people in photographs of her father's staff, confirmed those panels in the Great Hall which were made in her father's studio and provided the photograph in Chapter 7 of her father at work. Her husband, Tony Benyon, has taken particular interest in the Bristow panel described in Chapter 9 and has been very helpful in his assessment, not only of that panel, but also of the window from which it came and of the other early glass at the Hall.

Mr Alan Brooks stimulated initial research into 'the Apothecary' window in the Great Hall and was instrumental in suggesting that Simon Spear, Francis Spear's son, should donate the original drawings of the window to the Society. Simon Spear also provided the photograph in Chapter 6 of his father at work.

The late Professor Brian Ellis, a retired urological surgeon with a lifelong interest in photography, exhibited inexhaustible patience and ingenuity while photographing every aspect of heraldry and glass at the Hall. Most of the illustrations are the result of his expertise. The authors' only regret is that he did not live to see the result of his work. The authors also wish to thank Ian Lomas who took over the photography duties in the closing stages and whose flexibility and technical excellence in creating the missing images was crucial to meeting the deadline.

Dr Henry Oakeley, a Garden Fellow at the Royal College of Physicians in London and Dr Timothy Cutler, also a Garden Fellow at the College and Curator of the Physic Garden at Barber-Surgeons' Hall in London, have given much valuable information about the various plants illustrated in the windows at the Hall.

Christine Stevenson, Secretary of the Parochial Church Council of St Lawrence, Ayot St Lawrence, has been very helpful regarding the whereabouts of the various parts of the Bristow window described in Chapter 9.

Darrell Buttery, Past Governor of the Company of Merchant Adventurers of York and Past President of the York Civic Trust was instrumental not only in finding a lost heraldic stray of the Society's Arms in Yorkshire, but also in identifying its maker.

Thomas Woodcock, Garter King of Arms, and Dr Peadar O'Mordha, Member of the Court of Assistants of the Society, have provided much information concerning the Heraldry at the Hall from the records of the College of Arms.

Jacques Ruijterman, glass engraver at Arundel, has given technical details of his work on a panel described in Chapter 10, and on a second panel in the Hall.

Sue Medway, Curator of the Chelsea Physic Garden, has kindly provided details of the various Apothecary Arms at the Garden.

The authors are also very grateful to the archivists of a number of organisations: Vicky West at the Barbers' Company, Vicky Haig at Christ's Hospital, Alastair MacQueen at the Joiners' Company and Kate Higgins at the Mercers' Company.

The clerks of a number of City companies have been most helpful with information about the heraldry of their companies. The authors would like to thank Peter Durrant and Malachy Doran of the Barbers, Alison Evans of the Glaziers & Painters of Glass, Greville Bibby of the Grocers, Helen Perkins of the Spectacle Makers, David Homer of the Tallow Chandlers, Alex Robertson of the Turners and Georgina Brown of the Wax Chandlers.

The authors received details from a number of stained glass artists about their work for the Society and wish to thank Alfred Fisher, Mel Howse, Mac McHugh, Leonie Seliger, Richard Scowen and Stella Timmins.

The authors have received much help from a number of libraries and museums, particularly apropos publication of images in the collections: Eva Oledzka and the staff at the Bodleian Library in Oxford, Elizabeth Labres and the staff of the Bradford Museums, Beatriz Waters, head of British Museum Images and Alexia Kirk and the staff of the Victoria and Albert Archive of Art and Design.

The authors acknowledge help from Dr David Starkey, Professor James Carley, the Rt. Hon. the Lord McColl of Dulwich and the Rt. Hon. the Lord Ribeiro of Achimota and Ovington.

Finally, the authors wish to express profound thanks to the Friends of the Archive at Apothecaries' Hall and to the Court of the Society for their continuing interest in this project and their most generous support, without which this publication would not have been possible

The publication process has been both instructive and enjoyable for the authors. This has been entirely due to the professional input and relaxed forbearance of the staff at Philip Wilson Publishers. The authors are particularly grateful to Clare Martelli and Christopher Bromley for their interest, their guidance and reassuring encouragement throughout.

Foreword

Apothecaries' Hall offers the visitor a rich visual experience – and not just because it is the oldest livery hall in the City of London. The tone is set by a great coat of Arms that hangs magnificently over the entrance from the street. Inside the building there are splendid armorial bearings and other heraldic features in all the principal rooms; and there is fabulous stained glass in most of the windows. The dazzling colours, the exquisite carving, the delicate artistry: they are all captivating, and they lend a sense of grandeur and history to the Hall. The Society of Apothecaries recently celebrated its 400th anniversary; and it is immediately apparent to the casual observer that its four centuries are reflected in these striking armorial and decorative artefacts. But how to interpret them? Why were they made; and what is their precise significance in the history of the Society and of the City of London in general? This timely and comprehensive book addresses these important questions.

The authors are uniquely qualified to lead us through this compelling story. William Shand is a Past Master of the Society, and an accomplished practitioner in the art of making stained glass. As Clerk of the Society Andrew Wallington-Smith was closely involved in the care of all the artefacts in the Hall. Both authors have a deep interest and expertise in heraldry. Together they have assembled a definitive guide to these important treasures.

The reader is led through the history of the Society's Arms, the displays of them within and outside the Hall, and the different versions of the Royal Arms seen throughout the building; and there is a detailed analysis of the many personal armorial windows, and of the other important stained glass in the various rooms. In each chapter the authors relate the striking and beautiful imagery to the history of the Society and to its professional and charitable purposes.

This book will be of immense value to members of the Society, and to anyone interested in heraldry, stained glass or the history of livery companies. With their expert insight the authors present a detailed and fascinating survey, using helpfully annotated illustrations, and interpreting the historical evidence. The Society is deeply grateful to them for their work in producing this remarkable and meticulously researched volume, which will be an invaluable resource for years to come.

Professor Charles Mackworth-Young, CVO, MD, FRCP
(Quatercentenary Master 2017–2018)

Identification of Windows and Panels in the Great Hall

The following scheme for identification of panels in the Great Hall will be used throughout the book. The six main windows are labelled as shown in Diagram 1.

Viewed from inside, the windows on the west wall are labelled, from left to right, West 1, West 2, West 3 and West 4; and on the east wall, East 1 and East 2.

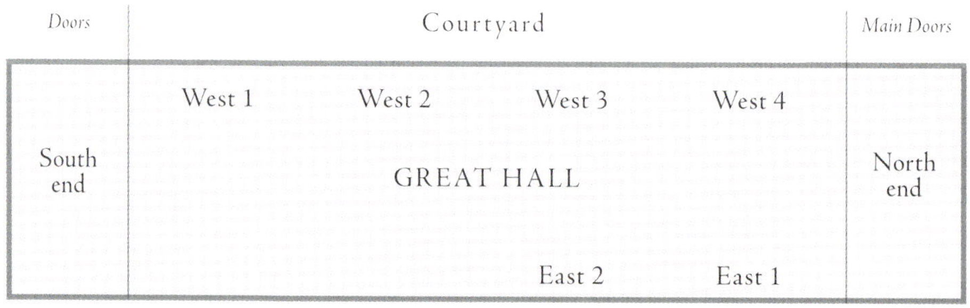

Diagram 1

Looking at each of the six windows, the panels are numbered from left to right and from top to bottom as shown in Diagrams 2 and 3.

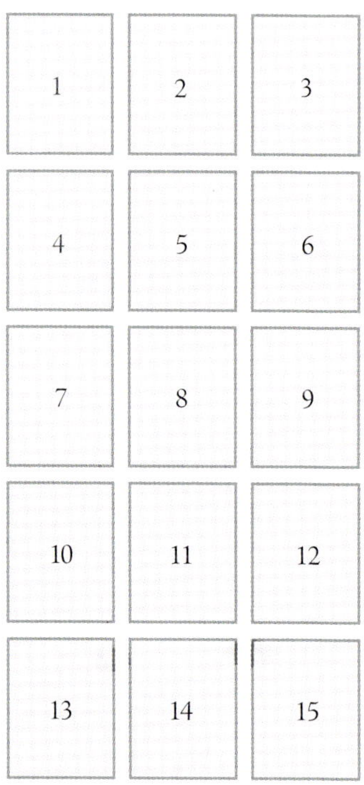

Diagram 2. Panels viewed from inside the Hall

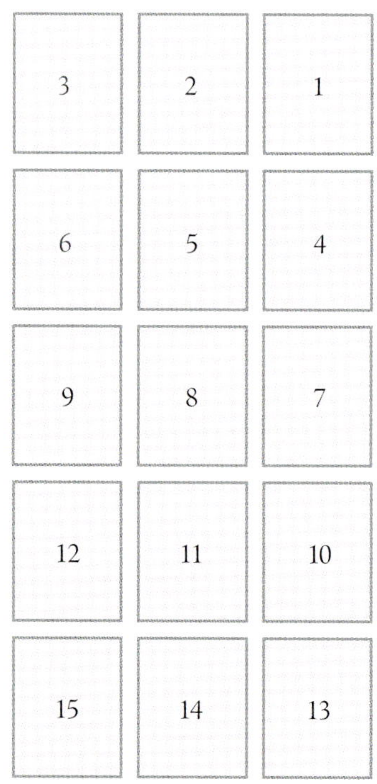

Diagram 3. Panels viewed from the Courtyard

Introduction

The Worshipful Society of Apothecaries of London was founded on 6 December 1617 by the granting of a Royal Charter or Letters Patent from King James I of England and VI of Scotland. Until that time the Apothecaries had been part of the merchant Company of Grocers, but had never been fully integrated into that Company. Separation was achieved largely through the good offices of Gideon de Laune (1565–1659), one of the Royal Apothecaries, and also by others such as the King's Physicians, Sir Theodore de Mayerne and Henry Atkins. Gideon de Laune lived and worked in the district of Blackfriars and was much favoured by the Queen, Anne of Denmark.

However, after the granting of Arms by Letters Patent from the College of Arms, opposition to the separation from various quarters, notably by the Company of Grocers, continued, until in 1624 the King declared: 'I myself did devise that corporation, and do allow it. The grocers, who complain of it, are but merchants; the mystery of these apothecaries, were belonging to apothecaries, wherein the grocers are unskilful; and therefore I think it fitting they should be a corporation of themselves.'[1] As a result, the new Company became firmly established as part of the City Livery scene, with the Company described in its charter as a 'Society' – a title that remains unique in the City of London to this day.

In 1632 the Society purchased its first Hall, a property originally owned by George Brooke, 9th Baron Cobham, and known as Cobham House. It had previously been the guesthouse, kitchens, pantry and buttery on the west side of the cloister of the Dominican or Black Friars Priory, which had stood on the site until the Dissolution of the Monasteries. The Hall was largely destroyed in the Great Fire of London in 1666 and no glass or heraldic device survives from the pre-fire period. The present Hall was rebuilt on the old foundations immediately after the fire, being finished by 1672. The Great Staircase and principal rooms remain much as they were when completed, the Hall having sustained only a broken window and skylight in the First World War, and then some bomb damage to the north wall and fireplace of the Parlour, together with broken windows, in the Second World War.

Between 1952 and 1972, one of the tenants at Apothecaries' Hall was a stained glass artist of international renown. The studio which he established at the Hall had a strong connection with a company known originally as 'Whitefriars Glass', which had been founded in the seventeenth century on the site of a Carmelite Priory, a London house of the White Friars, on the west side of the River Fleet in Magpie Alley – making a tenuous but nonetheless interesting connection between the White Friars of Magpie Alley and the Black Friars of what was much later to be known as Black Friars Lane on the east side of the river. During this period, many important windows were produced, both in this country – including those of Apothecaries' Hall – and abroad.

Over the years, the Hall has become a repository for a broad spectrum of heraldry in a variety of media, including stained and other glass. The Society's Arms appear in several designs around the Hall – on such diverse items as silverware and writing paper, for example. Royal connections have also provided a source of heraldic decoration in various media, including stained glass, but the Hall is particularly renowned for its collection of glass relating to the heraldry of the Arms of its Masters and Honorary Freemen, together with one Warden, one Secretary and one Registrar and Clerk, mostly to be seen in the windows of the Great Hall. All this is well known to many members of the medical, dental and pharmaceutical professions, but in the view of the authors the collection deserves to be brought to the attention of a wider audience, which, apart from collating in one volume all the information about heraldry and glass associated with the Society, is the prime purpose of this book.

CHAPTER 1

The Heraldry of the Society

The Achievement of Arms: A Statement of Intent

The Society was granted its Charter by King James I and VI (1566–1625) on 6 December 1617. Just five days later, on 12 December, William Camden (1551–1623), Clarenceaux King of Arms, granted the Society its armorial bearings by patent. This would seem to indicate that the design of the Arms had already been prepared and was simply awaiting the grant of the Charter. The speed of the transaction contrasts very markedly with the thirteen subsequent years of argument and delay before the Society had its Charter enrolled and was then granted livery by the Court of Aldermen of the City of London in 1630.

Payment to the College of Arms from the Society for the commission did not occur until April 1620. In his book The History of the Society of Apothecaries, despite acknowledging the 1617 date in the patent, C. R. B. Barrett makes the extraordinary claim that the Society did not apply for a grant of Arms until 1620,[1] almost certainly confusing the issue of the grant with payment for it by the Society.

The original grant hangs in the Brande Room at Apothecaries' Hall (Figure 1.1), but there is also a contemporary copy on the main staircase in the Entrance Hall. The blazon given, in the original spelling, is as follows:

> *In a Shield azure, Apollo the inuentor of phiſique Proper, with his heade Radiant, holding in his left hand a bowe & his Right hand an Arow dor, Suplanting a Serpent Argent; aboue the Shield an Helme therevppon a mantle gules, doubled Argent, and for their Creast vppon a Wreath of their Colours, a Rhynoceros proper, Supported by too Vnicorns, or, armed and vngulated arzent; vppon a Compartiment to make the Atchieuement complete, this motto,* OPIFERQVE PER ORBEM DICOR: *the which Armes and Creast, Supporters and whole Atchieuement, I the forſayd King of Armes do give graunt ratify and confirme to the sayd Bodie incoporat of the Apothecaries of London by the aſſent and conſent of the Commiſſioners for the Office of the Earle Marshall of England.*

This original grant is annotated in the margin as approved in the Visitation of London in 1634 by Sir Henry St George, Richmond Herald.

The Shield

Figure 1.2 shows the Arms in greater detail to assist with the interpretation of what they represent and therefore how they came to be chosen.

Implicit in the Charter was the understanding that the Apothecaries should be subservient to the College of Physicians and that their only function was to dispense the prescriptions of physicians. However, the new Society was full of independently minded gentlemen who had their own ideas of their worth and work, but it is impossible to tell whether the Society made any contribution to the design of its armorial bearings.

The grant says 'Now wheras the afforenamed Master, Wardens and Companie haue requested me, William Camden Clarenceaux, to deuiſe [devise], aſſigne [assign] and

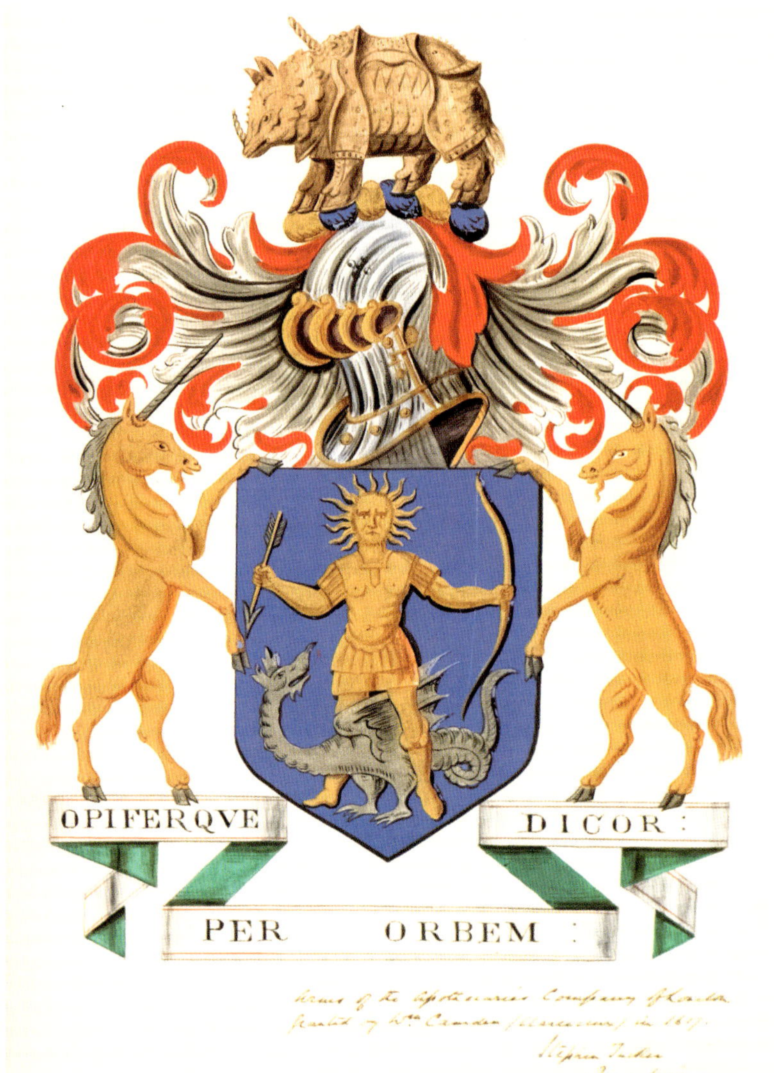

1.2 Drawing of the Society's Arms held at the College of Arms authenticated by Stephen Tucker, Rouge Croix Pursuivant (1872–80)

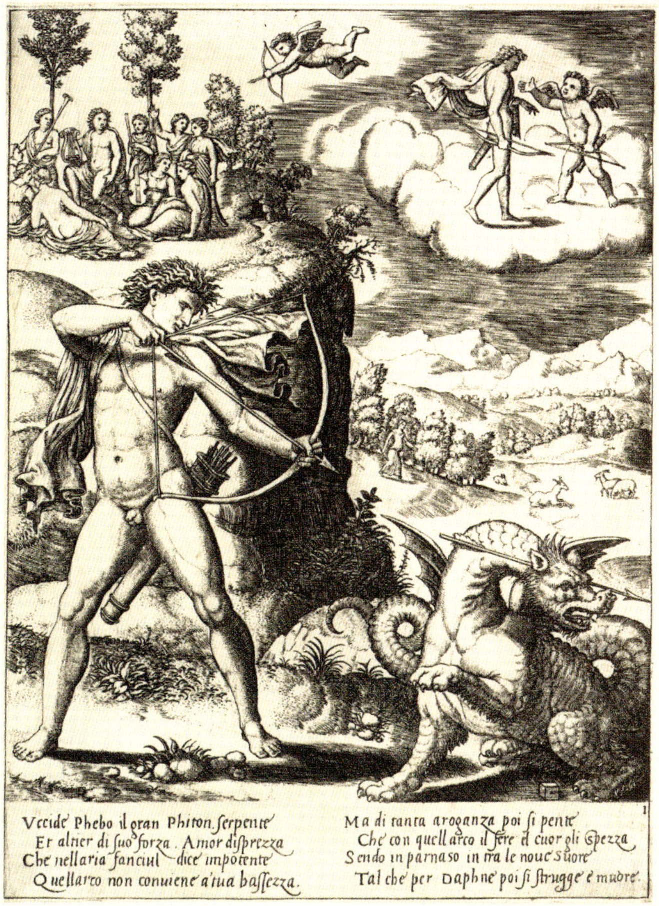
Vccide Phebo il gran Phiton serpente
Et altier di suo forza. Amor disprezza
Che nellaria fanciul dice impotente
Quellarco non conuiene a tua bassezza.
Ma di tanta aroganza poi si pente
Che con quell arco il fere el cuor gli spezza
Sendo in parnaso in tra le noue Suore
Tal che per Daphne poi si strugge e muore.

1.3 Master of the Die (Italian, active Rome, c.1530–60), engraving after Baldassare

emblazon Armes, Creast and Supporters fitt for their Seale, I could not but condeſcend to their reaſonable request therein and haue accordingly aſſigned to them for their Armes', which suggests that the design was all Camden's work.

Unfortunately, to this day, the Heralds do not record any explanation of why a particular design has been chosen for Arms, and so a considerable exercise in deduction is required to decipher compositions.

In the Society's Arms the main charge is usually referred to as Apollo killing the dragon of disease. Herein lie difficulties. The blazon describes Apollo as 'supplanting a serpent'. How has the serpent become a dragon? Why is the dragon associated with disease? What are Apollo's medical qualifications?

Camden describes the god as being 'the inventor of physic', in support of which the original Hippocratic oath began 'I swear by Apollo the Physician, by Asclepius, by Hygieia, by Panacea, and by all the gods and goddesses, making them my witnesses, that I will carry out, according to my ability and judgment, this oath and this indenture…'.[2]

The principal god of medicine, however, was not Apollo but his son Asclepius, who was slain by Zeus to prevent the human race becoming immortal under his care. Greek mythology tells us that Apollo and his twin sister Artemis, the huntress, were the offspring of a dalliance between Zeus and Leto and that his most important role was that of sun god, the producer of light, indicated by his radiant head, but that he also had sidelines in music, poetry, art, dance, prophecy, archery, knowledge and finally healing. It seems clear that it was Apollo's healing ability that Camden wished to highlight by showing him striking down disease.

A further problem is that Apollo's bow and arrow was used to spread plague, especially into the Greek encampment during the Trojan War, and this would seem a most inappropriate attribute to emphasise when promoting the characteristics of a medical institution. On the other hand, it may have been Camden using prophetic powers, as the arrow might now be said to represent, for example, the technique of using a needle to inject an engineered viral vector (disease) in order to promote an immune response in the treatment of advanced malignant disease!

As the deity in charge of prophecy, Apollo was the patron of Delphi where he was venerated for slaying Pytho, the serpent or earth-dragon which lived at the centre of the earth. Pytho had been sent by a jealous and furious Hera, Zeus's wife, to kill Leto. Apollo intercepted Pytho and killed him with a volley of arrows. As Pytho was a child of Gaia, the primal mother-earth Goddess, Apollo was required by Zeus to perform penance not only for slaying Pytho but also for the sacrilege of doing so in the precinct of the oracle at Delphi. So, he instituted the Pythian Games which were held two years after each quadrennial Olympic Games and which included art and dance, these being two of his responsibilities. It is, of course, the slaying of Pytho by Apollo which forms the main charge of the Society's Arms.

Camden, who was an antiquary and a historian, may have been influenced by sixteenth-century engravings. Figure 1.3 is an Italian engraving from the story of Apollo and Daphne, which shows Apollo standing on the left shooting Pytho with an arrow; above on the left are the muses, and on the right on a cloud Eros approaching Apollo. The virgin huntress Daphne can also be seen in the middle distance. In the artist's caption, Pytho is called 'Phiton Serpente' but the beast is drawn as a dragon, notably with four legs. Also in the caption reference is made to Phebo – Phoebus being Apollo's chief epithet, literally meaning 'bright' as the god of light. Figure 1.4 shows a German engraving of 1581 in which Apollo's clothing is not dissimilar to that on the Society's Arms and, again, the dragon has four legs.

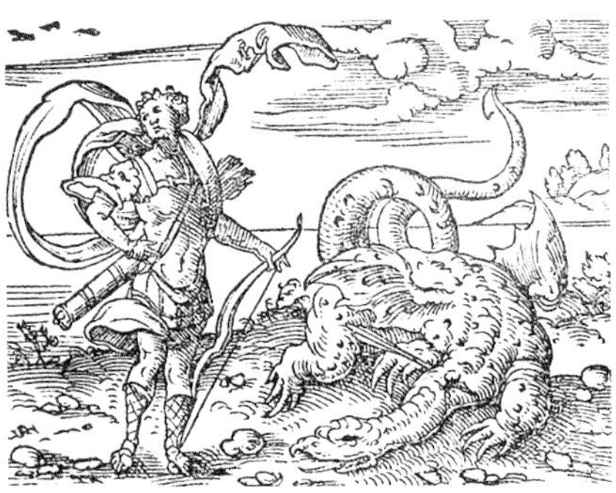

1.4 Virgil Solis (1514–1562), engraving for Ovid's *Metamorphoses*, Book I, published in 1581

Thus, in antiquity and the early Middle Ages the words 'serpent' and 'dragon' were used interchangeably.[3] Perhaps influenced by engravings such as these, Camden certainly sees the serpent as a dragon, as he has drawn him as such. Unfortunately, the dragon as drawn in the Society's Arms has only two legs, which makes him heraldically a wyvern – just to confuse matters!

As recently as the twentieth century in a remote Lucanian village in southern Italy, there persisted a folklore tale of a dragon which killed peasants, carried off their daughters, filled the land with its pestiferous breath and destroyed crops.[4] The important part of this description is the noxious breath. In the early Middle Ages, there were many myths related to dragons; for example, in 589 CE an epidemic of plague in Rome, following floods, was attributed to the breath of a dragon seen in the River Tiber, with Pope Pelagius himself falling victim to this plague.[5] St George's dragon was also notorious for poisoning people with its breath. The main consistencies of all dragon folklore were that the creatures lived in marshy areas, prevented access to pure water and that their insides and exhalations were lethal.[6] The swampy habitation and pestilential breath are key here. From their habitat and activities, dragons were associated with diseases that we know now as cholera, smallpox, plague and malaria, for example.

Dragons were therefore considered a cause of environmental disaster and could be used as a simple, but dramatic, allegory of epidemics and contagious disease, while crops were destroyed because there was no one left to tend them. Maidens were often included in the tales for salacious interest too. Thus, although Pytho himself apparently had no connection with disease, by the early Middle Ages these creatures were certainly thought of as dragons of disease.[7]

The Motto: *Opiferque Per Orbem Dicor*

The Roman poet Ovid seems to be conversant with Apollo's medical competence. The motto of the Society is taken from his *Metamorphoses*, a poem in fifteen books which chronicles the history of the world until the deification of Julius Caesar. The words come from verse 455 of the first book, 'The Divine Comedy', where Apollo is unsuccessfully attempting to court Daphne. This has come about since Apollo, in the pride of his victory over Pytho, has insulted Eros because of his puny bow and small stature, as seen in Figure 1.3. In retaliation, Eros shoots Apollo with a golden arrow inflicting love, and shoots Daphne, a virgin huntress, with a lead-tipped arrow which makes her hostile to love. The full verse runs as follows:

> *Inventum medicina meum est*
>   The medical art is my discovery,
> *OPIFERQUE PER ORBEM DICOR*
>   And I am called throughout the world the bringer of aid.
> *Et herbarum subjecta potentia nobis*
>   The potency of herbs is at my will.
> *Ei mihi, quod nullis amor est sanabilis herbis*
>   Woe to me, because love is curable by no herbs,
> *Nec prosunt domino, quae prosunt omnibus artes*
>   Nor by the skills which benefit all but their master.

While this verse as a whole indicates Apollo's frivolous failure as a medical man to entice love, the choice of the second line as the Socety's motto reinforces the wider ambition to overcome the dragon of disease.

It is pertinent to recall that a famous apothecary who qualified with the Licence of the Society of Apothecaries (LSA), Sir Ronald Ross (1857–1932), won the Nobel Prize for Medicine in 1902 for his work on the transmission of malaria, an important example of fulfilling the Society's motto.

As an epilogue, the lovelorn Apollo turns Daphne into a laurel bush (*Daphne mezereum*), a shrub that produces mezereon bark which was listed in the British Pharmaceutical Codex until 1934 and used as a stimulant and a vesicant.[8]

The Supporters

The unicorn supporters of the shield, to which the Society is entitled as a chartered body, almost certainly come from the Scottish Royal Arms as a tribute to King James I and VI, who granted the Charter. There may be a further connotation as, on the Continent there was already a connection between unicorns, signifying purity, and apothecaries – this can still be seen in the unicorn symbols which adorn apothecaries' shops in Germany.

Traditionally, when beasts are used as supporters they face each other and are rampant so as to present a formidable appearance, but this is rarely specified in the blazon. Heraldic painters and carvers have on occasion, either through ignorance or to make the achievement fit the space available, been known to use their own creativity. Thus, in some representations of the Society's Arms the unicorns appear as guardant or couchant, as will be seen later in Chapter 2. There is also the question of sex. All unicorns are male and sometimes this is very obvious but at other times, perhaps for Victorian audiences, it is rather more discreet. With no female unicorns, the image of the animal became one of idealised masculinity and romance.

Unicorn mythology essentially stems from Eurasia and China where, until the late Pleistocene era, the Elasmotherium existed. This predecessor of the rhinoceros had a dramatic single projecting horn.[9] It was later conflated with a wild ass or an antelope or oryx in profile, to become a horse-like creature. As the legend progressed from east to west the unicorn was attributed with all manner of fabulous abilities: in the East as a judge of right or wrong and as a tomb guardian; in Persia and Babylon, the horn was considered to have magical properties which could cure disease; and it became a totem of Zoroastrianism; in the West it symbolised innocence and purity, and finally was swept up into Christian allegory and connected very much with the Virgin Mary.

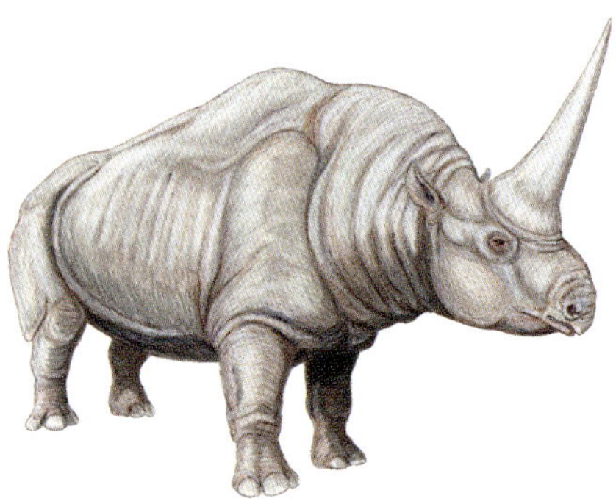

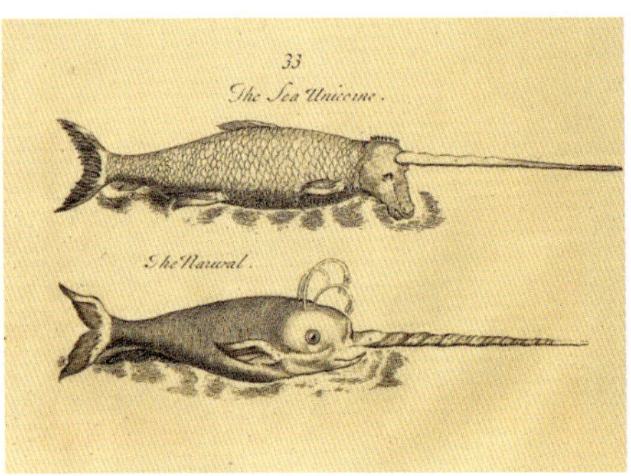

1.5 The Elasmotherium

1.6 Illustration of the Sea Unicorn and the Narwhal from the English translation of *Histoire Générale des Drogues* (a Compleat History of Drugs) by Pierre Pomet (1658–99)

As it came through central Eurasia,[10] the story was further muddled with the introduction of narwhal 'horns' (*Monodon monoceros*). A natural history treatise of 1694 by the French apothecary Pierre Pomet, chief druggist to King Louis XIV, illustrates a narwhal next to a mythical 'Licorne de Mer', or sea unicorn, with a horse-like head. Narwhal 'horns' in practice fulfilled the role of imaginary unicorn horns and were certainly owned by James III's Queen, Margaret of Denmark, and also by Mary, Queen of Scots.[11] Indeed, the Society too has one on show in the Great Hall.

Despite the Venetian traveller-explorer Marco Polo's thirteenth-century expedition to seek the unicorn failing (he only managed to see a Sumatran rhinoceros), the legend lived on. When the Hebrew Old Testament was translated into Greek, the term *re êm*, a beast unknown to the translators but possibly denoting a wild ox, became *monokeros* or unicorn.[12] Through further translation into Latin by St Jerome, the term became either *unicornus* or *rhinoceros* used indiscriminately and when the King James 1611 Authorised Version of the Bible was written, all references to 'rhinoceros' were changed to 'unicorn'.

Essentially then, the unicorn is a stylised version of the rhinoceros (which also features on the Society's arms and will be discussed below). As a result of all these embellishments, the beast we now see is an elegant horse with a delicate horn – it is no surprise that this most beautiful of all fabulous creatures was appropriated for use in heraldry.

The courtly romantic aspect of the unicorn was used by King James I of Scotland (1394–1437) during his eighteen-year captivity in England when he wooed Joan Beaufort to be his Queen.[13] He later established unicorns into the Scottish Royal Arms, these

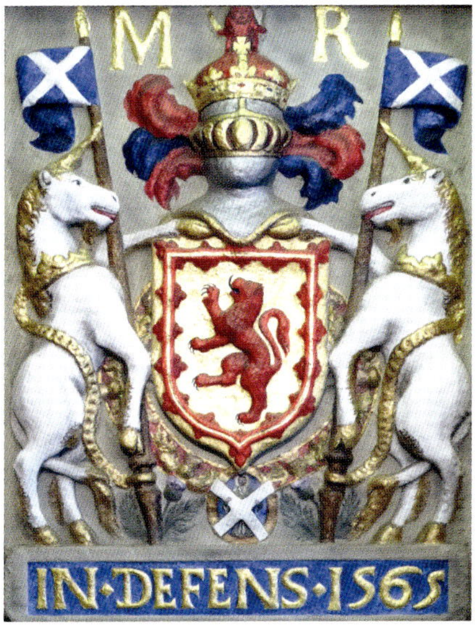

1.7 The Arms of Mary Queen of Scots, formerly incorporated into Leith Tolbooth (1565), and now in the vestibule of South Leith Parish Church

being chained and gorged with an open crown symbolic of the bonds of love, not as a captive symbol; by 1426, he had introduced a new officer of arms, Unicorn Pursuivant.[14] The two unicorns remained in the Scottish Royal Arms (Figure 1.7) until 1603, when James VI became King of England and merged the two royal coats of Arms with the one lion and the one unicorn as supporters, as used today (see Figure 8.3).

The Helm and Mantling

The helm is a peer's helm,[15] which is a silver helmet with five gold bars and shown in profile. The Society shares the privilege of a peer's helm with three other livery companies – the Fishmongers (Arms granted 1512), the Goldsmiths (Arms granted 1571) and the Clockmakers (Arms granted 1672). It is also depicted in the City of London Arms (see Figure 5.13), which were in use before the founding of the College of Arms in 1494. As the style of helm is not included in any of these blazons, it is not clear why a peer's helm was chosen or allowed.

The Society's mantling is Gules doubled Argent, which were the standard tinctures for nearly all mantlings in the sixteenth and seventeenth centuries. Towards the end of the seventeenth century, this custom changed and mantlings, like the wreaths, became 'of the colours', which in the Society's case would have been Azure doubled Or.[16] In some of the Arms seen in the Hall, this change of the colours has been used – although, strictly speaking, it is wrong.

The Crest

The Society's Arms contain the only example of Dürer's Gomda (Indian rhinoceros) in heraldry and it is used as the crest. The obvious questions are why was a rhinoceros chosen at all and why this one with a dorsal horn in addition to its nasal horn?

There is a longstanding connection, sometimes confusing, between the mythical unicorn and the genuine rhinoceros. Indeed, in Linnaean taxonomy the Indian rhinoceros is called *Rhinoceros unicornis*. Both the rhinoceros and the unicorn feature in the Society's armorial bearings, perhaps in part because of this confusion. However, a third unicorn as the crest would have spoilt the subtley of the achievement and maybe that is why the next-of-kin rhinoceros was chosen instead. Both beasts are relevant as, for a lengthy period, the horn of each was thought to have medicinal properties.

Powdered rhino horn had long been used in Asian countries, particularly China, and it is likely that its use became better known in Europe due to the activities of the Honourable East India Company, which had received its charter in 1600. In traditional Chinese medicine the horn was mainly employed to treat fever, rheumatism and gout. The ancient Greeks and Persians believed that rhino horn could be used to purify water and that a rhino horn vessel could be used to detect poison – a belief that persisted into

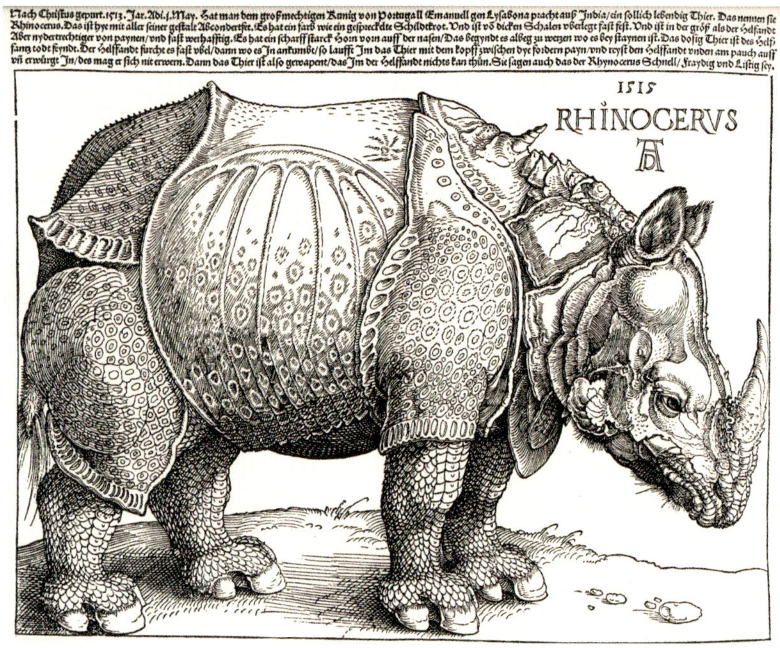

1.8 Albrecht Dürer (1471–1528), 1515, woodcut of rhinoceros

the eighteenth century among royal courts of Europe. There may be some truth in this theory that rhino horn is alexipharmic, because it is composed very largely of the protein keratin (other animals' horns have a bony core covered by only a thin layer of keratin); poisons, which are strongly alkaline, may react chemically with the rhino horn and thus be rendered ineffective.

In 1618 the Royal College of Physicians published the first formal pharmacopoeia of drugs in common use, the *Pharmacopoeia Londinensis*,[17] but rhino horn was not included until the 1639 edition. Subsequently, assortments of publications in the late seventeenth and early eighteenth centuries suggest a variety of uses for the horn. These include that it is 'good against Poyson, Plague and all Pestilential Diseases and is an excellent sudorifik' (a sudorific being something that produces sweating).[18] The same source states that it is 'often used instead of Unicorns Horn' and recommends that the powdered skin of rhinoceros is 'good against Malignant disease'. Fifty years later, Robert James states that rhino horn may be used 'to supply the want of the Unicorn's Horn',[19] but interestingly, he also considers all reports of a quadruped with a single horn to be 'fictitious, except [for] the Rhinoceros'. He commends it for 'contagious Poisons and other Distempers which require Sudorifics'.[20] Culpepper also recommended unicorn horn as an aphrodisiac (in accordance with the masculinity-enhancing attributes discussed above). So, with rhinoceros horn cited as a suitable substitute for unicorn, it is not surprising that it later came to be regarded as an aphrodisiac too, as well as being the source of a valuable medicinal product against poisons and other disorders.[21] As an alleged wonder drug of its time, this would have made it a suitable emblem for the *à la mode* apothecaries.

Scientific studies have been commissioned to test the supposed curative properties of rhino horn. Testing was carried out in 1983 by researchers at Hoffmann-La Roche,[22] and followed up twenty-five years later with a study at the Zoological Society of London.[23] Both studies arrived at the same conclusion: rhinoceros horn has no medicinal properties whatsoever. Additionally, research conducted in 1990 at the Chinese University of Hong Kong was unable to produce any evidence to support the wild claims of rhinoceros horn's curative power.[24]

Turning now to the question of why an inaccurate drawing of a rhinoceros with a dorsal horn was used as the Society's crest, we need only look at Dürer's famous woodcut as illustrated in Figure 1.8. Although the rhinoceros had been used in Roman public entertainments, none had been seen again in Europe until 1515. This slightly whimsical woodcut by Dürer, drawn in that year, became the standard representation of the rhinoceros until the late eighteenth century, when its true features were properly known. Even after 1746, when a rhinoceros calf called Clara was exhibited throughout Europe by an enterprising Dutch sea captain called Douwe Mout van der Meer, the old fanciful representation retained its popularity.[25]

In 1515 King Manuel I (1469–1521) of Portugal was given an Indian rhinoceros for his menagerie by the Sultan of Cambay (modern Gujarat) as a diplomatic gift. It caused a sensation on its arrival in Lisbon and descriptions were sent all over Europe. In order to test Pliny the Elder's theory, in his treatise *Naturalis Historia*, that elephants and rhinoceros have a natural antipathy to each other, the king arranged a fight with a young elephant from his collection. The elephant panicked with the noise of the crowd and no blows were exchanged.

After this fiasco, King Manuel gave the rhinoceros to Pope Leo X (1475–1521) in order to curry political favour and to add to the Indian elephant which he had presented the previous year. The rhinoceros sailed in late 1515 via Marseilles where King Francis I (1494–1547) wished to view the animal.[26] On resuming its voyage, the ship was wrecked north of La Spezia and the rhinoceros was drowned as it was chained to the deck. The carcass was recovered and the stuffed hide sent on to Rome.

The first person to create an image of this rhinoceros was the Florentine Giovanni Giacomo Penni as an illustration for a poem in 1515, the only known copy of this being held by the Institución Colombina in Seville.[27] This is a rather primitive drawing and has no hint of a dorsal horn.

Another description of the rhinoceros from Portugal, along with a sketch, reached Albrecht Dürer in Nuremberg. Its unknown artist had added the following notes:

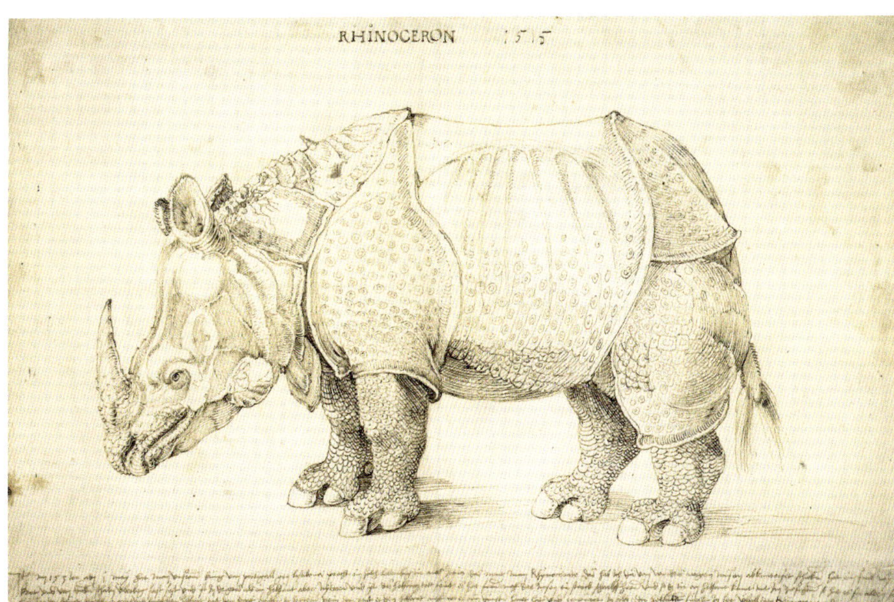

1.9 Albrecht Dürer, 1515, drawing based on the Portuguese sketch, bequeathed to the British Museum by Sir Hans Sloane in 1753

> *Because it is such a marvel I considered that I must send this representation. It has the colour of a toad and is covered all over with thick scales, and in size it is as large as an elephant, but lower, and is the deadly enemy of the elephant. It has on the front of the nose a strong sharp horn: and when this animal comes near the elephant to fight it always first whets its horn on the stones and runs at the elephant with his head between its forelegs. Then rips the elephant where its skin is thinnest then gores it.*[28]

A much-embellished sketch by Dürer (Figure 1.9), based on this Portuguese sketch, since lost,[29] shows the rhinoceros with hard plates over its body like sheets of rivetted armour, a gorget at the neck, chainmail covering the legs and a small dorsal horn behind its head. Dürer simply reversed this picture in producing his famous woodcut print (Figure 1.8).

There are several possibilities as to why a more lifelike animal was not drawn: perhaps the rhinoceros was dressed in armour for the fight with the elephant;[30] Dürer, living in the armour-making centre of Nuremberg, may have seen the thick folds of skin as armour-like and been inventive;[31] or the rhino may simply have been in poor condition, having suffered from the trials of his voyage. The dorsal horn is known only from this drawing and woodcut.

In his 1953 essay on the Dürer Gomda and its artistic reproductions, F. J. Cole remarks:

> *If something can be said in extenuation of Dürer's imposing coat of armour, which after all is only an artistic elaboration of the plicae of the skin, it must be conceded that the small dorsal spiral horn is entirely and gratuitously fictitious … He had presumably heard of a two-horned rhinoceros … The Portuguese sketch showed only one, and Dürer, perhaps anxious that his figure should not be found wanting in so striking a feature, ventured to invent an inconspicuous second horn on the withers, where it might easily have escaped the notice of his predecessors.*[32]

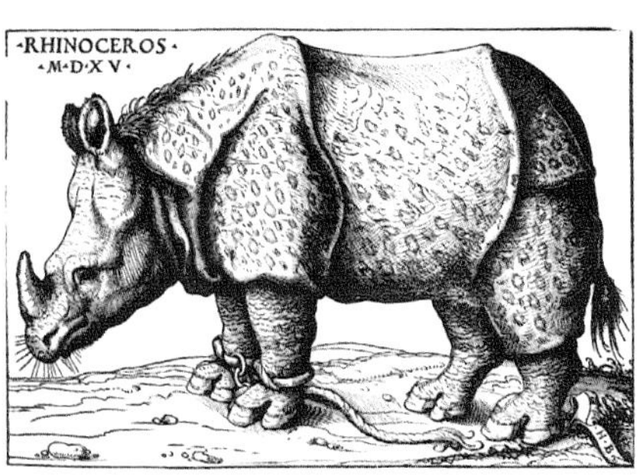

1.10 Hans Burgkmair the Elder (1473–1531), 1515, woodcut of the Lisbon rhinoceros

Another woodcut (Figure 1.10) was made by Hans Burgkmair in Augsburg at the same time as Dürer produced his in Nuremberg. Burgkmair was in touch with merchants in Lisbon but it is not known what descriptions or sketches he used as a source.[33] Although broadly similar to Dürer's woodcut, but without the dorsal horn, his image is truer to life and includes the shackles and chain which restrain the animal. Yet the simple fact is that Dürer was more influential than the others and it was his image that remained powerful for so long, with eight editions of his block being cut.

In confirmation of this, in the sixteenth century alone the following authors produced direct copies or variants of Dürer's woodcut: Conrad Gesner (1516–1565) in 1551, Bishop Paolo Giovio (1483–1552) in 1556, Pierio Valeriano (1477–1558) also in 1556, Ambroise Paré (1510–1590) in 1573, André Thevet (1502–1590) in 1575, Marcus Gheeraerts the Elder (1520–1590) in 1583 and Joachim Camerarius the Younger (1534–1598) in 1595.[34]

For use as the Society's crest, Dürer's Gomda has again been reversed from the woodcut to conform to heraldic practice that animals face to the dexter.

Conclusion

Traditonally, the emergence of the apothecary as the doctor to the poor is ascribed to the Great Plague of 1665 but this inevitable development must already have been going on for some time, with the plague merely accelerating this enlarged role.

A great number of other livery companies' Arms display a symbol of the tool or materials used in their trade – the Fishmongers' fish, the Vintners' and Brewers' barrels, the Barbers' fleams, the Saddlers' saddles, the Carpenters' compasses, the Farriers' horsehoes and so on. The Grocers, from whom the Apothecaries split, have cloves as part of their Arms to signify origins in the spice trade. The universal sign over the apothecary's shop was the pestle and mortar, such as the eighteenth-century example in the Courtyard at Apothecaries' Hall which was given in 1984 by Dr Douglas Whittet (Master 1982–83). Although this obvious symbol does feature in the circular window at the southern end of the Great Hall (see Chapter 6), it was not included in the Society's Arms. The Arms of the Society would therefore seem perhaps to be illustrating a deeper meaning.

There is very little in the mythology of Apollo which describes his healing activities, his pursuit of Pytho being merely revenge for the intended assault on his mother. His position as the sun god, of course, did give him the naturally prophylactic powers of sunshine, predicting perhaps the modern day use of light therapy for treating seasonal affective disorder, but ignoring on the other hand the scourge that is melanoma.

So, for all Apollo's imperfections, the Society's achievement of Arms, and particularly the motto, perhaps conveys a sense of the higher role of practising medicine rather than merely dispensing to order. The lofty ideals of the whole composition perhaps tell us that the Master and Wardens, or indeed Camden himself, were emphasising the fact that the Apothecary's transformation from pharmacist to general practitioner was well under way by 1617. These Arms, which have an element of St George and the Dragon imagery, can therefore be regarded as a statement of intent by a confident new company.

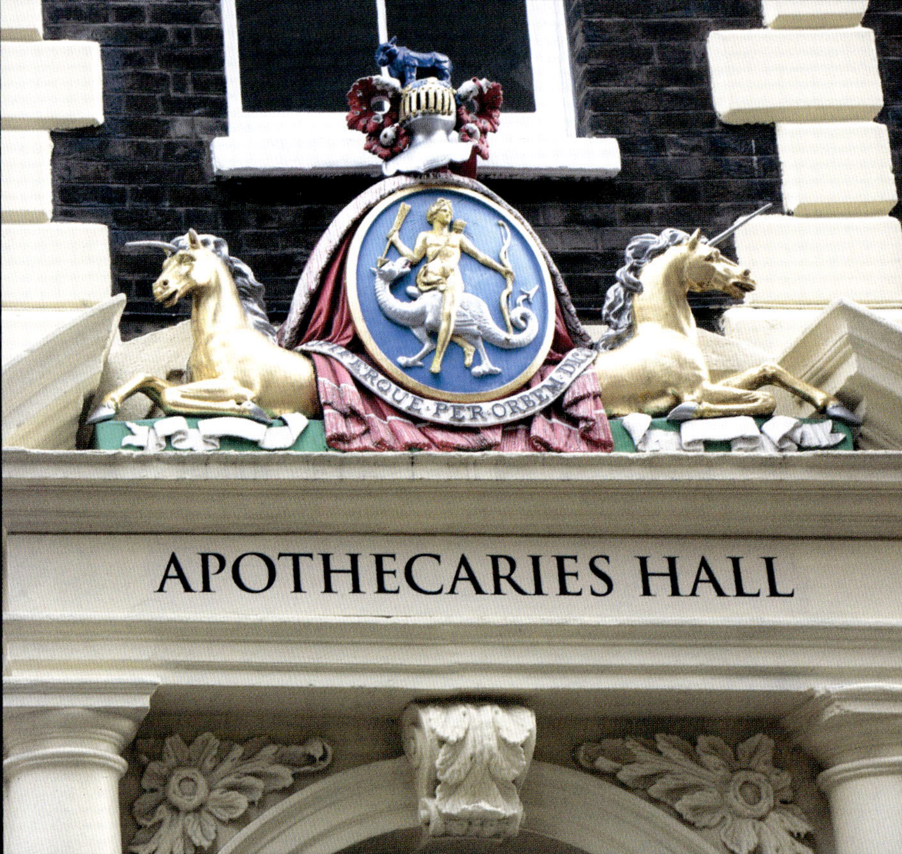
APOTHECARIES HALL

CHAPTER 2

Principal Displays of the Society's Arms

With the grant of such notable Arms, it is not surprising that the Society wished to display them wherever possible but it is only on close inspection of the Hall that one realises how very many there are. This chapter examines the wooden, plaster and vexillological representations of the Society's Arms.[1] The versions in stone, glass, textiles, ceramics and jewellery will be considered in Chapter 3 or in their own specialist sections.

External Arms

The first representation of the Arms which a visitor to the Hall will see are those over the archway of the main entrance in Black Friars Lane (Figure 2.1). Prior to 1785, the forecourt was separated from Water Lane (now Black Friars Lane) only by railings and an iron gate. Over this gate was set the Society's Arms which, on 14 March 1751, the Clerk reported had 'completely fallen down and was broken to pieces'.[2] In 1760 the Immediate Past Master, William Gataker, presented Arms to be set up over the gate,[3] presumably to replace those which had fallen down nine years earlier.

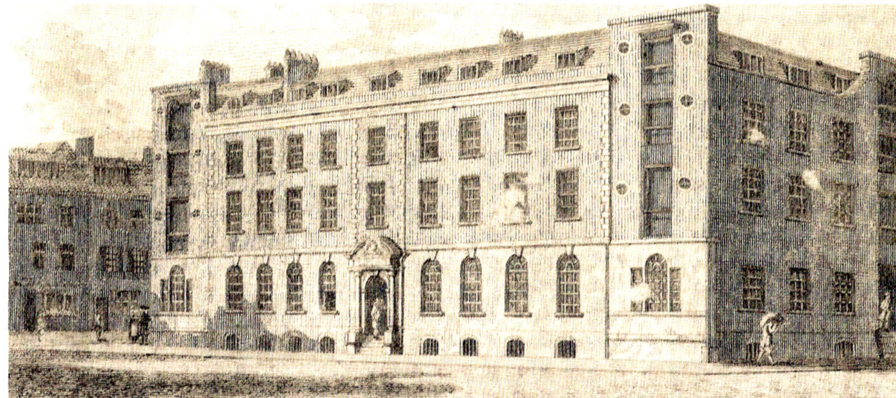

2.2 The new West frontage of the Hall drawn by John Carter, published in the Stationers' London Almanack for 1787

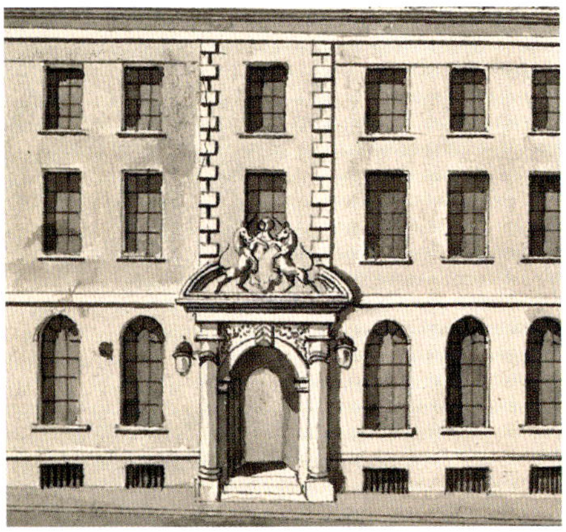

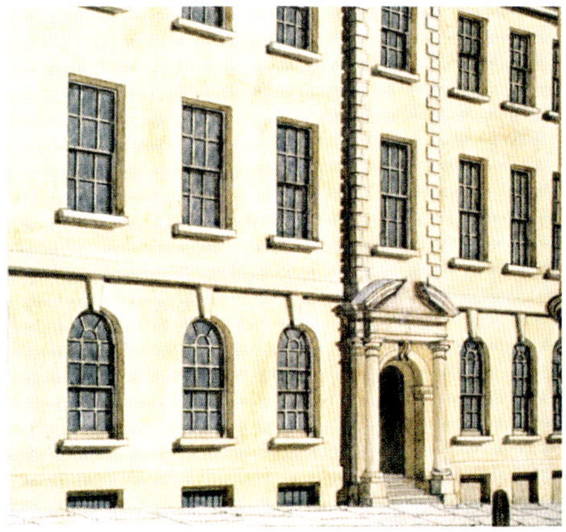

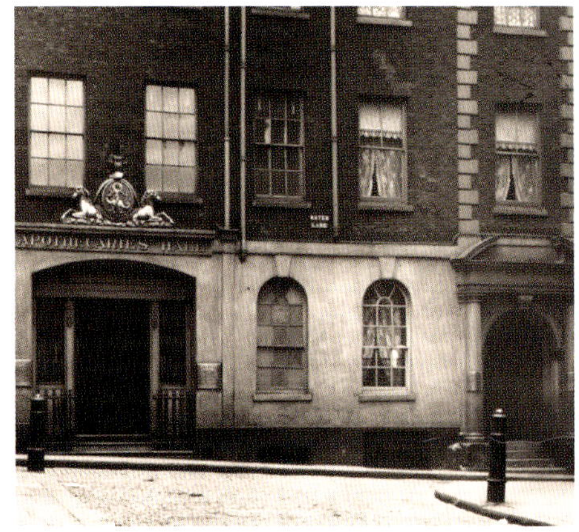

2.3 Anonymous sketch of the West frontage, *c.*1800

2.4 The West frontage by Valentine Davis, 1806

2.5 The Arms over the old shop door in 1915; the main archway entrance to the Hall is on the right

In 1786 the western range of the Courtyard buildings was completed with the imposing archway we see today. Figure 2.2 shows these works a year later but it is not clear from the engraving whether there are Arms over the Archway.

An anonymous sketch of the new frontage dating *c.*1800 does show some Arms (Figure 2.3) but these lack any detail and may therefore be fanciful, as a more detailed drawing of the frontage by Valentine Davis in 1806 clearly shows the broken pediment to be empty (Figure 2.4).

It would appear that it was not possible to transfer Gataker's Arms to the new entrance and these have been lost. So when were the current Arms made? Although they are early Georgian in style (cf. the Chelsea Garden ticket of 1785, Figure 3.31), it is likely that they were made specifically to be placed over the retail shop entrance when it was formed in the third and fourth windows to the left of the Archway in 1823 (Figure 2.5). A watercolour by T. H. Shepherd in 1855 of the Hall frontage (Figure 2.7) clearly shows a very comparable version of the current Archway Arms, with the unicorns facing outwards, over the shop entrance. Whatever their origin, these wooden Arms remained over the shop entrance until its closure in 1922, when they were transferred to their current position over the Archway.

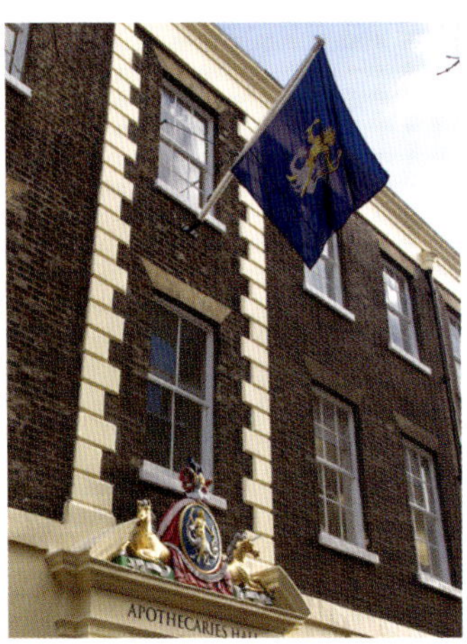

2.6 The Society's banner flying over the entrance to the Hall

These Arms (Figure 2.1) are very striking and certainly make an impression, but the Georgian style with an oval shield gives no real sense of cohesiveness. The most obvious deviation from the patent is that the unicorns are no longer rampant, as supporters should be, but have been stood easy, that is to say they are couchant and facing away from the shield they should be supporting, with the result that the helm, mantling and poor rhinoceros are perfoming a very precarious balancing act. Interestingly, this is also the case with the supporters of the Wax Chandlers' Arms at the entrance to their Hall in Gresham Street. To cover the unicorns' dereliction of duty, an elaborate tasselled drape has been added in approximately the colours of the mantling. The helm is also improper as it has almost become a sovereign's helm, now being affronté, whilst the crest remains in profile – all a bit of a heraldic mess! The Arms were last fully re-gilded in 1988 and have been touched up in each of the Society's periodic external redecorations.[4]

On Society red-letter days such as the Master's Day Service, Court meetings or Livery Dinners, the Society's banner flies from a small flagstaff high above the Archway (Figure 2.6).

The banner only displays, as a banner should, the charge from the shield, namely Apollo and the dragon, unlike the barge banner in the Hall which displays the full achievement of Arms (Figure 2.19). This banner, together with the flagstaff, was a gift from Past Assistant John Missen in 2003.

In a City of London landscape of tall buildings and narrow lanes it is always difficult to site a flagstaff effectively and it has already been moved once, in 2005.[5] Ideally, it should be vertical but, on the Hall, this would mean that the banner could not be seen. Hence this compromise above the Lane, which has the disadvantages of having to disturb the tenants whenever it is hoisted and, because of the swirling winds of the narrow street, the banner frequently fouling its pole.

2.7 T. H. Shepherd, 1855, watercolour showing the Arms over the shop entrance

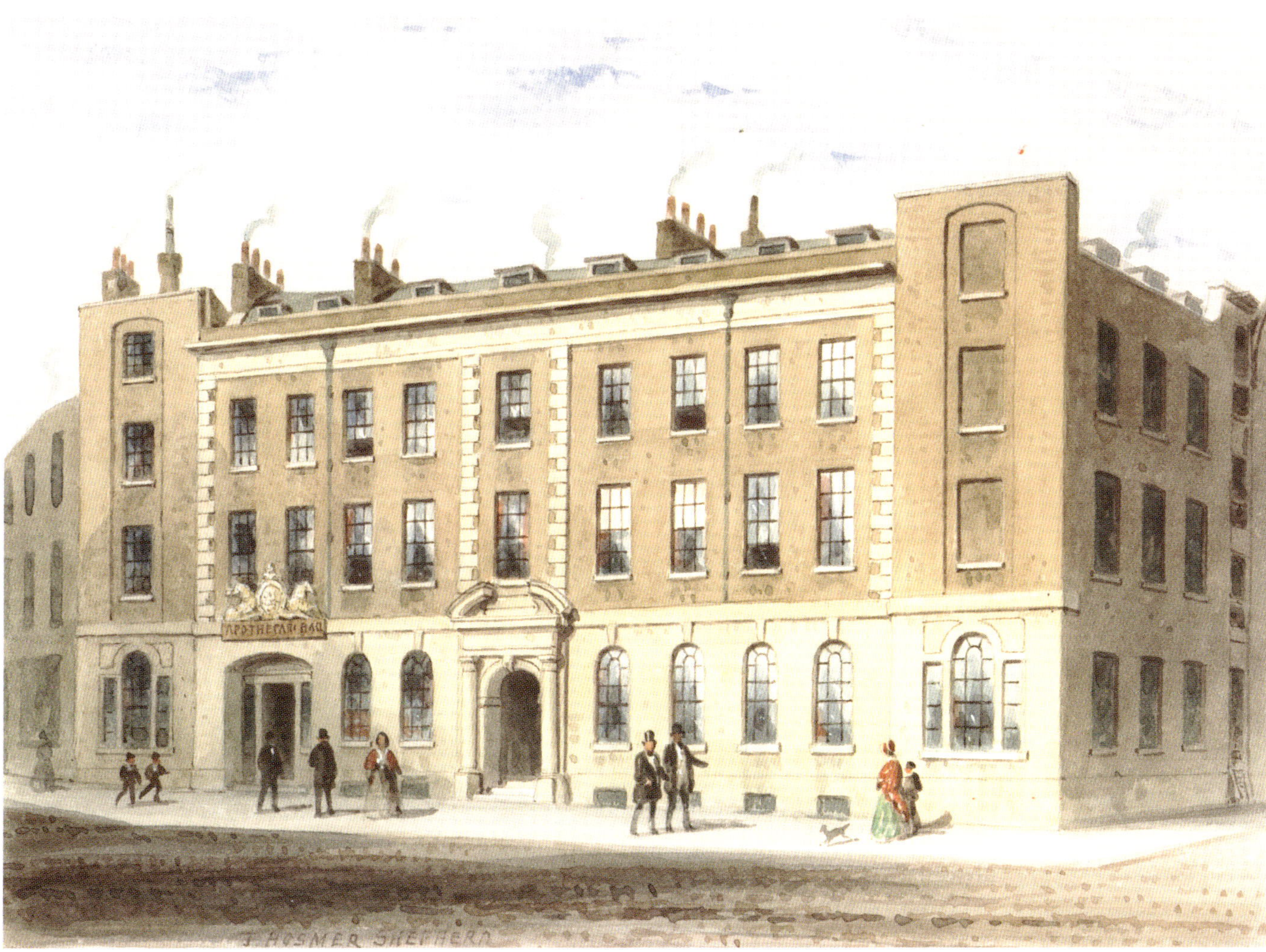

The Courtyard

The court minutes tell us that on 18 January 1670, Mr Young the stonecutter sent the drafts of the front door-case to the Hall with the Company's Arms and that the plainest version was chosen at a cost of £30.[6] This was in the days of the Courtyard opening directly onto Water Lane and so it is presumed that the door-case would have been that on the old main entrance at the top of the stone steps in the Courtyard. In which circumstance, these stone carved Arms would have been placed over this entrance but, as there is no further record of them, nor is it known what they looked like, nor where precisely they were placed, nor when they were taken down, there is nothing more to be said.

2.8 The Arms on the Courtyard East wall in 2010 and after restoration in 2016

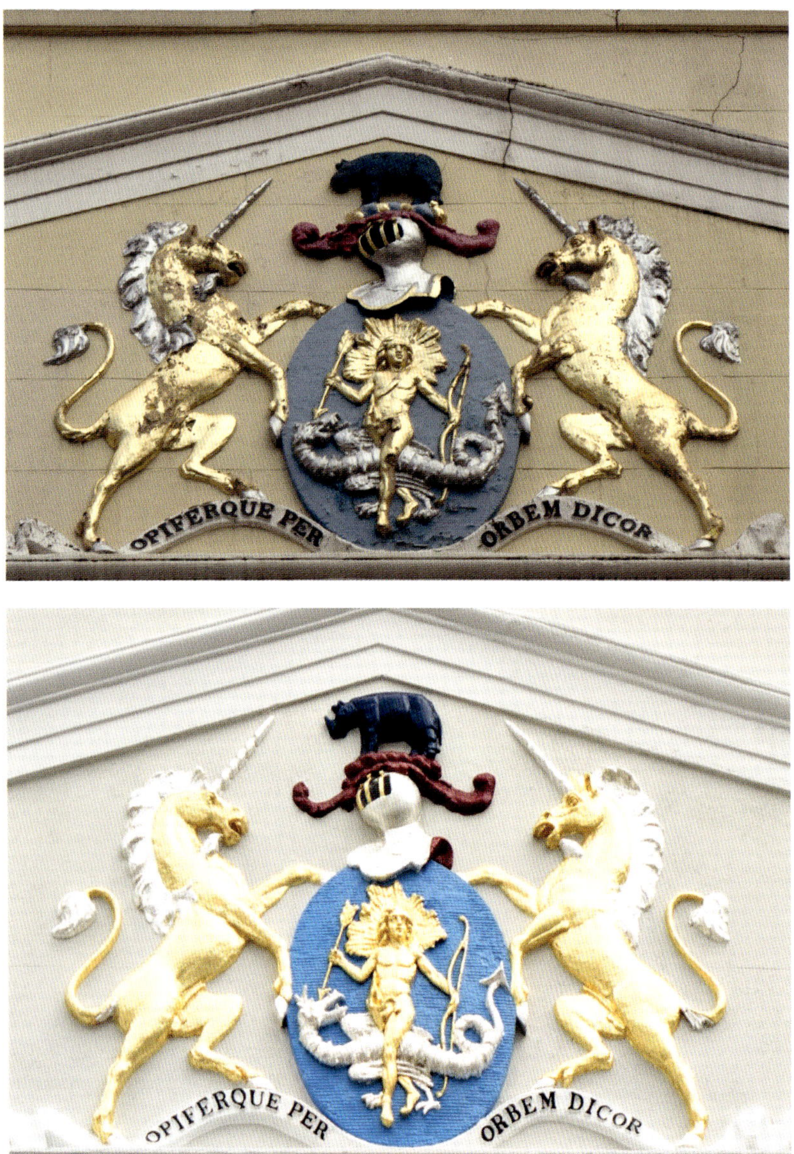

On entering the Courtyard, the Arms which catch the eye are those above the clock, high on the east wall (Figure 2.8). This part of the east wall was originally topped with balusters and coping. This was replaced wth a coped pediment,[7] and on 15 March 1785 the Court ordered that the wall be stuccoed and that Arms be erected thereon, also in stucco.[8] This was carried out by Messrs Adam, the firm of the famous Scottish neoclassical architect Robert Adam (1728–1792). Interestingly, the first four times these Arms were painted they were finished in a plain stone colour and it was only on the fifth repaint, probably in the late nineteenth century, that colour and gilding were introduced.[9]

Again, the shield is oval but this time the unicorns are very splendidly doing their duty. The helm is much more securely seated on the shield and is facing the correct way, with a much happier rhinoceros on the wreath but the mantling is a bit mean. On the other hand, Apollo is very radiant, his dress closer to the traditional portrayals of him and the dragon looks a more dangerous opponent.

The Society's Arms in wood also appear in the Courtyard in the broken pediment over the double doors in the north wall leading to the Entrance Hall (Figure 2.9). The origin of these Arms has proved to be somewhat enigmatic. By 2015 the Arms were in a very sorry state (Figure 2.11); both supporters had lost their horns and the sinister unicorn his whole face. The woodwork was in an extremely precarious condition,

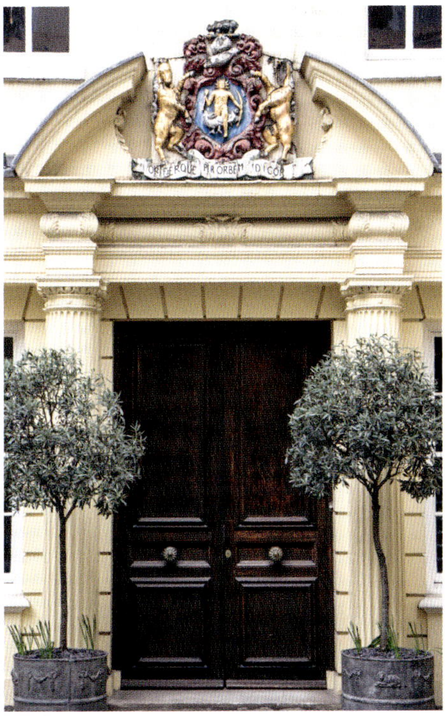

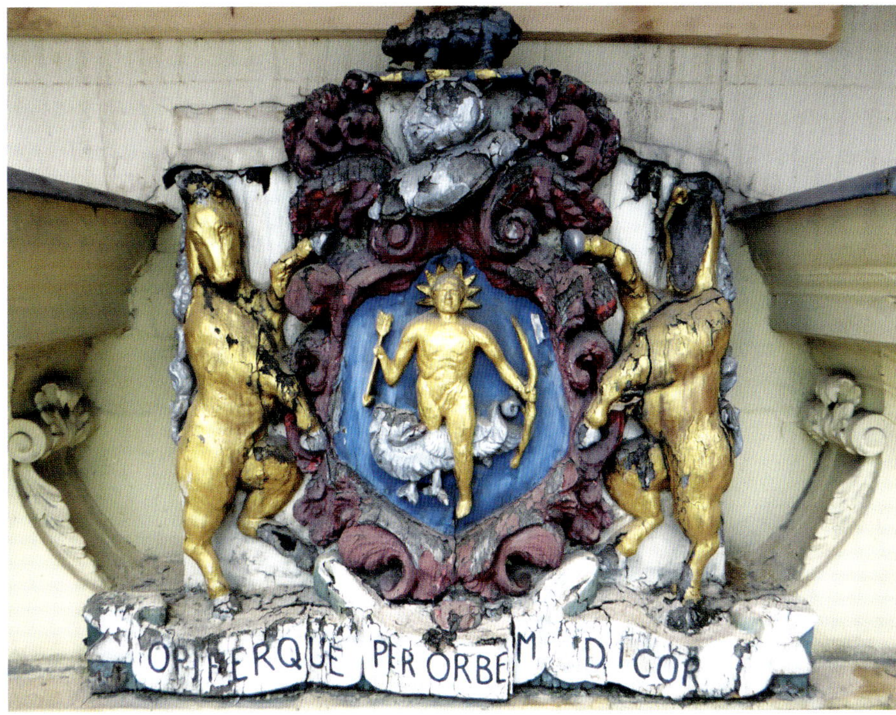

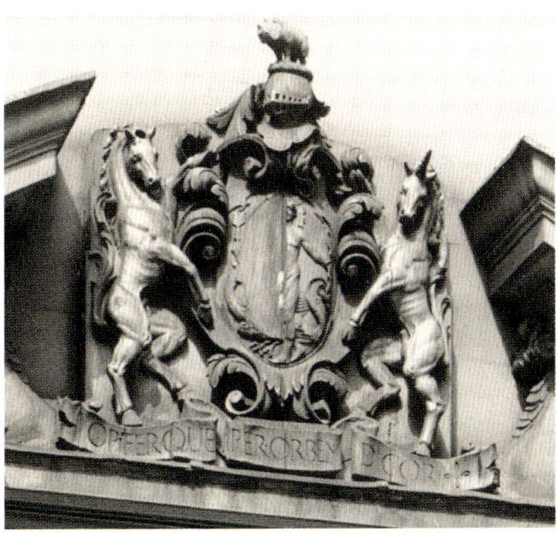

2.9 (top, left) The Arms over the Courtyard doors in the North wall

2.10 (above) The Arms over the Courtyard doors, c.1960

2.11 (top, right) The Arms over the Courtyard doors, 2015

with wet rot and fungal growth penetrating the structure. This had come about because of disagreements with the heritage supervisory bodies about what restoration was appropriate for such 'ancient' Arms. It had been required that no refurbishment work was to take place, that the Arms were to be taken down and preserved in this state and that a new copy be carved – all of which the Society was unwilling to do.

For many years, given the vertical nature of the Arms and their apparent age, it was suspected that they may have come from the stern of the third barge, which was discarded in 1817. Closer reading of Barrett, however, reveals that when that barge was sold 'only two small pieces of carving and two streamers were the sole relics'.[10] The pieces of carving referred to are probably the cartouche and the small Arms now displayed in the Court Room. Whilst Barrett is not entirely reliable, as four banners survived in addition to the two streamers, a relic the size of these Courtyard Arms would surely have been remarked upon.

The doorway and pediment on which the Arms are placed were only made in 1928–29 during the modifications to the Hall which enclosed the Entrance Hall. The question arises as to where these Arms came from. If these are surviving barge Arms, where were they between 1817 and 1929? Or were new Arms carved for this position?

Examination of Figures 2.10 and 2.11 shows the Arms in *c.*1960 and in 2015; despite their dilapidated states, it is quite clear that these are different sets of Arms. The helm and crest in the 1960 Arms are much more prominent, being raised and turned through 45 degrees, and higher than the mantling. The scrolling of the mantling is of a similar style but different in detail and the unicorns are also different in detail.

The Society's Year Book for 1960–61 states categorically that 'Mr Park is now to carve a coat of Arms in oak to be erected over the doors opening from the Courtyard to the Entrance Hall.' To pay for the wood and the cost of tincturing, £100 had been given anonymously. The Year Book for 1962–63 states that these Arms had duly been erected over the doors. Liveryman William Park FRCS was a general surgeon with an interest in wood carving. He also carved a matching pair of crested wooden clocks for committee rooms at the Royal College of Surgeons in Lincoln's Inn Fields.[11] The conclusion must be that the 1929 Arms were indeed replaced by new ones in 1962 and the reason must have been the decaying state of the 1929 Arms. Figure 2.10 shows that the dexter unicorn has lost his horn and the dexter side of the shield is almost blank, although half of Apollo with his bow is still visible on the sinister side. The Archive is silent on the erection and dismantling of the 1929–61 Arms and it is impossible now to state their origin with any certainty. It remains unlikely, however, that they came from the last barge.

The final mystery is why both sets of Arms deteriorated so badly in only about thirty-five years, while the wooden Arms over the Courtyard Archway entrance from Black Friars Lane, already described, have not suffered thus despite being nearly 200 years old. Possibly it is to do with the atmospheric conditions in this somewhat damp corner of the Courtyard, comparing unfavourably with the blustery drying winds of Black Friars Lane.

DBR Conservation was responsible for the refurbishment of the Arms in 2016 and the results can be seen in Figure 2.12. This restoration was generously paid for by the Heritage of London Trust and by Messrs Farebrother, the Society's surveyors since 1825,[12] as part of the Society's 400th anniversary celebrations.

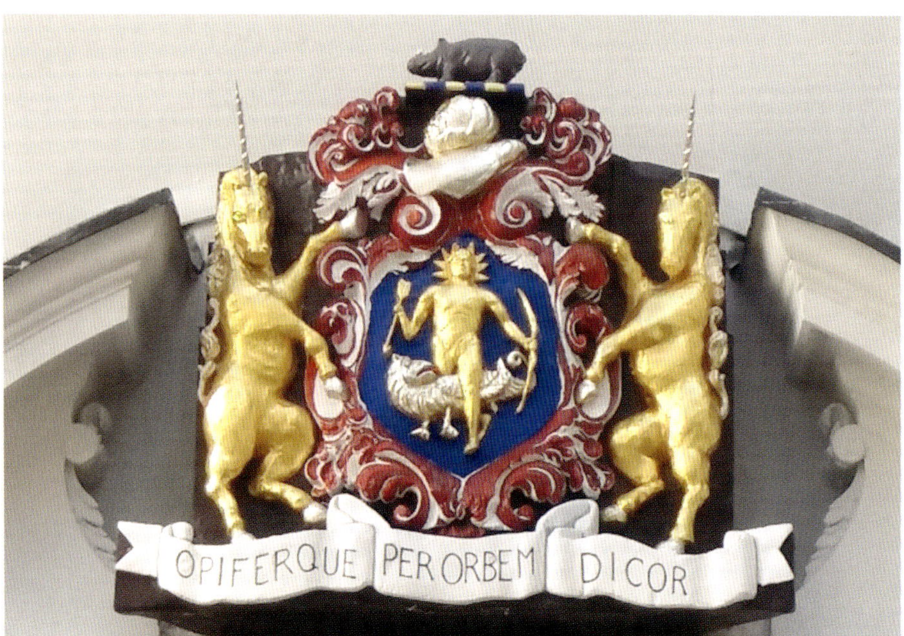

2.12 Restored Arms over the Courtyard doors, 2016

The Arms are a fairly faithful reproduction of the Camden original; the mantling is excessive but not unattractive. The carver has not done badly with Apollo, but his opponent looks about as dangerous as a household pet. The most obvious change is that the unicorns are in an unconventional attitude, being rampant and also guardant, as they were in the 1929 version of the Arms. This may have been necessitated by the space available in the broken pediment, but the whole effect is very successful.

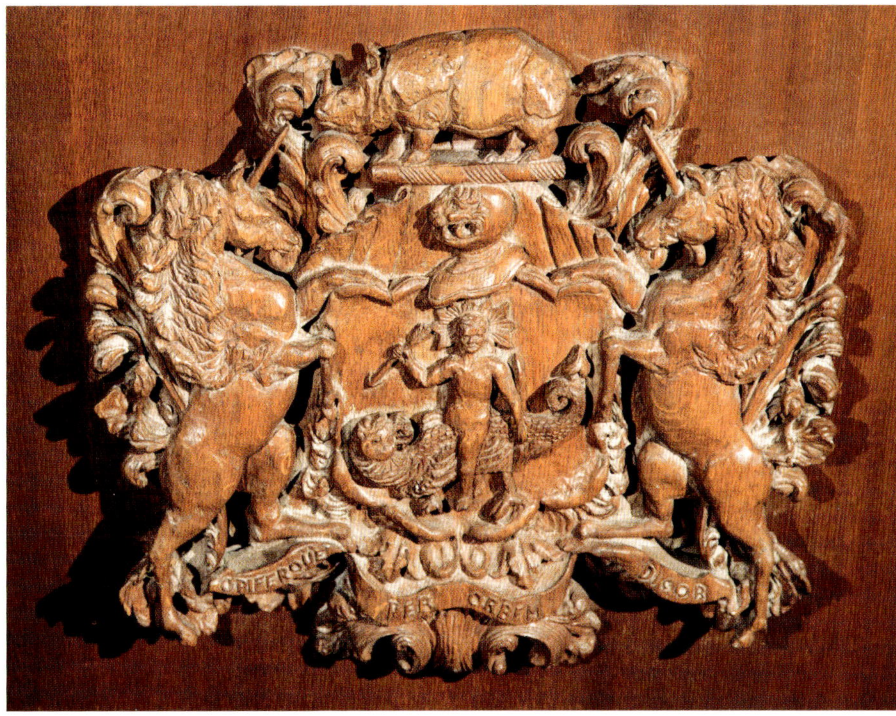

2.13 The Arms under the staircase

The Entrance Hall, Stairs and Landing

On coming into the Entrance Hall, there is a coat of Arms which is elaborately carved on the underside of the second flight of the staircase (Figure 2.13). These were carved in oak and placed there in 1960 by Liveryman William Park before he embarked on the more ambitious project of carving the large Arms over the Courtyard doors. It is a good likeness of the Camden Arms for a small piece and the carving is meticulous but quite unlike the style of his Courtyard Arms.

The next three displays of the Arms to be encountered are all in stained glass and will be illustrated and described more fully in their respective chapters.

The first, seen on ascending the stairs to the first-floor landing, is the oldest representation of the Arms in the Hall. The window was installed in 1671 at the rebuilding of the Hall after the Great Fire of 1666. Originally, this would have been an external wall but owing to subsequent building it is now internal and therefore the window is backlit. It can easily be missed if it is not illuminated (this one is discussed in detail in Chapter 5).

On reaching the first-floor landing, two further representations of the Arms in glass are encountered in the pair of windows overlooking the Courtyard (considered in Chapter 10).

The Court Room

On entering the Court Room, the most dramatic version of the Arms anywhere in the Hall is displayed in the glass of the right-hand window (discussed in Chapter 7).

Turning around and looking up, there is another set of Arms over the door to the landing from the Court Room (Figure 2.15). These were undoubtedly carved for the Society's barge; Wall says that they are seventeenth century.[13]

The Society has had three barges in its time. This first was commissioned in 1673 and sold in 1713. The second saw service from 1727 to 1764, and the third barge was in use between 1765 and *c.*1813, when the last herbarising expedition took place by river.[14]

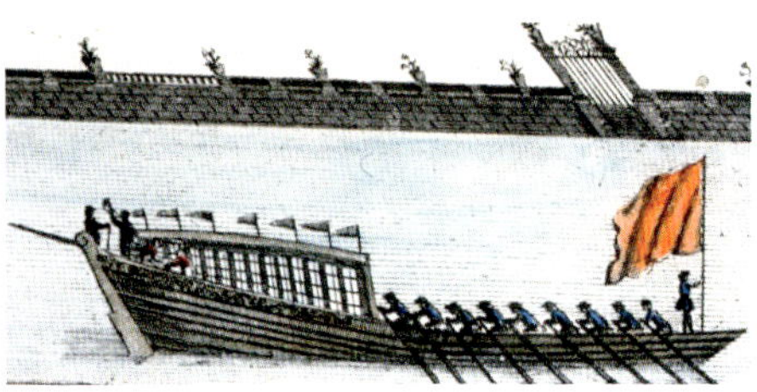

2.14 A typical Livery Company barge of the eighteenth century (with the wall and gate of the Chelsea Physic Garden in the background)

In July 1673, the Court accepted an estimate from Nicholas Wheatley of £110.0.0d to build the Society's first barge. Wheatley had just completed a barge for the Company of Mercers and in the contract it stated that Mr Cleere, who had carried out the Mercers' carving, was to do the carved work for the Apothecaries and 'no other person'. There were two brothers Cleere, William (d.1690) and Richard (Master Joiner & Ceiler 1676[15]) both members of the Joiners Company, active at this time. Correspondence with the Mercers' Company reveals that it was Richard Cleere who carried out the barge work for the Mercers.[16]

If Wall is right about the dating, these Arms must have been carved in 1673 by Richard Cleere. The contract with the Society states:

> *and to differ nothing from the [Mercers'] barge save only some extraordinary carved work, as instead of the Maidenhead, the said Mercers' Arms, two Unicorns to be carved in good oak or elm timber and set on each side of the door into the house of the said barge and a Rhinoceros carved in like manner and set over the same entrance and also the coat of Arms of the Company of Apothecaries with the supporters and crest well carved in like manner and set at the stern of the barge with screws to take on and off.*[17]

The unicorns and the rhinoceros around the door have disappeared but the Arms survive, with their screw-holes clearly visible. The date of the carving, and the Arms' continued existence, would seem to confirm that they were displayed on all three barges. However, details for the second barge, which was contracted to the shipwright John Hall for £230 in 1727, confuse the issue. The specification for this barge states:

> *The inside of the house, being wainscot, was to be varnished, the great carved shield gilded and painted in proper colours, the carved trail boards gilded on each side. The waist board was to be ornamented with the King's, the City's and the Company's Arms and Crest … Two large carved figures afore the house and two ditto abaft to be gilded.*[18]

Can the Arms in the Court Room be considered to be 'a great carved shield' which appeared to be fitted inside the [deck] house? Probably not, but remember that these smallish Arms were designed to be detachable and perhaps therefore were saved, whereas a larger artefact might not have been. Neither were the four large carved figures, nor any of the finely decorated heraldic waist and trail boards saved.

No specification exists for the third barge, so it is impossible to know what carved decoration was saved from the previous barges or made anew for this one. It must be presumed that the mobile Court Room Arms were once again put into service in this barge.

Despite extensive research by Liveryman Col John Nicholls-Palmer in the 1980s, the Society can find no illustration of any of its barges. Frustratingly, George Bowman, the Society's Surveyor at the time, presented a drawing of the third barge which was framed and hung in the Hall but which has disappeared without trace. The barges must have looked something like Figure 2.14, which appears in the margin of a plan of the Chelsea Physic Garden dated 1732.

The artistically difficult charges of the Court Room Arms are very finely carved and the detail is exceptional. They have indeed been 'well carved' as specified in the contract and are a very reasonable reproduction of the Camden Arms. The rhinoceros is rather poorly represented and is unique in that he seems to have two dorsal horns and no nasal horn! The carver has made a small, and rarely spotted, mistake as he has

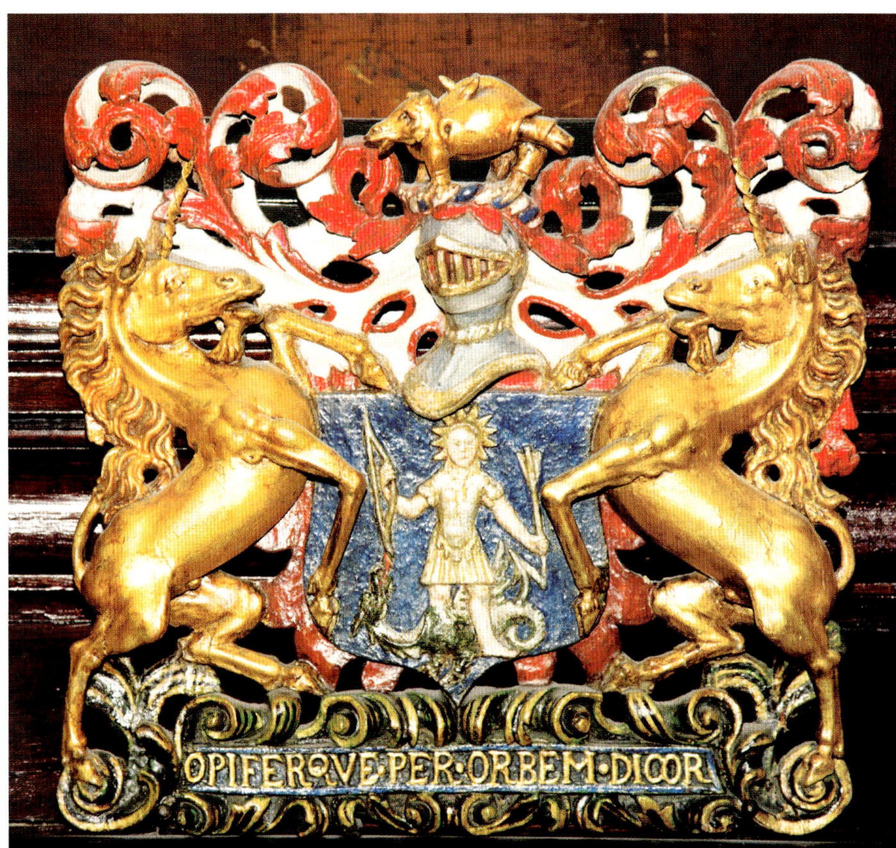

2.15 The 1673 Arms over the main door in the Court Room, showing the screw holes in the tails of the unicorns

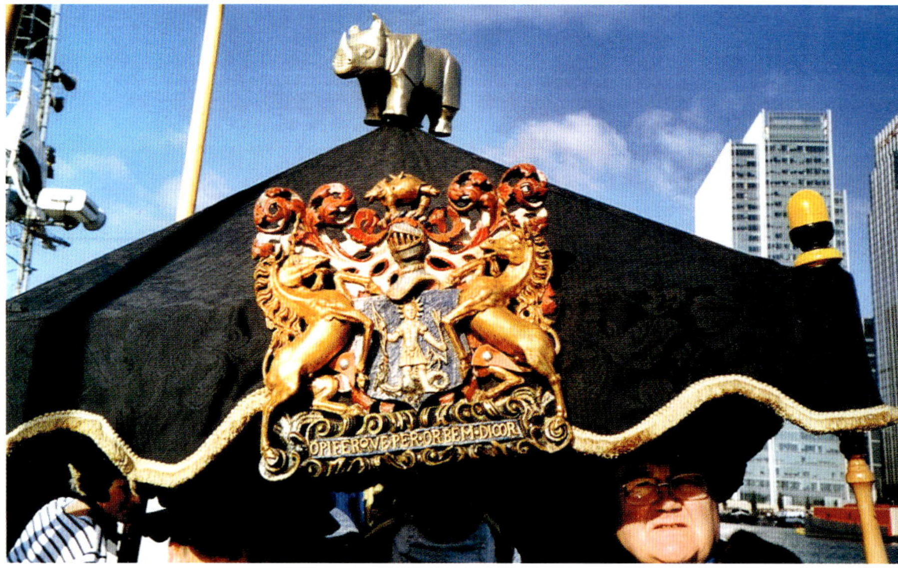

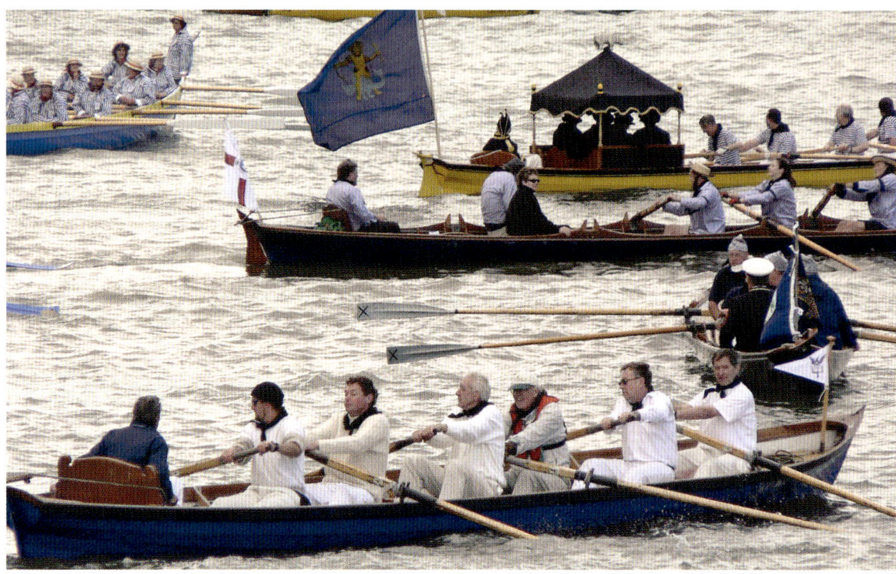

2.16 The 1673 Arms attached to the 2005 re-enactment cutter's canopy with the Master, Prof Brian Livesley, sitting on the port side

2.17 The Society's cutter, with yellow hull, participating in the 2005 re-enactment

reversed the hands in which Apollo carries his bow and arrow. Unusually, the forelegs of the unicorns protectively encroach upon the shield. These Arms were last cleaned and restored in 1989.[19]

Probably the last time the barge was used formally was on 8 January 1806 when the Society, with other City barges and many other small craft, escorted Lord Nelson's body upriver from Greenwich to Westminster in a large procession as part of his state funeral before burial at St Paul's on 9 January.

To mark the 200th anniversary of the Battle of Trafalgar this procession was re-enacted in September 2005, and as one of the original participants, the Society was allocated a place. No longer owning a barge, one of the modern livery cutters was hired and decked out in the Society colours and emblems, including the Court Room Arms which were attached to the forward end of the canopy (Figures 2.16 and 2.17). As far as can be determined, this was the only artefact which featured in both processions.

The Great Hall

In the Great Hall there are two representations of the Arms. The larger but least visible is part of the screen and panelling at the south end of the Hall (Figure 2.18). The whole screen is carved out of dark Irish oak and was completed on the rebuilding of the Hall. It is possible that the Arms and capitals of the columns were originally gilded, which would have had a very dramatic effect.

In 1957 it was debated whether these Arms should be painted and gilded;[20] the views of the Victoria and Albert Museum, the Society for the Protection of Ancient Buildings and Mr Carl Edwards were sought. All the consultees vigorously advised against such a project and Mr Edwards commented:

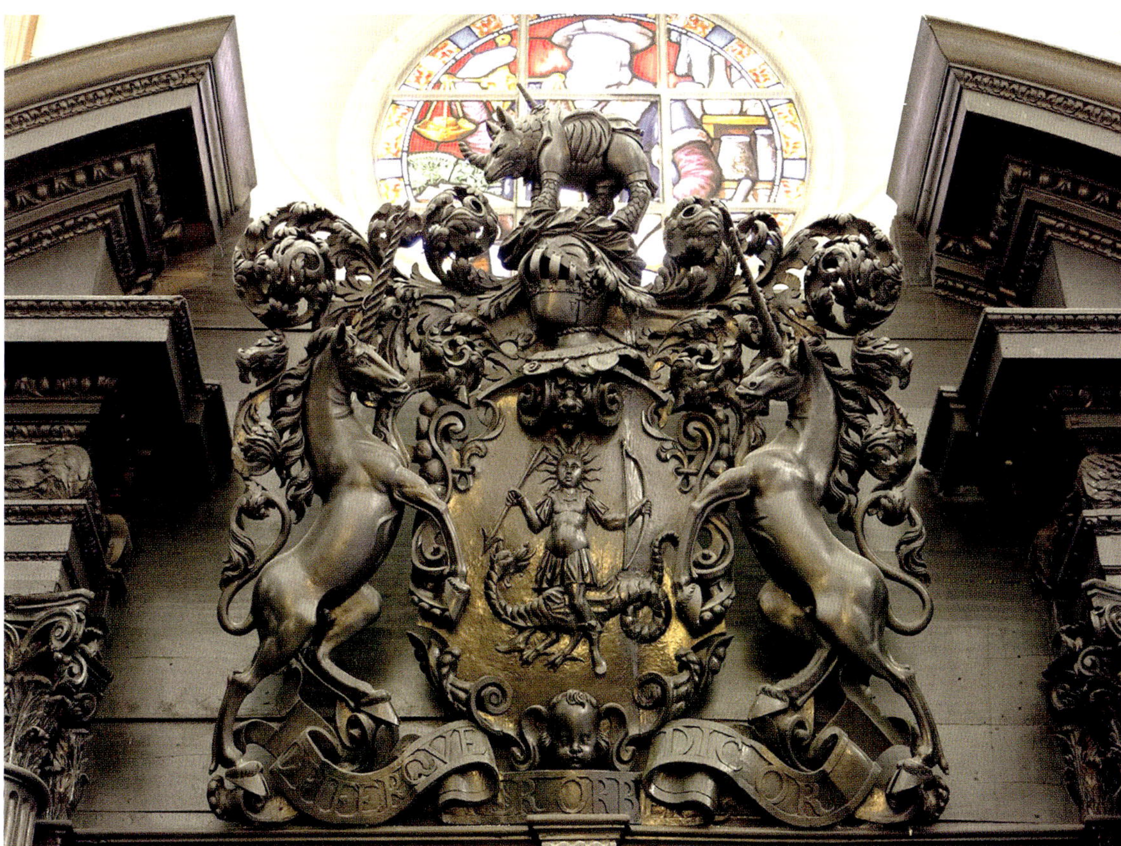

2.18 The large oak-carved Arms in the Great Hall

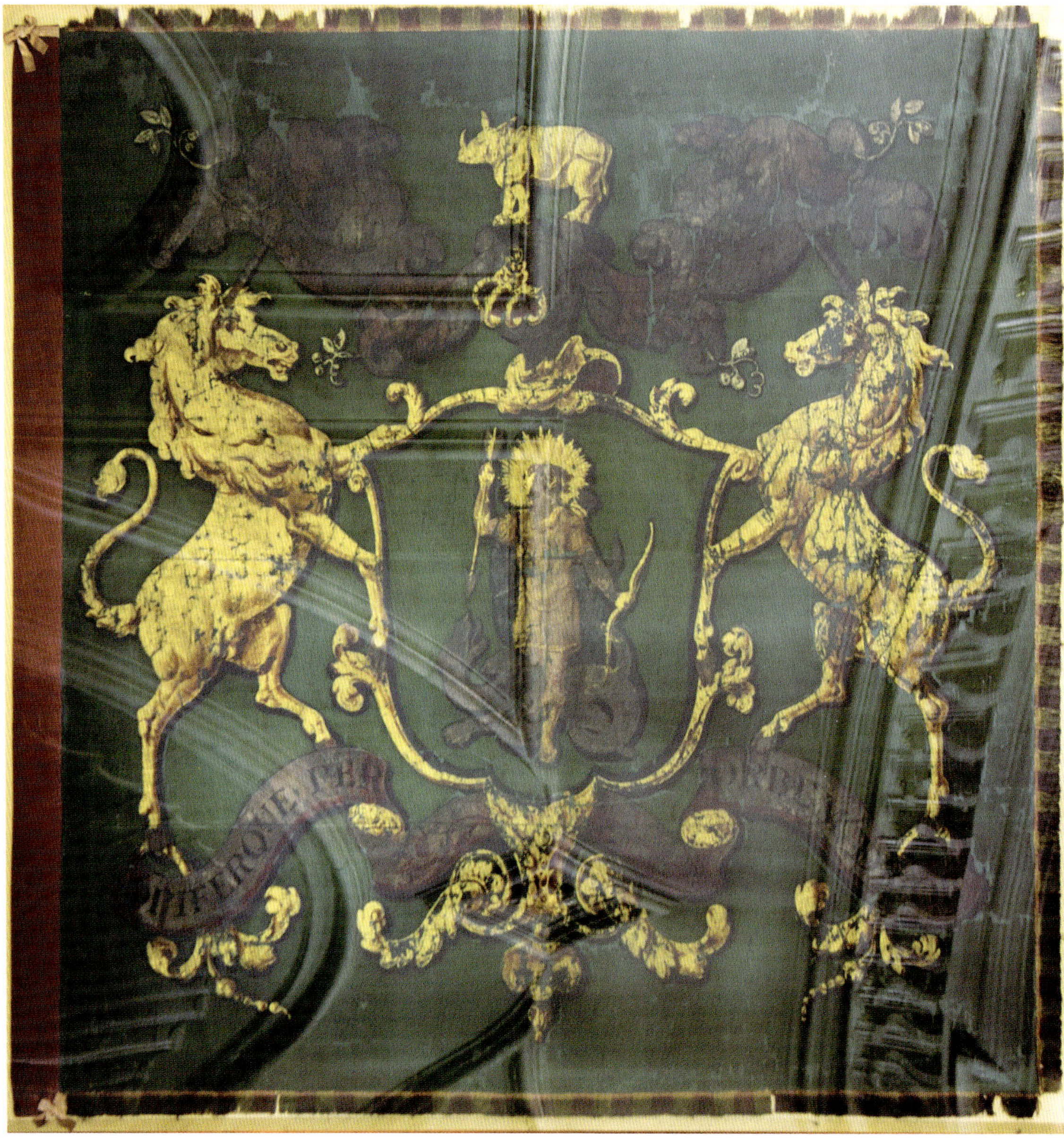

2.19 The restored barge banner Arms in the Great Hall

> *While painting will without doubt bring out the larger shapes and help to make the general design easily understood it will, on the other hand, destroy the more subtle forms. This is because a number of coats of paint would have to be used to achieve a good result and also because colour tends to destroy delicate contours. For these reasons the painting of sculpture in the round is an exceedingly difficult art which, in my view, is lost today … In conclusion … if the result was unsuccessful it would be very difficult to remove the paint without injuring the carving.*

Accordingly, at the March 1957 meeting of the Court, it was decided not to proceed with painting but to investigate better lighting.

As built, this screen was some 10 feet further forward than at present and the archway under the Arms was open, the main entrance to the Great Hall being via the stone steps from the Courtyard. In 1793 the whole screen with the Arms was moved back against the south wall of the Great Hall as the Court perceived that this would be more commodious for the Assistants' table than having it at the north end.[21] The panel currently filling the archway was one of the side panels and its pair is now beneath the Musicians' Gallery at the north end of the Hall. The screen was made by the master joiners Burges and Davyes between 1671 and 1674 and the Arms were carved in 1671 by Henry Phillips, for which he received £36.0.0d in 1673.[22] Phillips was the King's Master Sculptor and Carver in Wood from 1661 until his death in 1693, when he was succeeded by Grinling Gibbons.

The second representation of the Arms in the Great Hall is the barge banner high on the south wall (Figure 2.19). The first mention of banners for a barge is in the Court minutes of 20 July 1630, when banners and streamers were to be provided for Lord Mayor's Day. It is not until the next year, however, that Society banners or colours were specified. On 29 August 1631, Mr John Tailor, an apothecary named in the Charter in 1617, undertook 'to provide three banners, one with the King's Arms, another with the City Arms and a third with the Company's Arms, and two long streamers, with staves to bear them and rowling staves and papers in which to wrap them, and to paint the bearing staves, for which he is to have £38-0-0'[23] – a not inconsiderable sum.

In fact, this was so expensive that in the end only the streamers were purchased. The banners had to wait until 1634 when a subscription for them had been raised.[24] These barge colours were transferred to the second barge and lasted until 1761.

On 28 August 1761, a new set of flags and streamers was ordered for the second barge at a cost of £48.0.0d from John Stock & Co. It consisted of four banners: the King's Arms, the Company Arms with crest and supporters, the City Arms with crest and supporters and the Company Arms without supporters in a compartment. Two streamers were also made with the City Arms and the Company Arms with proper ornaments.[25]

The banners and streamers seen in the Hall today are the successors of these latter ones. In 1797 new colours were required and were ordered from Mr Sharp,[26] but the

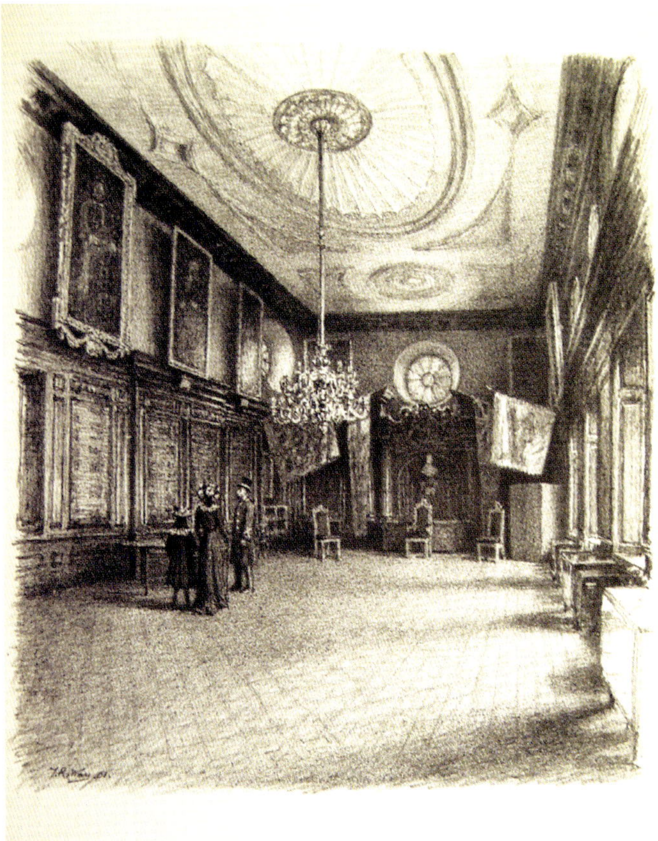

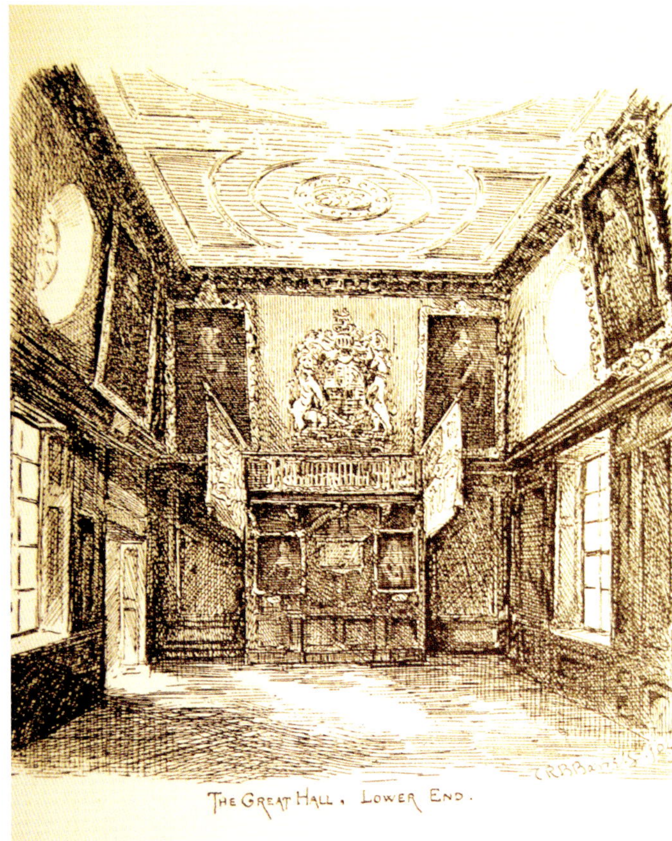

2.20 (left) The South (the City & St Luke banners and the streamers) and (right) North (the Society & Royal banners) ends of the Great Hall, with the banners and streamers displayed in 1905

Society did not participate in the Lord Mayor's Day procession that year as the banners were not ready. The new suit of colours consisted of the King's Arms, the City Arms, the Society Arms, a representation of St Luke, the patron saint of physicians, and two streamers featuring the City Arms and ornaments and the Union Flag with Society ornaments. In 1801 the union canton of the Society streamer was altered to include the cross of St Patrick following the Act of Union with Ireland.[27] When the barge fell out of use, the banners and streamers were displayed at each end of the Great Hall on poles, the crutches of which can still be seen on the Musicians' Gallery (Figure 2.20).

In 1987 the banners and streamers were found to be in poor condition and a programme of conservation was planned.[28] Over five months in 1987–88 the Arms banner was conserved at a cost of £2,208 and placed in a glazed elm case. This banner was lent to the National Maritime Museum in Greenwich for the Royal River Exhibition in 2012.[29] The St Luke banner and the two streamers were also encased, but the other two banners were in too poor a condition to be conserved and remain in storage in the Hall.

Summary

Neither the Library nor the Parlour has any fixed coats of Arms and the table below gives a summary of the Arms mentioned in this chapter, with the addition of the Arms on the wall of Cobham House (discussed in Chapter 3).

DATE	WHERE	PURPOSE	MATERIAL	ARTIST
1671	Stairs	Window	Glass	prob Richard Dutton (c.1636–1686)
1671	Great Hall	Screen Display	Wood	Henry Phillips (d.1693)
1673	Court Room	Barge Arms	Wood	Richard Cleere
18th C.	Landing	Window	Glass	Unknown
1785	Courtyard	Wall Display	Plaster	Messrs Adam
1797	Great Hall	Barge Banner	Fabric	Mr Sharp
1823	Archway	Entrance Display	Wood	Unknown
19th C.	Landing	Window	Glass	Unknown
1915	Cobham House	Wall Display	Stone	Unknown
1960	Entrance Hall	Understairs	Wood	William Park (1912–2004)
1961	Courtyard	Doorway Display	Wood	William Park (1912–2004)
1967	Court Room	Window	Glass	Carl Edwards (1914–1985)

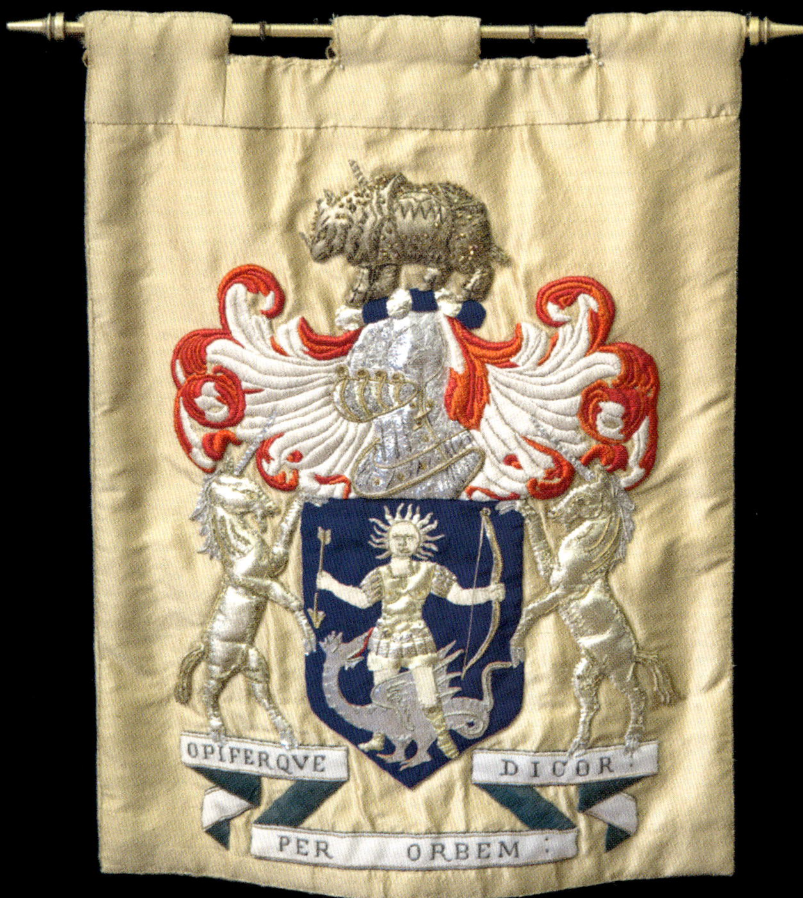

3.30 The embroidered lectern Arms

CHAPTER 3

Other Uses of the Society's Arms

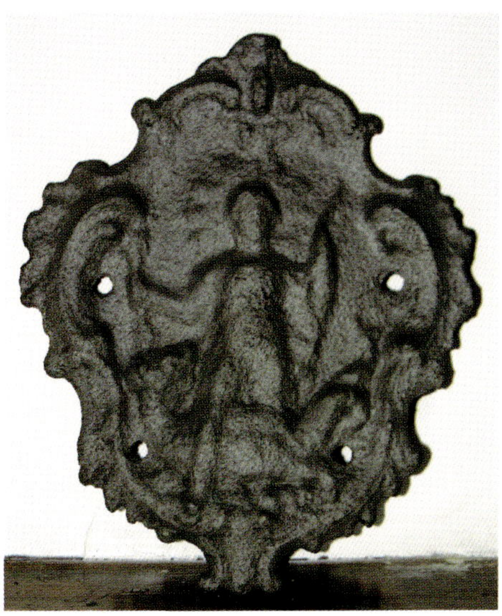

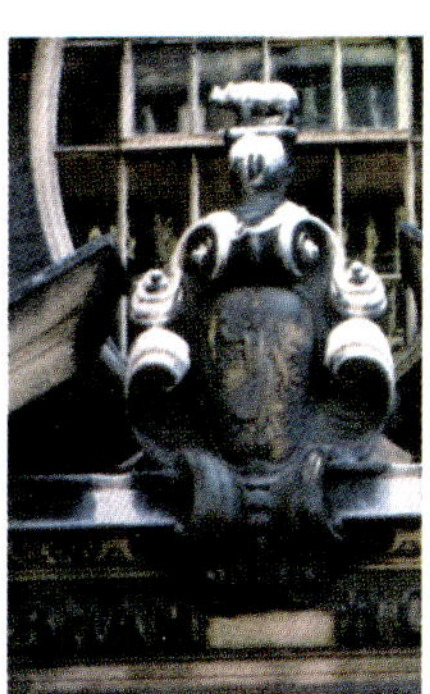

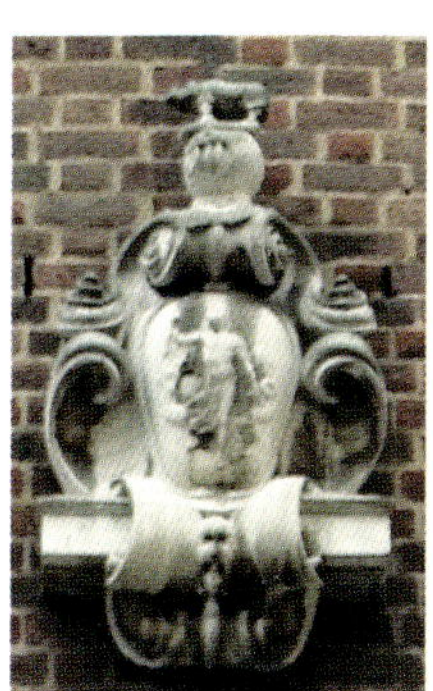

3.1 A sand-cast metal blazon of Arms of the Society, c.1800

3.2 The stone Arms set up over the Cobham House entrance in 1916, photographed in 1974

3.3 The Cobham House Arms after the 1985 redevelopment

A coat of Arms, apart from stating who or what you are, can also be used to indicate belonging or possession. When Arms are granted to individuals they usually include a badge, normally a variant of one of the main charges on its own and also a standard to be flown, both of which can be used to indicate belonging, possession or presence. The Society was granted neither of these extras and so, to overcome this omission, the Arms have been used in various ways over the years: either the full achievement of Arms; or just the shield; or just the crest – the latter two displays technically illegal in the eyes of the College of Arms.

Stone and Metal

The Court Minutes of 13 October 1757 record an order for a dozen metal plates bearing the Society's Arms to be cast and affixed to houses belonging to the Society.[1] This was not part of the fire insurance schemes which were springing up at the time but simply the marking of the Society's property. The Society has one rather weather-beaten example (Figure 3.1) in the Archive and none remain anywhere on the Society's estate.

In a similar way, however, when the Society's Mill and Engine House on Water Lane to the north of the Hall was developed for letting in 1915–16, it was renamed Cobham House and a stone coat of Arms was set up in a pediment over the entrance door (Figure 3.2). The site was then let to a firm of blouse manufacturers and a newspaper exporter.[2] When Cobham House was redeveloped in 1985, these Arms were moved to the wall of New Cobham House overlooking Black Friars Lane (Figure 3.3). It is not known who carved these Arms and having weathered badly the detail is not easy to see. The Arms consist of the shield, helm and crest without mantling or supporters and are placed on a small stone shelf. This leaves the rhinoceros unsupported but looking pretty steady nonetheless.

In the Brande Room there is a dramatic wrought-iron version of Society Arms (Figure 3.4). It is large, 3' x 2' 6", and looks as if it should have been the fireback to the

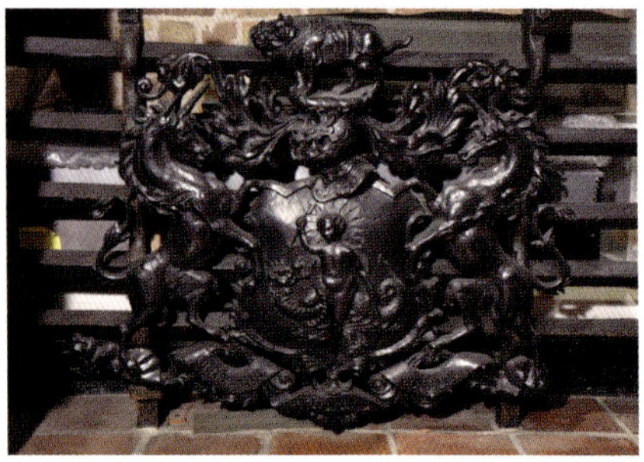

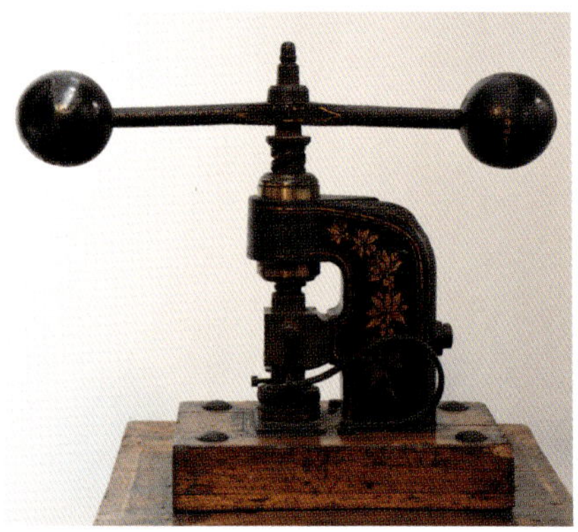

3.4 The 'fire grate' Arms

3.5 The Society's Corporation Seal Press

old kitchen fireplace which is in the Brande Room but it is modern and its provenance is not known. It is a good and well balanced representation of the Camden Arms. With the refurbishment of the Brande Room in 1994 the intention was to display these Arms above the fireplace but, with the placing of the Charter and Patent of Arms in that position, it was decided to attach them to the fire basket instead and they are now largely hidden behind miscellaneous boxes of archives.

Ceremonial: Corporation Seal, Leading Staff and Master's Chair

James I and VI's Charter of 1617 created the Society into a corporate body. The Charter directed that the Society

> *may have for ever a Common Seal for the Causes and Businesses of them and their Successors whatsoever, to serve for all things by them to be done. And that it shall and may be lawful for the same Master, Wardens, and Society of the Art and Mystery of Apothecaries of the City of London, and their Successors, the same Seal, at their pleasure from time to time to break, change, alter, and new make, as to them shall seem best.*

To this day, all of the Society's yeomanry, livery and freedom certificates, diplomas and licences, and deeds, leases and covenants are sealed with the Society's Corporate Seal. In March 1755 this seal was reported to be defective and a new one was ordered to be fashioned. The new seal was engraved by a Mr Garden and the old one was broken.[3] It is unlikely that the current seal (Figure 3.5) dates from 1755 but no mention of a new seal appears in the records since then. In 2012 the table on which the seal is mounted was restored by Mr Paul Ash and the seal itself was reconditioned and a new collar fitted by Mr Grant MacDonald. The seal is engraved with the full achievement of Arms of the Society.

In an inventory of all the Society's possessions compiled by Israel Wolfe, the Renter Warden for 1626–27, the 'Companyes Seale' is recorded, together with, inter alia, a chamber pot and a brush, but there is no mention of a leading staff. The leading staff or mace carried by the Beadle (Figure 3.6) was presented in 1658 by Michael Markland,[4] Master 1659–60, and unlike the longer staffs-of-office used by most of the other companies, is hand-held like a truncheon. It has a wooden shaft and a chased silver head bearing the Arms on an ornate oval face supported by a single but imposing unicorn (Figure 3.7). If the necessity arose, it could be reversed with the silver head forming a sword-like basket handle and the wooden end, which is turned, a club.

In 1941 the Society received a bequest of £1,200 from the late Algernon Dutton Brenchley, Master 1924–25, in which he suggested that part of this sum might be used to acquire a new silver-gilt mace,[5] but this suggestion was not acted upon and in 1962 the

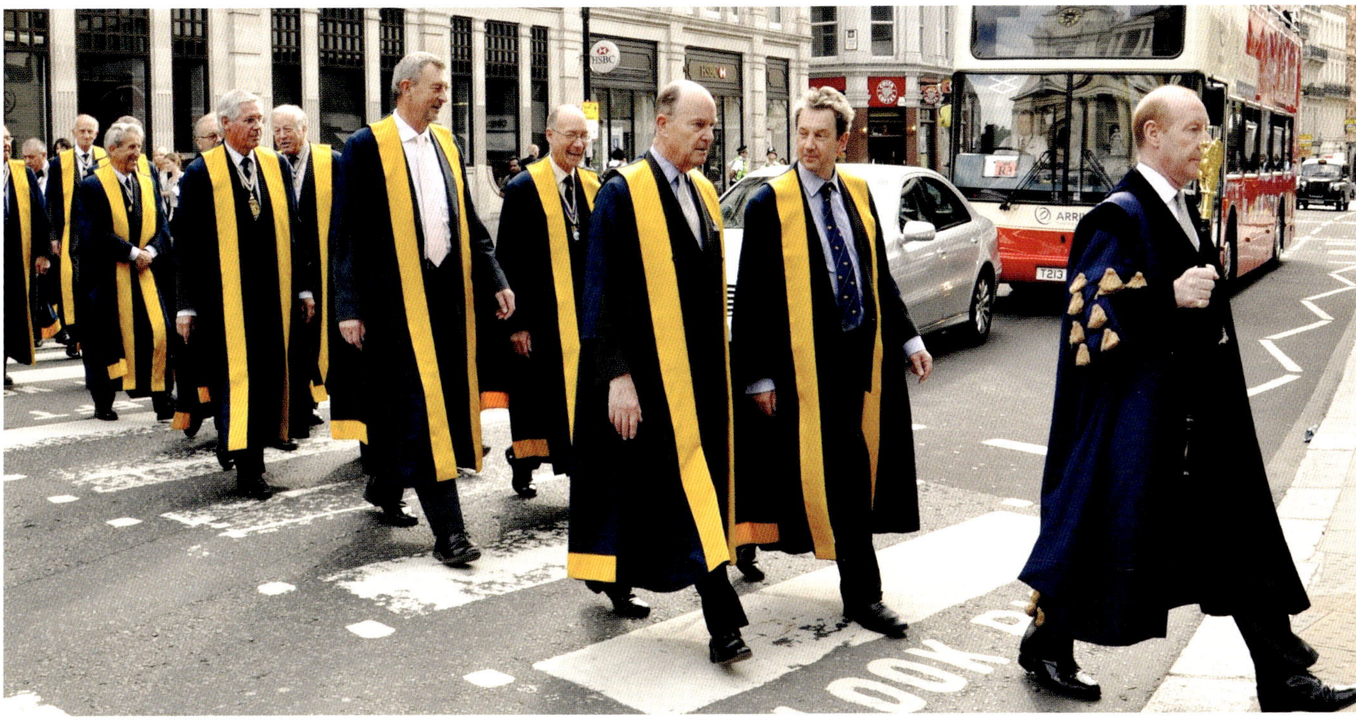

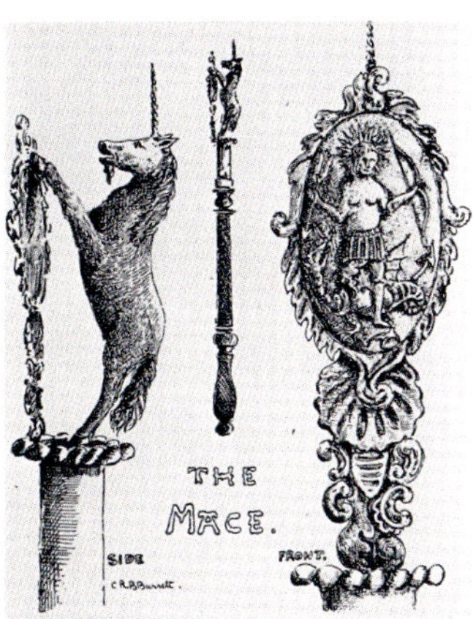

3.6 John Williams, Beadle, with mace, leading the Court in procession in 2011

3.7 The Society's mace

Master, Redvers Ironside, paid for the staff to be repaired and re-gilded.[6] Further repairs in 1987 were funded by Court Assistant F. L. W. Collings.

The Society Arms in unusual form also appear on the Master's Chair (Figure 3.8). This was made in 1812 from broken branches of the cedar trees planted in the Chelsea Physic Garden in 1683.[7] The accompanying Wardens' chairs were made from the same material in 1847. The back of the Master's Chair is surmounted by a large carved wooden Gomda (rhinoceros). It has been as fancifully carved as Dürer drew it, but suffers from the frequent accidental loss of its nasal horn! Below it is a roundel displaying Apollo and the dragon with the motto encircling it. The whole representation is unconventional but satisfactorily adapted to the design of the chair.

Ceremonial: Court Jewels

There is no record of when Court jewels, sometimes described as badges, were first introduced. On 13 March 1894 the Court minutes record that 'Consideration about whether or not the Society should have a Badge was postponed sine die'. In the Archive there is an incomplete collection of formal photographs of Masters in their gowns. The first photograph of a Master in a gown with a badge is Joseph Stewart Burton, Master 1898–99.

It is further documented that in 1901 William Shillito, Master 1886–87, presented a jewel (Figure 3.9) and the Court Minutes of 7 May 1901, records that this jewel is to be

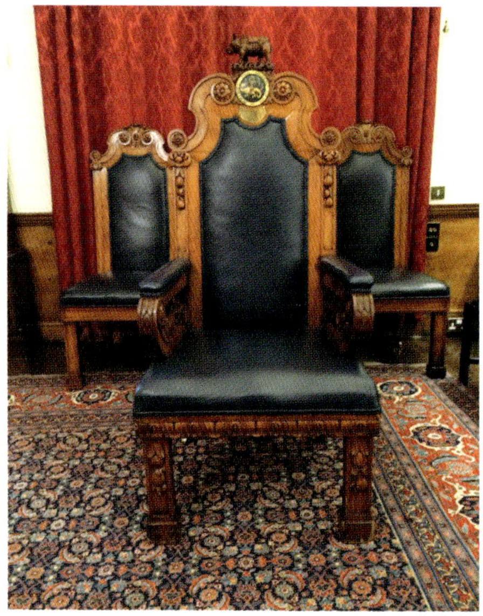

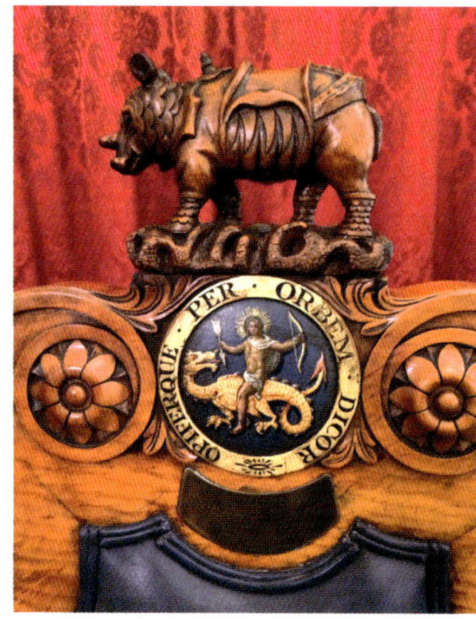

3.8a The Private Court cedar chairs

3.8b Heraldic detail on the Master's chair

worn 'by the Master for the time being' and furthermore 'that the badge presented by Dr Griffith be worn by the Deputy Master for the time being'.

It is presumed that it was Dr Samuel Clewin Griffith, Master 1897–98, who presented the 'Griffith' badge probably at the end of his Master's year and therefore the photograph of Burton must be with the Griffith jewel. There is no surviving description of the Griffith jewel but the jewel worn by Burton is virtually identical to Figure 3.9, which raises the question of why a new jewel was needed in 1901.

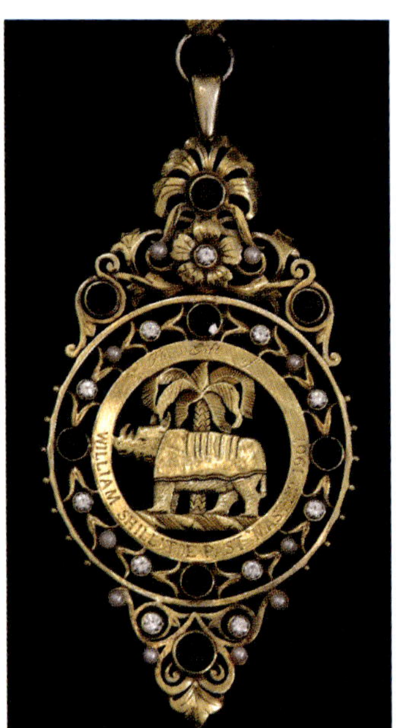

3.9 The Immediate Past Master's jewel, replicated in 1989

In 1920 the Shillito badge was downgraded to be the Immediate Past Master's jewel, the fate of Dr Griffith's badge, if it still existed, being unknown. The Shillito Immediate Past Master's jewel was stolen, with other items, in a burglary in 1987 (see below) and was replicated by Alan Mudd of Clerkenwell in 1989. This current jewel is a silver-gilt rhinoceros and tree set in a circle with imitation pearls and red and white simulant stones, and bears the inscription on the circlet commemorating William Shillito's gift.

In 1920 the Master, Samuel Osborn, who had been Master Haberdasher 1910–11, presented the rather more ornate style of Master's jewel which is used today. The Master's jewel consists of the Society's Arms depicted in enamel, gold and silver and set upon an elaborate pierced fleur-de-lys scrollwork in gold studded with diamonds. The supporters are modelled in high relief in gold and the shield is of blue enamel with the charges thereon also depicted in high relief (Figures 3.10 and 3.11).

The original jewel was made by Messrs Garrard & Co Ltd and it had a somewhat chequered career. It was completely broken up, with parts lost, in a robbery by the Hall's office boy on 13 September 1947.[8] The boy had abruptly stopped work on 5 September and then returned to steal goods valued at about £600. The jewel was recovered and repaired by Messrs Hicklenton & Phillips. It later emerged that the boy (who is nameless in the minutes and who had been taken on in January 1947) had had four previous convic-

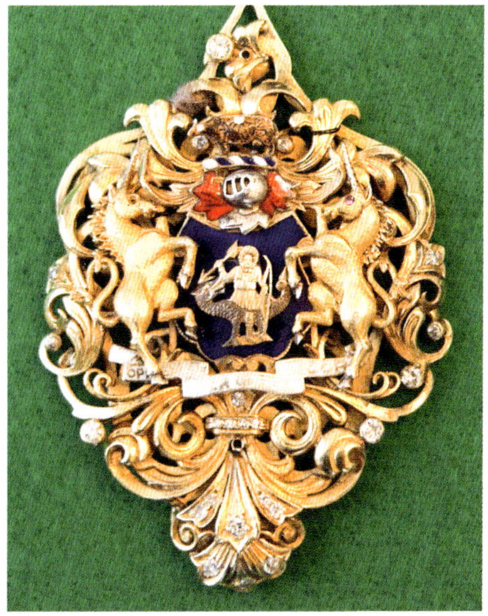

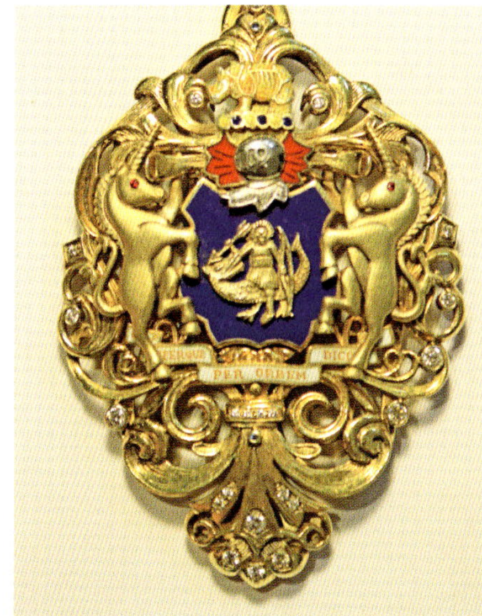

3.10 The Master's jewel 1988–2016

3.11 The Master's jewel 2017–present

tions for robbery and theft and had been bound over for one year by the Guildhall Juvenile Court subject to his joining the Navy!

The Master's jewel was stolen again forty years later in a burglary during a dinner on 24 February 1987,[9] which begs the question of why it was not being worn. The police were unable to solve the crime and the jewel was finally replaced by Garrards in May 1988 after some exasperation on the Society's part at the delay (Figure 3.10).[10]

In 2003, Sir John Chalstrey, Master 1994–95, on completion of his year as Lord Mayor, presented the shrieval chain which he had used as Sheriff in 1993–94 to replace the ribbon upon which the Master's jewel was hung. The chain is now used at the beginning of Society events and is subsequently surreptitiously changed for the ribbon before dinner so that the Master can remove his gown for the meal.

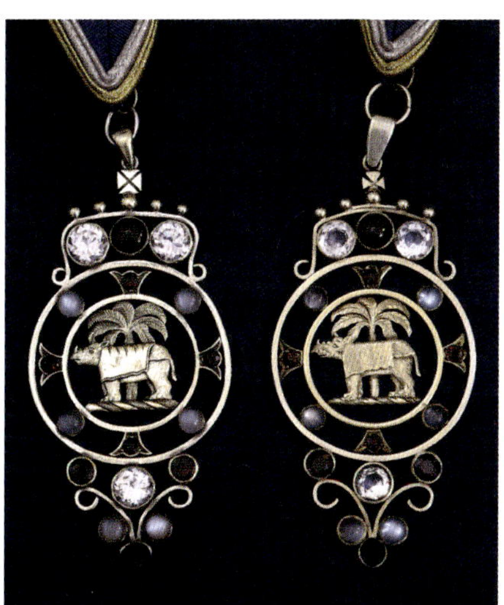

3.12 The near-identical Wardens' jewels

The jewel takes a significant amount of wear and tear as it is also worn at the many events which the Master attends to represent the Society outside the Hall. As a result, this replacement jewel was repaired and re-enamelled in 1994, 1998, 2003, 2012 and 2015. Consideration has been given to providing a duplicate, but cheaper, version for use on these outside occasions, as some other companies do, but this has not been undertaken.

Regrettably, this jewel was stolen after an external event in 2016 and a further replacement was commissioned from Grant Macdonald (Silversmiths) Ltd in 2017. The replacement is very similar to the previous jewel and is sterling silver gold plated with a central hand-painted enamelled coat of Arms surrounded by a pierced fleur-de-lys and scrollwork frame set with diamonds, rubies and sapphires (Figure 3.11).

The Wardens' jewels are less elaborate and feature simply a silver-gilt rhinoceros with a tree behind it, set in a surround with moonstones, rubies, garnets and imitation diamonds (Figure 3.12). It is unclear when Wardens' jewels were introduced but, because of their similarity to what is now the Immediate Past Master's jewel, it may have been in

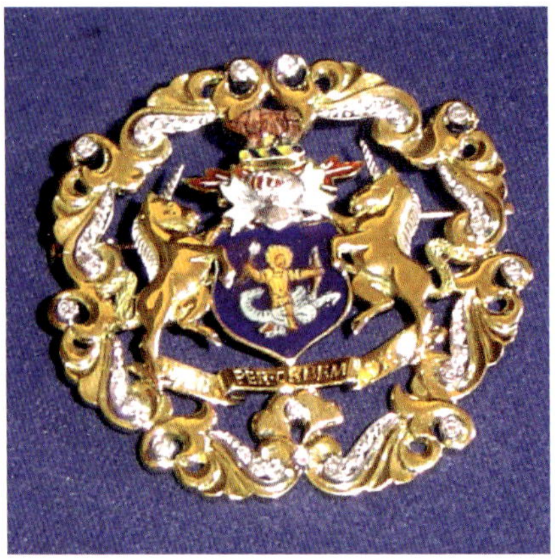

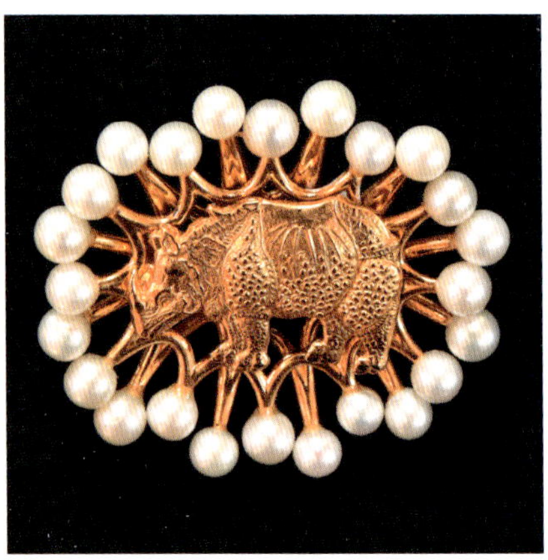

3.13 The Master's Lady's jewel

3.14 The brooch for Past Masters' Ladies

the period 1901–20. The tree may be an allusion either to the Company of Grocers, which often displays a camel and a palm tree as a device, or to the original cedar trees grown by the Society at the Chelsea Physic Garden. There is no significant difference between the two badges, except for the silver mark on the reverse of one. One of these jewels was stolen in the burglary of 1987 and a replacement was ordered from Messrs Garrard & Co Ltd, but after an eleven-month wait the commission was passed to Mr Alan Mudd who delivered the new jewel in May 1988.[11]

Ceremonial: Brooches and Badges

In 1997 a brooch to be worn by the Master's Lady during her year was proposed.[12] Three designs were considered and the design in Figure 3.13 commissioned from Alan Mudd, now of Norfolk. It was first worn in July 1998. The design is the full achievement of the Society's Arms surrounded by an ornate border in silver gilt and enamel. The brooch was lost in 2007 and a replacement made by Mr Mudd later that year, this time fitted with a preventer chain.[13]

In 2015 the Court approved a brooch for use as an official emblem by Past Masters' Ladies.[14] The design shown in Figure 3.14 was commissioned from Mr Grant Macdonald and consists of a silver-gilt Society rhinoceros surrounded by an orle of seed pearls.

In 1960 W. S. C. Copeman, Master 1958–59, presented a badge for use by the Chairman of the Society's Faculty of the History of Medicine, now the President of the Faculty of the History and Philosophy of Medicine and Pharmacy. The badge is a silver-gilt circle, chased and pierced with the Society's crest in front of a tree and was made by Messrs Garrard & Co Ltd. In 2015 a similar jewel was made for the President of the Faculty of Conflict and Catastrophe Medicine (Figure 3.15). They are very similar in style to the Immediate Past Master's jewel (see Figure 3.9).

Lesser badges, suspended from a blue ribbon edged in silver and gold, are die stamped in gilt-plated sterling silver, with two-colour vitreous enamel, and worn by the officials of the Society. The badge is circular with an inner circle of light blue enamel bearing the rhinoceros in silver gilt and an outer ring bearing the words 'Society of Apothecaries' and the official's title. On the ribbon they carry a device associated with their office. These badges (Figure 3.16) were established as shown opposite.

Past Masters wear a Society silver-gilt medallion suspended from a blue ribbon edged in silver and gold (Figure 3.17). On the obverse, the full Arms of the Society are stamped and the reverse bears the name of the Past Master and the years of his or her Mastership. These medals are often reused by later Masters with a family connection to the original user.

The same medallion but without the ribbon is awarded to those who give any of the Faculty Eponymous Lectures. It is also used as the Master's Medal, which was established

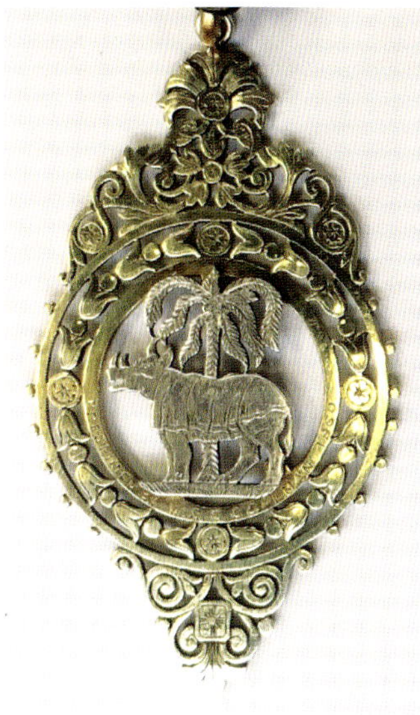

YEAR	OFFICIAL	DEVICE	DONOR
1979	Clerk	crossed quills	P. H. Willcox, Master 1978–79
1984	Chaplain	a cross	T. D. Whittet, Master 1982–83
1986	Chairman of the Livery Committee	a chair	the Livery Committee
1991	Assistant Clerk		D.T.D. Hughes, Master 1992–93
1998	Registrar	a register	(the Society)
2000	Archivist	a book	(the Society)
2014	Treasurer	crossed keys	Sir Colin Berry, Master 2003–04
2016	Beadle		(the Society)

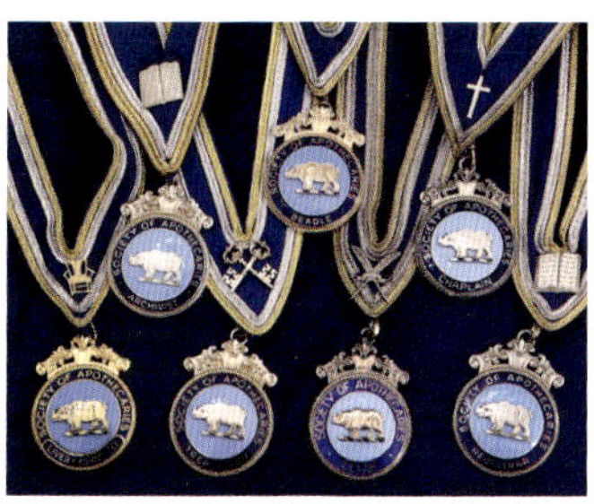

in 2005 in the Mastership of William Shand, to recognise people who have given exceptional service to the Society. To date, fifteen Master's Medals have been awarded.

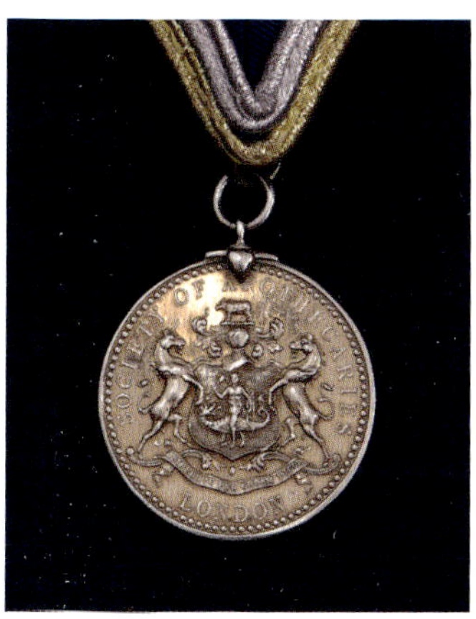

3.15 The Faculty Presidents' badge

3.16 The Officers' badges

3.17 The Past Master's medallion

Ceremonial: Clothing

The rhinoceros being such a recognisable symbol of the Society, it is no surprise to find it adorning the Society's ceremonial clothing. An embroidered gold rhinoceros has been displayed on the collar of the Court Assistants' gowns since the introduction of the parti-coloured gowns in 1969,[15] as illustrated in Figure 3.18. These gowns, which are blue with gold facings in addition to the collar, were last replaced in 2003.[16] The rhinoceros is also displayed on the collar of the Faculty Presidents', the Clerk's and the Registrar's gowns.

Interestingly, the Assistants' gowns used to be an awkward poncho style in black trimmed with mink, the Private Court gowns being rather grander versions of this. When the current colourful Assistants' gowns were introduced, there was a proposal by the Junior Warden of the day for the Master's and Wardens' gowns also to be replaced by ones with bright colours, perhaps to emulate the peacock designs of other companies. The Court, whilst agreeing to renew these gowns, decreed, however, that sober academic black was to be retained.[17]

The rhinoceros is not displayed on the Wardens' gowns but has featured on the right shoulder of the Master's gown (Figure 3.19) since 2012. This rhinoceros has an interesting history, as it was originally a distinguishing mark worn by members of 217 (City of London) General Hospital RAMC(V), which the Society had supported since its formation in 1967. The first Commanding Officer of 217 General Hospital was Colonel

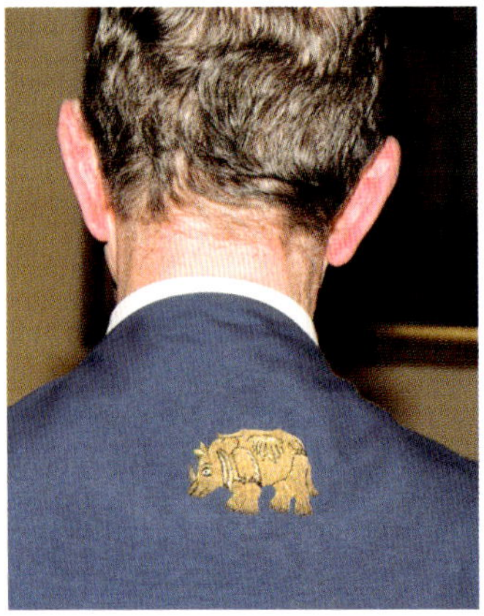

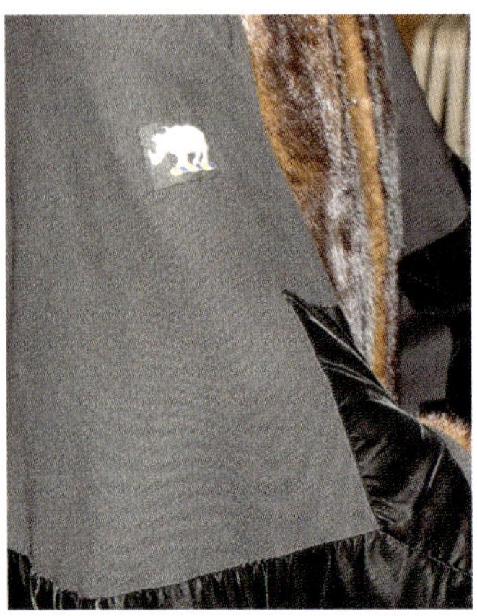

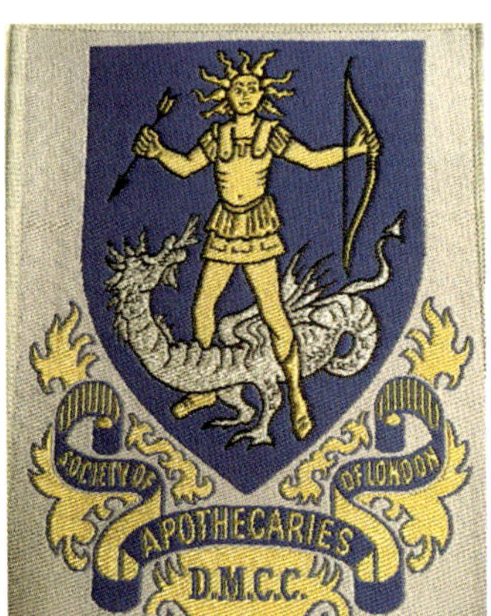

3.18 The collar of a Court gown

3.19 The rhinoceros on the Master's gown

3.20 The Diploma in the Medical Care of Catastrophes diplomate's badge of 1994

T. W. A. Glenister, Master 1991–92, and he proposed the use of the rhinoceros badge, inexplicably known in the unit as 'Percy', to mark the connection with the Society and this was authorised by the Ministry of Defence in 1970.[18]

In 1995, 217 General Hospital became part of 256 (City of London) Field Hospital RAMC(V) and the Society was allocated 'A' Squadron, whilst the other squadrons were supported by the Companies of Barbers and Cutlers. 'A' Squadron wore the rhinoceros emblem unofficially but with the reduction in size of 256 Field Hospital and the conversion of squadrons into detachments the practice ceased. In 2012 the unit returned the remaining badges to the Society and it was thought appropriate for one to be worn on the Master's gown to indicate the Society's continuing support for 256 Field Hospital.[19]

A badge for successful diplomates was introduced with the first Diploma in the Medical Care of Catastrophes examination in 1994.[20] The badge was an embroidered version of the Society's Arms for diplomates to wear on their working overalls in the field (Figure 3.20), rather as aircrew do, to demonstrate both the doctor's specialist qualification and the Society's educational activities in this important international area. For clarity only the shield was used and the motto was replaced in an ornate scroll, somewhat tautologically, with the name of the Society and the diploma, for those who were not heraldically conversant. The idea of the badge did not take off, however, and only half a dozen were issued – although the diploma itself has been very successful with 761 diplomates recorded in the twenty-five years to date.

Ceramics

Probably the most common source of the Society's Arms outside the Hall is on pill tiles or slabs, which occasionally come up for auction at sales of ceramics. The pill tile was initially a flat tin-glazed impermeable slab of plain pottery on which the mixture from a pill masser was placed and rolled by the apothecary in his shop.[21]

Subsequently, the pill tile became a decorative item showing the full achievement of Arms of the Society and thus indicating status as a master apothecary. To this end, it can be seen that the tiles illustrated in Figures 3.21, 3.22, 3.23 and 3.24 have two holes pierced in them at the top for hanging on the wall.

Existing pill tiles come in octagonal or heart shapes (although two rare ovals are known) and nearly all are white with cobalt oxide blue decoration and manganese dioxide purple-brown lettering. Extravagant mantling and festoons of foliage around the motto scroll are used to fill up the remaining space. The Society does possess one rare and spectacular polychromate tile, which is named for John Smithies and dated 1686 (Figure 3.23).

There are some twelve polychromate and a further ninety-seven blue and white decorative pill tiles known to exist. It is thought that all of these tiles were made in London at factories in Southwark, Lambeth, Mortlake and Limehouse between the

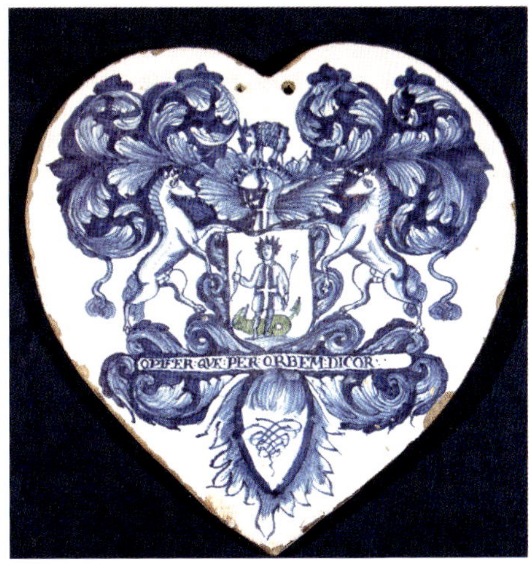

3.21 A Lambeth delft heart-shaped pill tile of c.1700, presented by A. M. A. Moore, Master 1961–62, in 1961

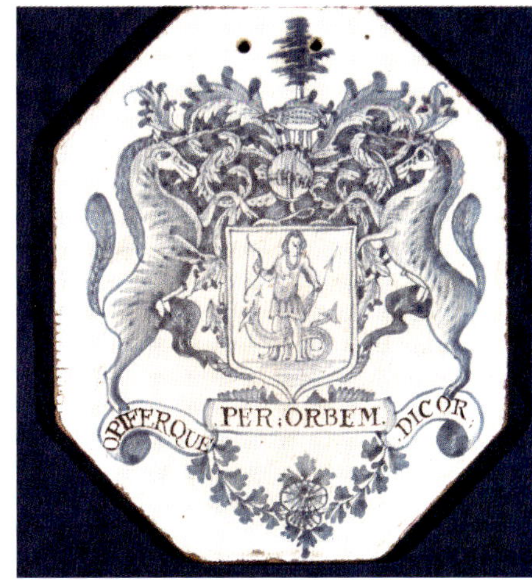

3.22 A Lambeth delft octagonal pill tile of c.1750 presented by Sir St Clair Thomson

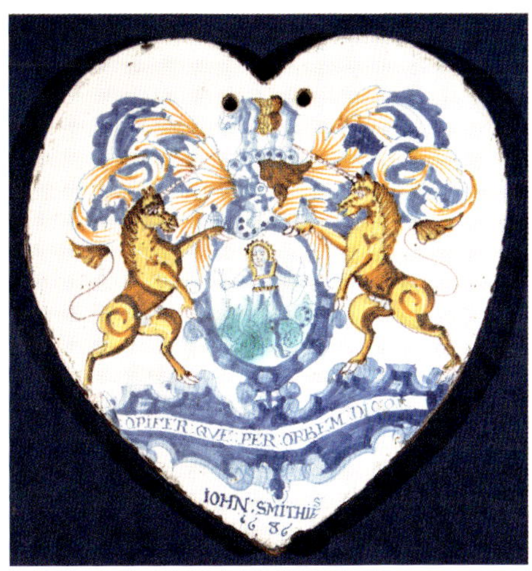

3.23 A Lambeth delft heart-shaped polychrome pill tile dated 1686 and named for John Smithies. Its acquisition by the Society is not recorded

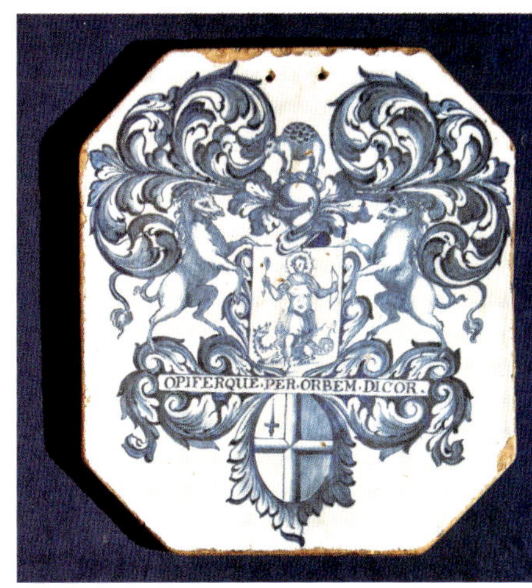

3.24 A Lambeth delft octagonal pill tile of c.1750 given by Sir Robert Gower in 1938

1650s and 1780s, which is why they are generally referred to as London Delftware. It is also likely that they were given by master apothecaries to their apprentices on the latter obtaining their freedom of the Society. This theory is reinforced by the Smithies tile, as John Smithies was made free in 1686 although he may have died young as nothing further is heard of him.[22]

One thing most of the tiles have in common is the often appalling representation of the Society's Arms. In many, Apollo looks unfit for any kind of combat, the dragon is more of a pet and the poor rhinoceros has become some sort of bug. Fortunately, the mantling camouflages the dismal artwork and the motto, which is often the most elegant part of the composition, identifies the Society. To be fair to the artists, it is extremely difficult to decorate delftware as it involves pouncing (tracing) a cartoon before painting freehand on wet glaze which dries instantly and is thereafter unchangeable. Clearly, some artists were better at it than others.

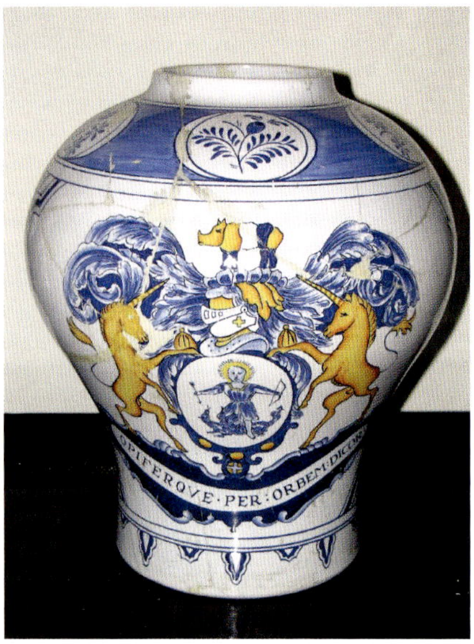

3.25 A polychromate tin-glazed earthenware reproduction drug jar

The tiles illustrated show a number of interesting idiosyncrasies:

– In Figure 3.21, the wyvern has become green and Apollo is wearing a large cross on his tunic; the green serpent also features in another tile held in the Museum of London.

– In Figures 3.21 and 3.22, Apollo is holding his bow and arrow in the wrong hand.

– In Figure 3.22, the gradations scratched on the left-hand edge of the tile indicate that it has probably been used for pill rolling and measuring.

– In Figure 3.22, the tree above the crest looks very much like a cedar and this is likely as the cedars of Lebanon, which came to be associated with the Society, were planted at the Chelsea Physic Garden in 1683; these trees also feature later in the Immediate Past Master's Jewel (see Figure 3.9) and in the Wardens' Jewels (see Figure 3.12).

– In Figure 3.22, this portrayal of the unicorns is often referred to as 'striped unicorns'. This is, however, merely an artistic variant.

– In Figure 3.24, an oval cartouche has been added below the achievement which displays the Arms of the City of London and indicates that the owner was a Freeman of the City.

The Society possesses one blue, ochre and white polychromate tin-glazed earthenware drug jar decorated with the Society's Arms, chinoiserie figures and bulrushes (Figure 3.25), which is very rare. Unfortunately it is heavily repaired and is, in fact, a post-war German copy of a jar in the collection of the Royal Pharmaceutical Society. None of the other drug jars in the possession of the Society displays any element of the Society's Arms.

Textiles, Needlepoint, Embroidery

There are examples of the Society's Arms on textiles in the Entrance Hall and in the Court Room.

The Entrance Hall and the four flights of stairs are furnished with a large Axminster wool carpet. The original carpet was laid in 1985 after the major refurbishment and was of a lighter blue colour. With the heavy footfall of the many Society events over the years, the stair sections of this carpet had to be renewed three times. The whole carpet was replaced in 2016 in a darker blue colour and with different detail. The stairs portion is dark blue with a lighter blue and gold border and is semée with gold rhinoceroses.

The centre of the main carpet, in the same background colour and design but without the field of rhinoceroses, contains a large and accurate depiction of the Camden Arms (Figure 3.26).

Also in the Entrance Hall there are two Queen Anne walnut chairs, one of which is an elbow chair with scroll elbows on down-swept supports. They both have a shaped crest rail carved with shell motif and a solid baluster splat. The trapezoid drop-in seats have been re-upholstered in gros-point needlework depicting the Society's Arms.

The Arms on the elbow chair (Figure 3.27) are a good representation of the Camden Arms in their correct colours. Those on the single chair (Figure 3.28) include the shield and motto but not the supporters, helm, mantling or crest. Neither the provenance of the chairs nor the embroiderer of the Arms is known and the suspicion must be that time or resolve ran out for the completion of the embroidery on the single chair!

In the Court Room, in front of the fireplace is a handsome mahogany fire screen (Figure 3.29) on cabriole legs with claw-and-ball feet and carved rhinoceros cresting. In the centre is a panel depicting the Society's Arms in petit-point, which was worked by Dr Margaret Vivian LMSSA, who presented the screen in 1935, when she also presented a rhinoceros-horn inkstand. At this stage, this was very much a working fireplace as Liveryman Mr Dennis Barrie, Registrar 1949–93, remembered providing coal to the Court Room when he joined the staff in 1946.

The Arms are also displayed on the lectern cover and the design is faithful to the Camden grant but with the rhinoceros crest slightly enlarged (Figure 3.30). These were

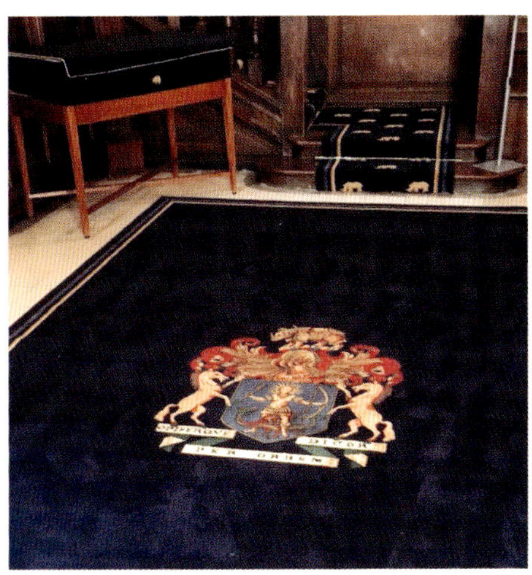

3.26 The Entrance Hall carpet

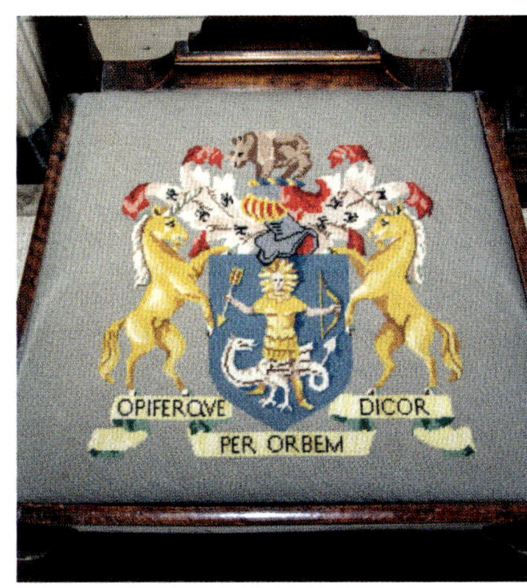

3.27 The walnut elbow chair with full representation of the Arms

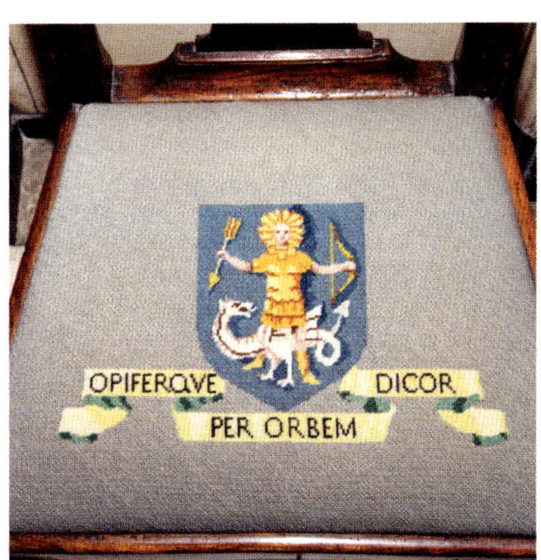

3.28 The walnut single chair with partial Arms representation

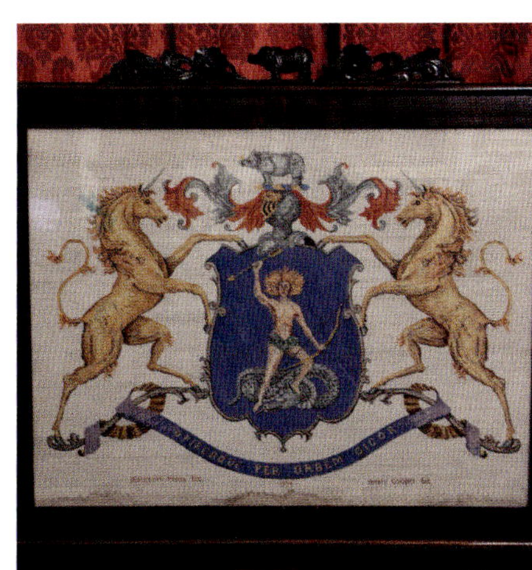

3.29 The mahogany fire screen with full representation of the Arms

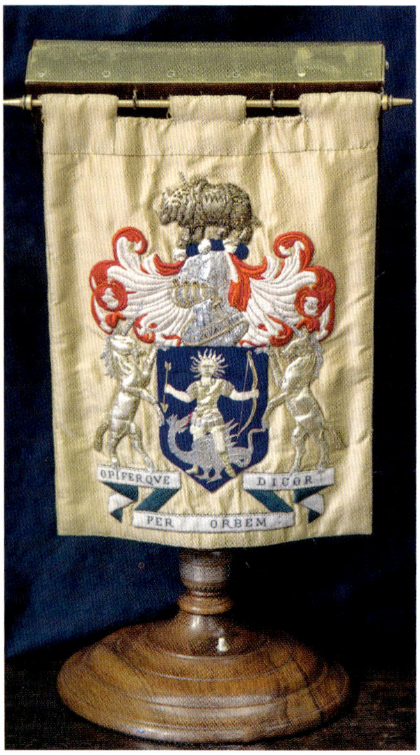

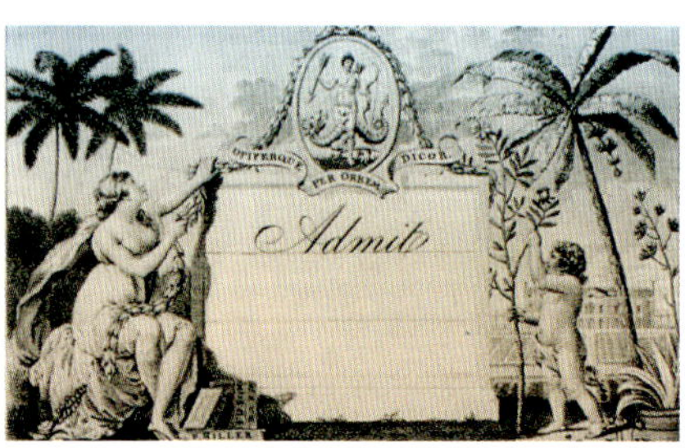

3.30 The embroidered lectern Arms

3.31 The Chelsea Physic Garden entrance ticket of 1785

embroidered in 1987 by Mrs Enid Taylor, Master 2002–03, the Society's first Lady Master.[23] She also presented a box in which to keep it and she renovated the work in 2007.[24] Not content with that, she also embroidered Arms for the Companies of Turners and Spectacle Makers for their use when using the lectern in the Hall.

Stationery

Printed handbills and papers for special occasions had become both possible and affordable in the late eighteenth century, and in December 1785 tickets for admission to the Chelsea Physic Garden were instituted. These were to allow liverymen entrance to the Garden as the gardeners were unable to recognise them all. The tickets were designed by Uriah Bristow, Master 1803–04.[25]

Figure 3.31 illustrates Dr Bristow's ticket; it is very much of the Garden, with the house, paths, formal beds and palm trees being conspicuous. Only the shield of the Arms is used and both Apollo and the dragon are vigorously portrayed, but it is not clear why the full achievement was not used, especially outside the Hall.

With the technological advances in printing presses, the improvement in the quality and supply of paper and the Victorian mania for etiquette, the introduction of printed stationery spread very quickly in the early part of the nineteenth century. Figure 3.32 shows various forms of the Society's Arms used on its letterheads. It is not clear why the design changed or why two variants were sometimes in use at the same time.

Artistic licence has been used mainly with the shape of the shield and the mantling, which in three examples has been replaced by greenery and swags. The unicorns and the motto are well treated throughout and generally Apollo is reasonably portrayed, but the rhinoceros is often forced into his familiar balancing act. The worst case of this is the 1822 LSA Diploma, which is an unusually severe image, possibly trying to echo classical works, and which illustrates why the Victorians could not be entirely trusted with heraldry!

On a rather grander note is the Court Summons from 1817 (Figure 3.33). The unknown apothecary's presence is desired 'at a Court of Aſsiſtants to be holden for the said Society at their Hall in Black Friars on Tuesday the 25th day of Novr by One of the Clock in the afternoon on special affairs'.

In the twentieth century, the Society settled on a close variation of the monochrome design introduced in around 1820 and this became the Society standard. It is not an unreasonable version, except that the mantling is mean and the helm is inadequate resulting in the wreath and rhinoceros looking precarious. This version of the achievement of Arms is used on diplomas, headed paper, menu cards, seating plans and invitations. On the latter, it is embossed in gold and presents a very stylish impression.

3.32 Examples of standard reproductions of the Society's Arms on stationery

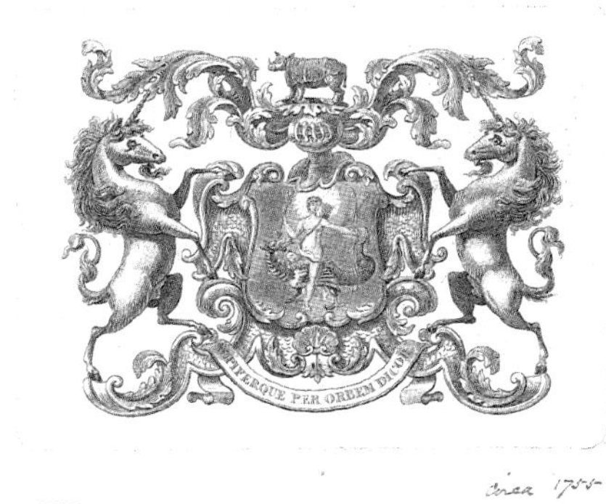

c.1755

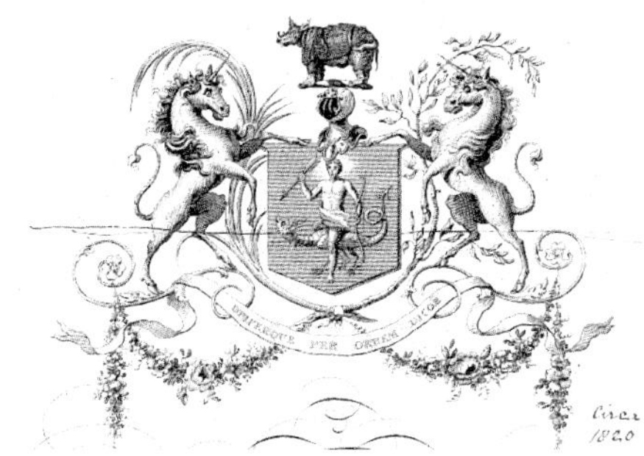

c.1820 & 1880

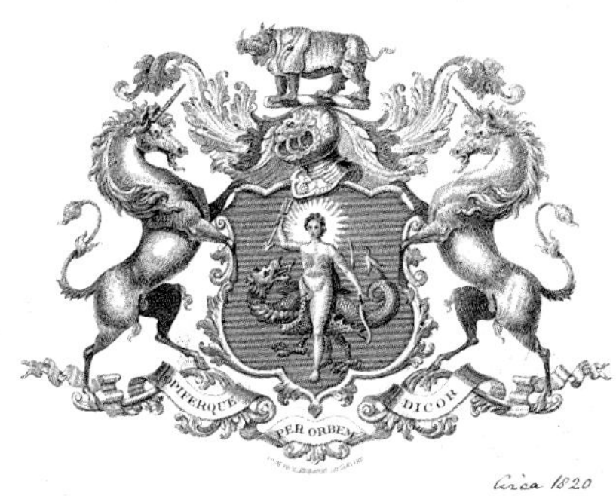

c.1820

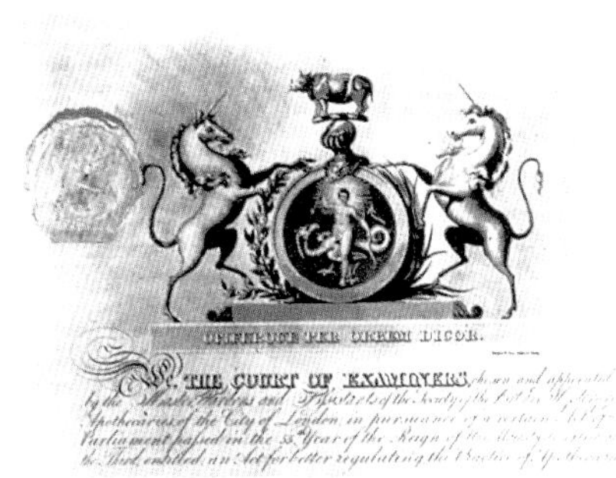

1822 LSA Diploma

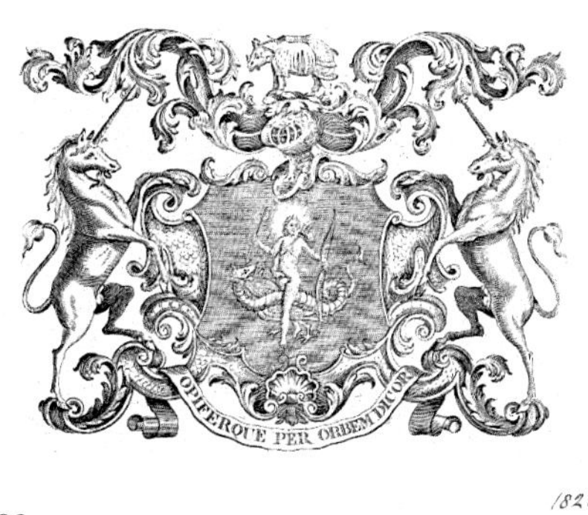

1826

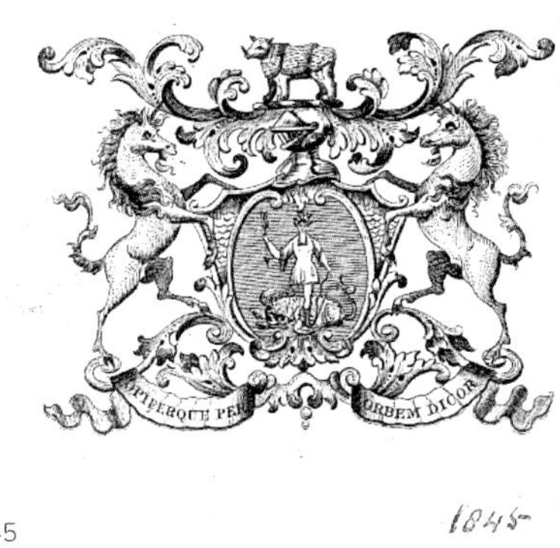

1845

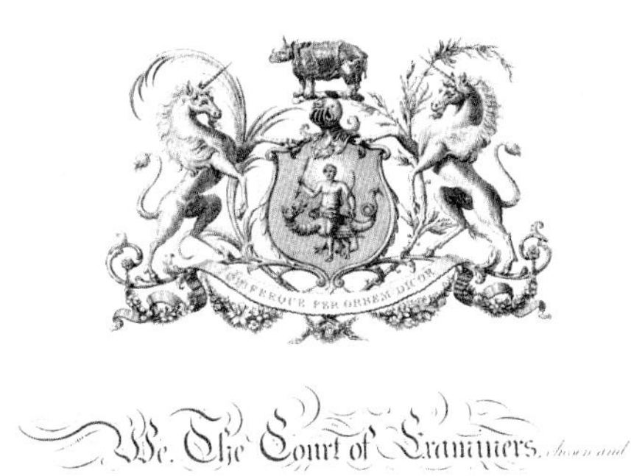

Court of Examiners

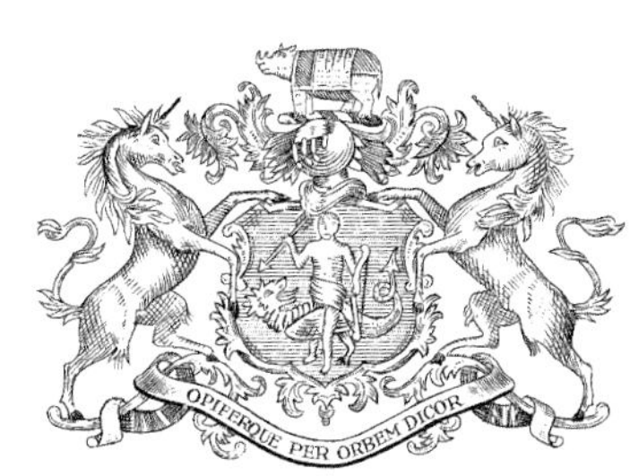

Twentieth century

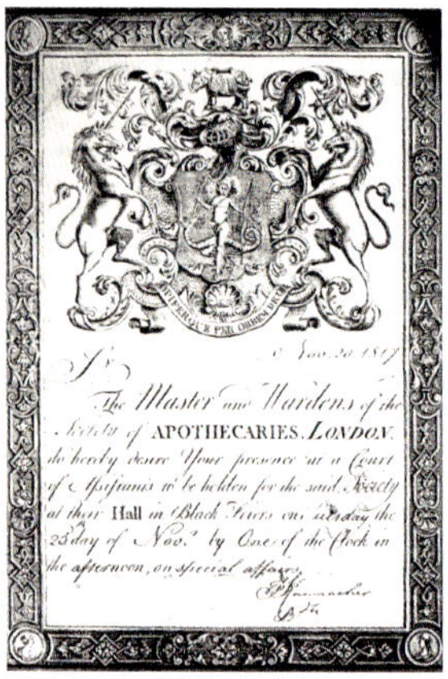
The Master and Wardens of the
Society of APOTHECARIES, LONDON
do hereby desire Your presence at a Court
of Assistants to be holden for the said Society
at their Hall in Black Friers on
25 day of Nov. by One of the Clock in
the afternoon, on special affairs.

3.33 A Court summons of 1817

Recently, this standard image has been replaced by the Camden original in full colour on livery and yeomanry admissions and promotions, important certificates, seating plans and the cover of the Society's magazine, *The Apothecary*.

Silver, Cutlery and Crockery

Another traditional use of heraldry is on the dining table. Much silverware, and the occasional gold items, have been donated to the Society over the years and the formal dinners provide an elegant backdrop for display of these treasures. The larger items (Figures 3.34, 3.35 and 3.38) include the Armada dishes, the loving cups and the Osborn salt, on most of which are engraved the full Arms.

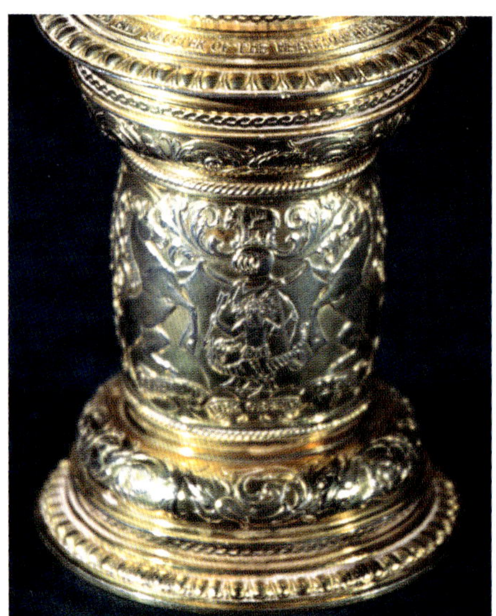

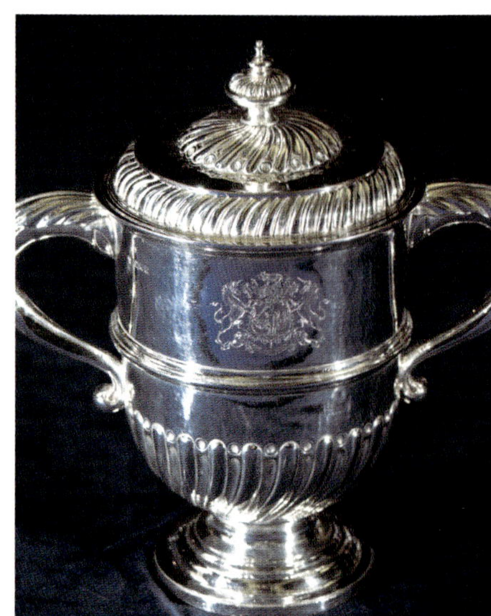

3.34 The Salt presented by Samuel Osborn, Master 1919–20, based on the design of one owned by the Company of Haberdashers

3.35 One of the Society's loving cups

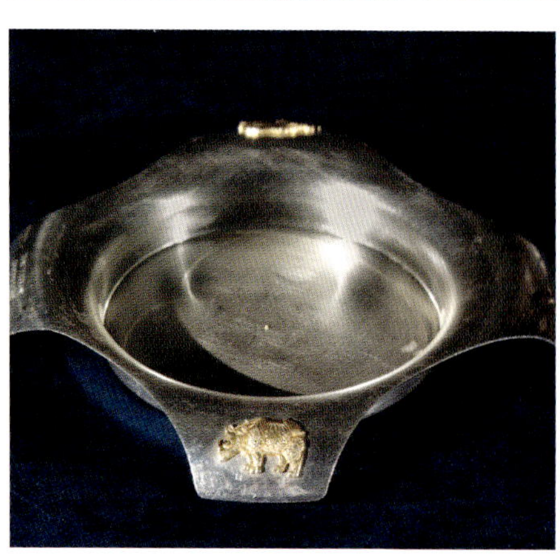

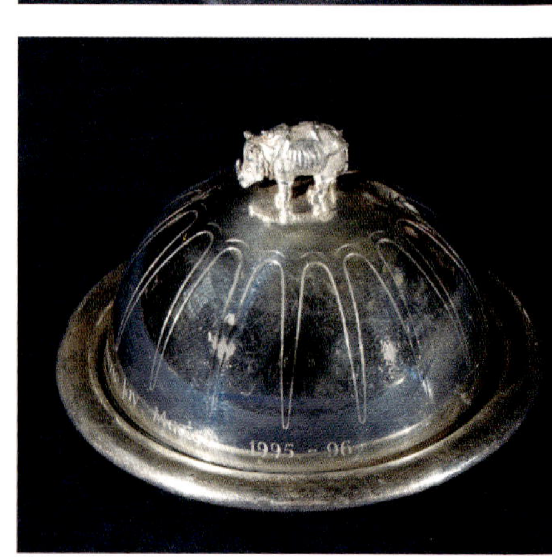
1995 – 96

3.36 The base of the 1997 butter dishes

3.37 The dome of the 1997 butter dishes

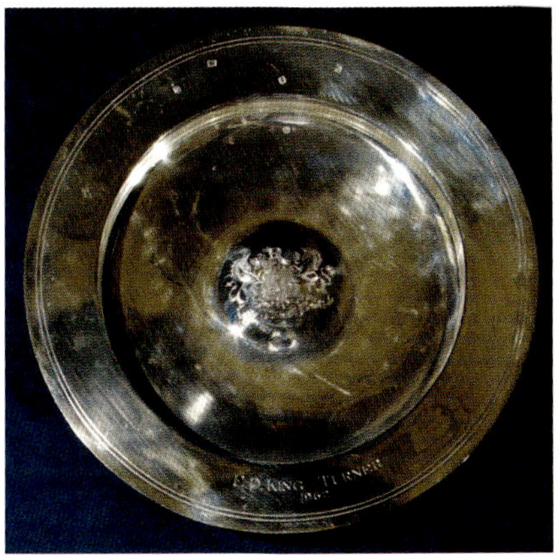

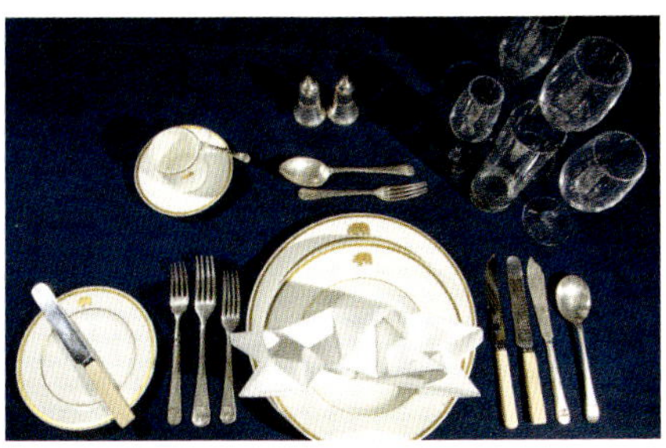

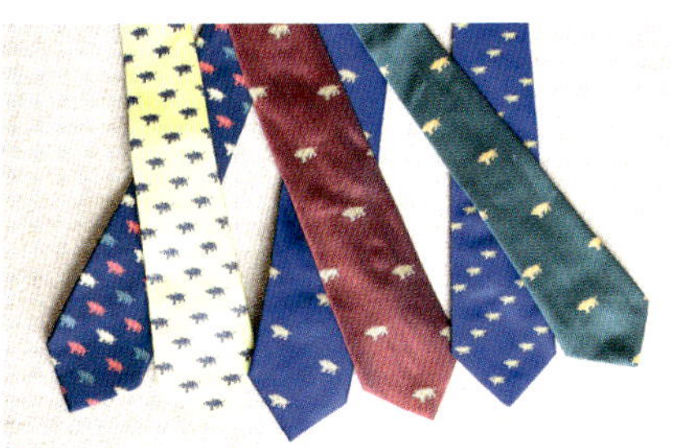

3.38 One of the Armada dishes with the full achievement of Arms engraved

3.39 The Court crockery presented by W. F. W. Southwood and the Society cutlery

3.40 Variants of the Society tie

More often it is just the rhinoceros crest which features on smaller items, for example the Society's cutlery. Amongst the more splendid examples, in 2003 W. F. W. Southwood, Master 1986–87, left a legacy which was used to buy a full set of gold band crockery (Figure 3.39) to be used at Court Dinners and this has a gold rhinoceros stamped on it. Between 1995 and 1998, liverymen presented thirty silver butter dishes which have two rhinoceroses in relief on the base and a larger standing version on the lid (Figures 3.36 and 3.37).

Social

The rhinoceros crest in differing colours and on varied backgrounds has formed the basis for a multitude of Society ties (Figure 3.40) and it has also been used for various items of jewellery male and female, and numerous objects of memorabilia which it would be tedious to itemise. This continues the heraldic story, showing the ongoing use of an ancient system to indicate belonging or possession in the modern age.

CHAPTER 4

Armorial Glass in the Great Hall

Introduction

The windows of the Great Hall contain a remarkable collection of armorial glass, a collection which continues to grow and which one day will fill all available window-space (Figures 4.1 and 4.2). It is the current practice for each Master at the end of their year of office to install a panel displaying their armorial bearings, but this is only a comparatively recent innovation for the Society, and one which has been somewhat intermittent over the years.

All the panels in the Great Hall are described in detail in Appendix 1; for the numbering system please refer to 'Identification of Windows and Panels in the Great Hall' at the front of the book. The oldest panel is likely to be sixteenth century in date but this was not acquired until 1980, and while they are now usually glazed with armorial bearings in chronological order, this has not always been the case. In addition, panels have been moved over the years, all of which adds to the complexity of describing in detail what is in effect a slowly evolving kaleidoscope of glass.

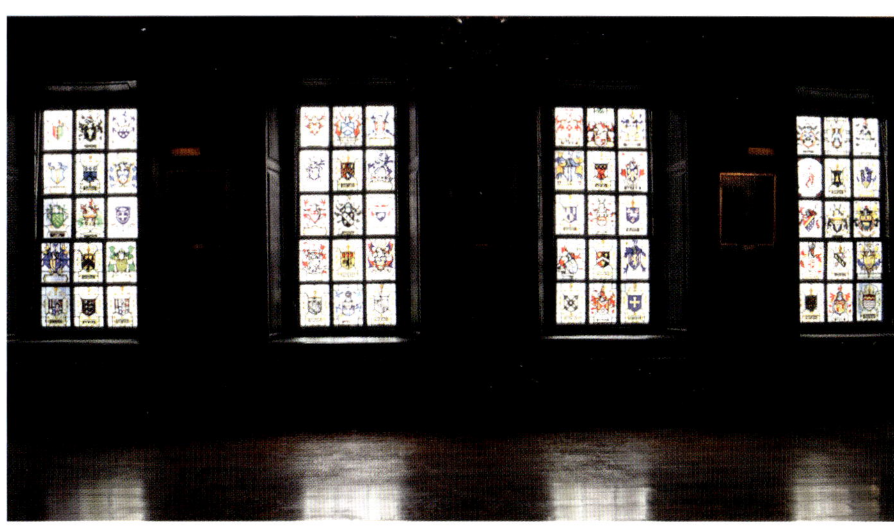

4.1 The west side of the Great Hall glazing scheme, completed in 2016

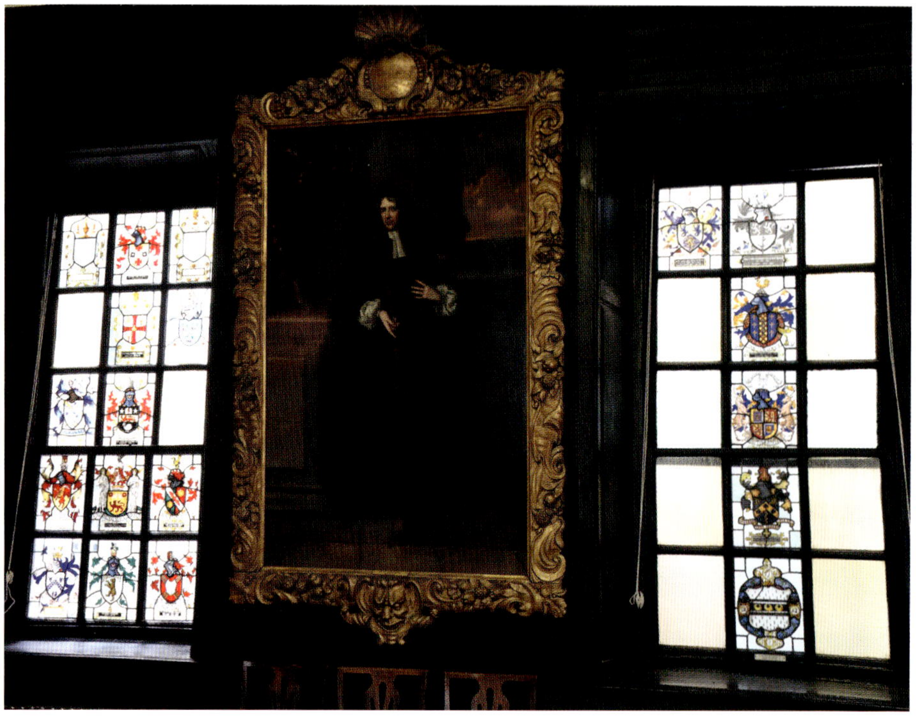

4.2 The east side of the Great Hall glazing scheme, ongoing in 2020

A print of the Courtyard at Apothecaries' Hall in 1814 by George Shepherd shows with reasonable certainty that at that time the windows on the west side of the Great Hall contained no stained glass. The frontispiece of C. R. B. Barrett's 1905 book *The History of the Society of Apothecaries* shows no stained glass in a drawing of what he calls the 'Upper end' (southern end) of the Great Hall, and later in his book a drawing of the 'Lower end' (northern end) again shows no stained glass.[1] In both drawings by Barrett, we do not see two of the windows, one on each side, but it seems reasonable to assume that there was no stained glass in the Great Hall in 1904, the date of the prints. In support of this assumption is the fact that Barrett comments on the stained glass in the windows on the Grand Staircase, as he calls it, and on other panels but makes no other reference to stained glass commemorating Masters.

As will be described below in detail, the first three commemorative panels were almost certainly installed in 1906. These and other early panels show the shield of the armorial bearings surrounded by one of two cartouche designs. In due course, the cartouche design was gradually abandoned so that the armorial bearings depicted fill the whole panel. Thus, there are seven panel designs which can be identified in the Great Hall windows as follows (Figures 4.3, 4.4, 4.5, 4.6 and 4.7).

At the time of writing, only two panels with blank cartouches remain, one of each design in window East 1. In due course, these too could be replaced with armorial panels so that the blank cartouche design would no longer be a feature of the Great Hall stained glass decoration.

4.3a Blank cartouche design A surmounted by a floral vase

4.3b Blank cartouche design B surmounted by a covered cup

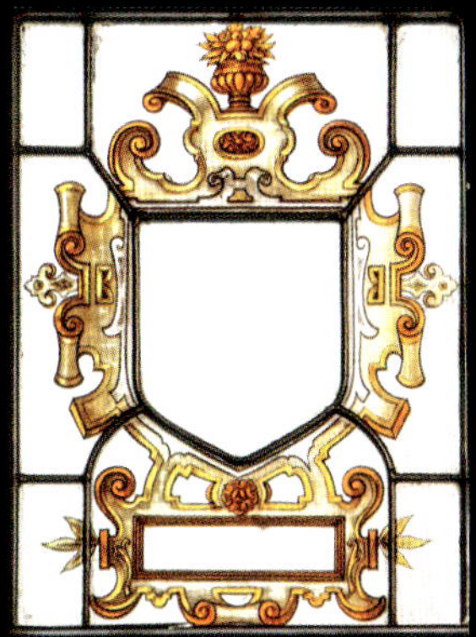

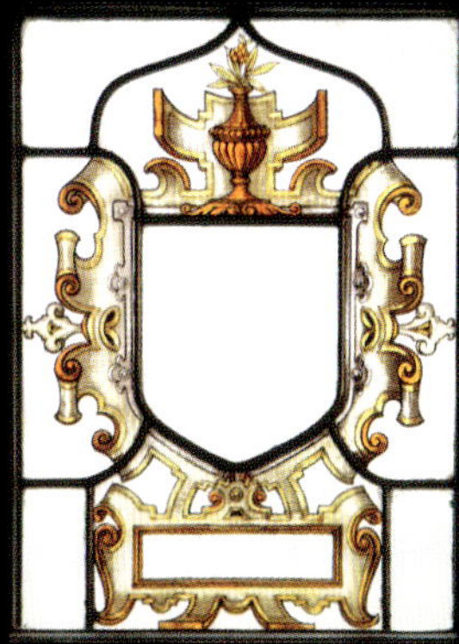

4.4a Cartouche A with Arms and personal details but no helm, crest, mantling or motto

4.4b Cartouche B with Arms and personal details but no helm, crest, mantling or motto

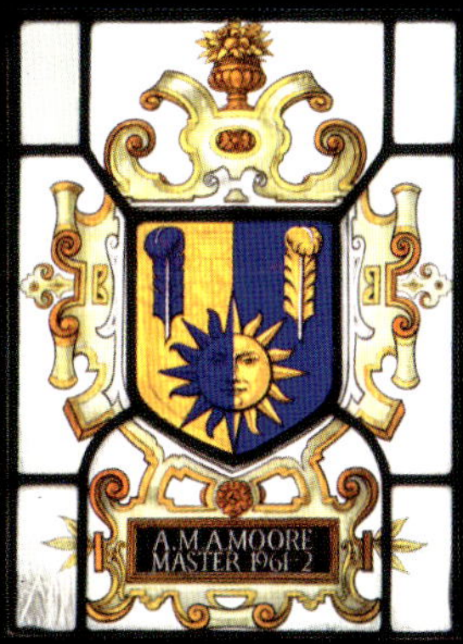

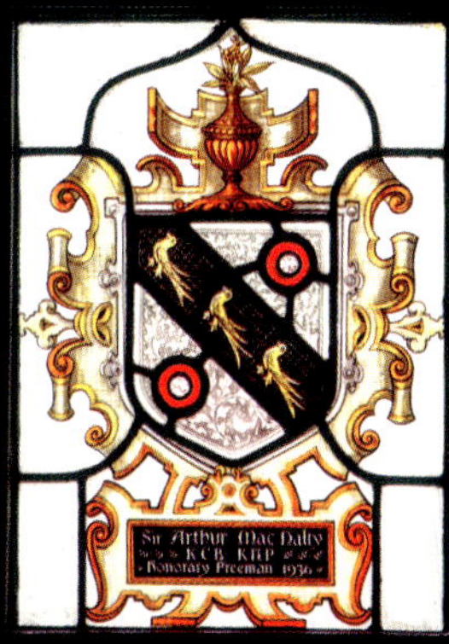

4.5 Full armorial bearings, including supporters if granted, and motto filling the whole panel

4.6 Armorial bearings for a lady which do not have a helm, mantling or a crest

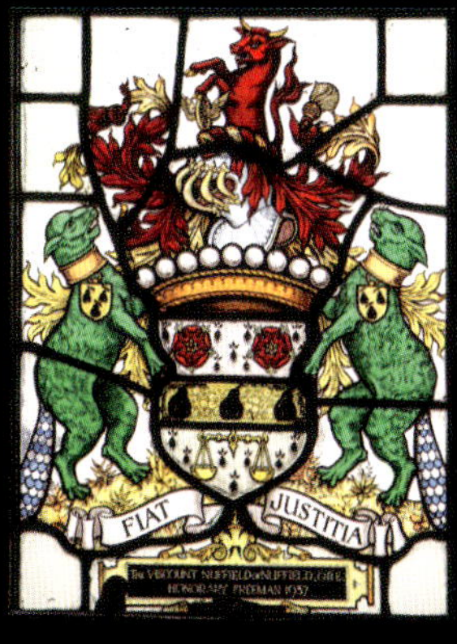

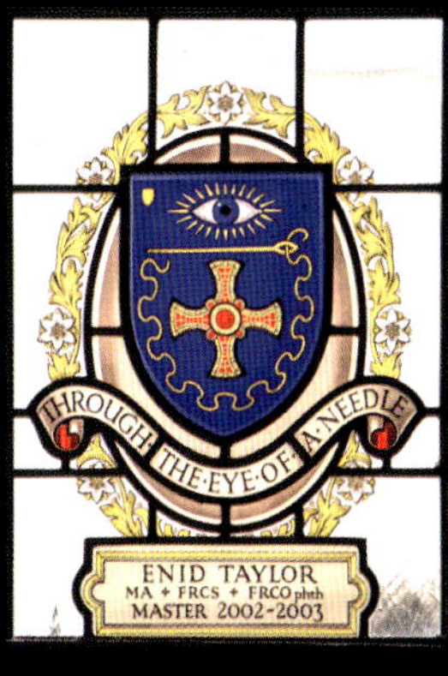

4.7 Crest only and personal details filling the whole panel

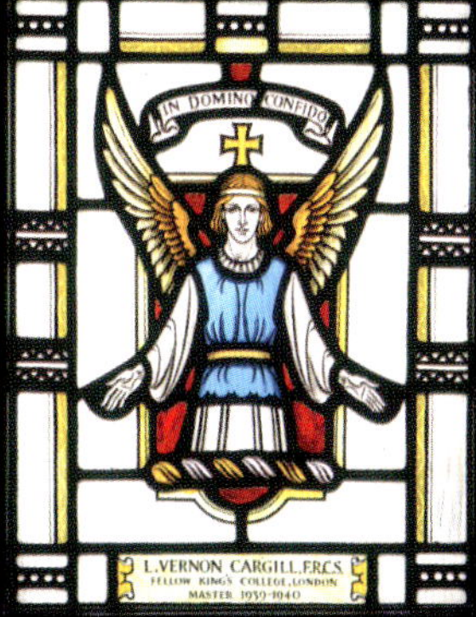

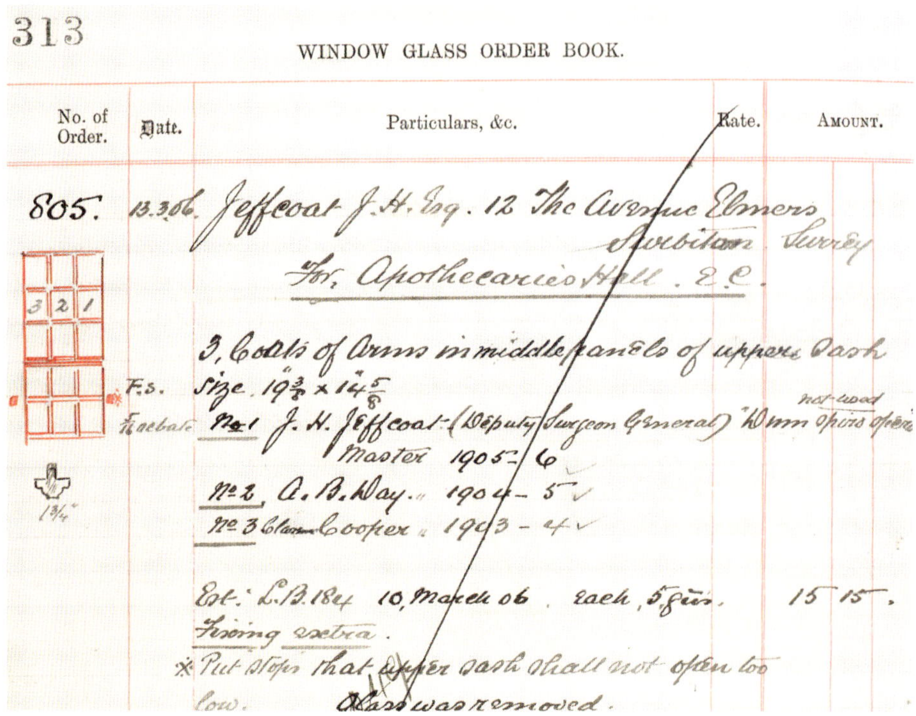
313

WINDOW GLASS ORDER BOOK.

No. of Order.	Date.	Particulars, &c.	Rate.	Amount.
805.	13.3.06	Jeffcoat J. H. Esq. 12 The Avenue Elmers Surbiton. Surrey For, Apothecaries Hall. E.C.		
		3, Coats of Arms in middle panels of upper sash		
	F.S.	Size. 19 3/8 x 14 5/8		
	Rebate	No 1 J. H. Jeffcoat (Deputy Surgeon General) Master 1905–6		
		No 2, A. B. Day. " 1904–5		
		No 3 Clarence Cooper " 1903–4		
		Est: L.B.184 10 March 06 each, 5 gns.		15 15.
		Fixing extra.		
		* Put stops that upper sash shall not open too low. Glass was removed.		

4.8 Entry in James Powell and Sons 'Window Glass Order Book (1904–1906)' dated 13 March 1906, showing the proposed positions of the Jeffcoat (1), Day (2) and Cooper (3) panels, as viewed from inside the Great Hall

West Side of the Great Hall

The Installation of the First Six Armorial Panels – An Inspiration

As already mentioned, the oldest armorial panel in the Hall (Uriah Bristow, Master 1803–04) was not installed until 1980 (window East 2, panel 14). The history of this panel and its installation is described in Chapter 9. The panel of the next most senior Master, Henry Morley (Master 1870–71), commemorated jointly with his great-grandson Henry Seaward Morley (Master 1953–54), was not installed until after the latter's year of office (window West 1, panel 2). The next, for Hugh Worthington Statham (Master 1881–82) was not installed until his granddaughter, together with the widow of his nephew Reginald Whiteside Statham (Master 1927–28), presented their two panels to the Society in the late 1930s (window West 1, panels 13 and 15).

The glass company James Powell & Sons (see Appendix III) was an important manufacturer of stained glass windows in London in the early part of the twentieth century, when the glazing scheme in the Great Hall was started. The company's extensive and detailed archive, now housed at the Victoria and Albert Museum's Archive of Art and Design, contains several entries relevant to the Society relating to this period.

In the company's 'Window Glass Order Book (1904–1906)', there appears an entry on 13 March 1906 recording an order for three panels of armorial bearings for J. H. Jeffcoat, A. B. Day and Clarence Cooper.[2] This is accompanied by a drawing of how the completed panels are to be installed, window not specified (Figure 4.8).

The window chosen by the Society for these panels was window West 3, the drawing showing how they would appear when viewed from inside the Great Hall, the Cooper panel on the left, the Day panel in the middle and the Jeffcoat panel on the right. The measurement of the panels is accurately recorded as being 19 $^{3}/_{8}$" x 14 $^{5}/_{8}$" and the cost is noted as £5.5.0d for the panel plus 5/- for fixing it in each case. A comment is also made that 'glass was removed'. This correlates nicely with the first photographic evidence of stained glass in the Great Hall, seen in a photograph of the west side of the Great Hall viewed from the Courtyard, taken in 1911 (Figure 4.10). The three panels, identified by their leading pattern, are panels 4, 5 and 6 in window West 3, panel 4 being Cooper's, panel 5 Day's and panel 6 Jeffcoat's. In each case, the shield is surrounded by one of the two cartouche designs illustrated in Figure 4.3.

The next record of relevance is an entry in the 'Journal Window Department (1905–1910)' book in the Powell archive, in effect a cash book, dated 8 June 1906, which records the payment by Jeffcoat not only for the making and fixing of his own panel but also for the Day and Cooper panels.[3] This suggests that Jeffcoat was the prime mover in initiating the glazing scheme, in his Master's year, although he was the junior member of the trio.

Returning to the 'Window Glass Order Book (1904–1906)', the next relevant entry on 20 October 1906 records an order for one armorial panel for 'Apothecary Hall' in the name of Griffith, S. C., MD (Master 1897–98).[4] The heraldic description of his armorial bearings is given in detail together with the details of the name label. The size of the panel, identical to the three above, is also recorded. The estimate for carrying out the work and for fixing the panel is the same as for the previous panels. In the 'Journal Window Department' book, the payment by Dr Griffith on 18 December 1906 is recorded and again it is noted that the panel has been installed.[5] In the 1911 photograph (Figure 4.10) this is seen to be panel 6 in window West 2.

On 11 March 1908, an entry in the 'Window Glass Order Book (1906–1909)' records an order for an armorial panel for George Wilks.[6] Again, the armorial bearings and the size of the panel are recorded, but in addition it is noted that the panel is 'to go next to Griffith'. This would have resulted in the Wilks panel being panel 5 in window West 2, but in the event the 1911 photograph shows it to be panel 5 in window West 4. In the photograph, the panel is partially obscured by the lamp in the middle of the Courtyard, but close examination of that part of the leading that can be seen puts its identification beyond doubt – a conclusion confirmed by a 1917 photograph of the west side of the Courtyard in a paper in the Society Archive entitled 'The Society of the Art and Mistery of Apothecaries

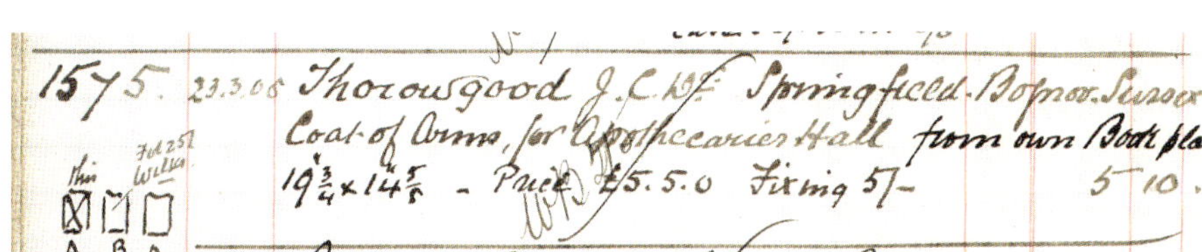
1575. 23.3.08 Thorowgood J. C. MD Springfield. Bognor. Sussex
Coat of Arms, for Apothecaries Hall from own Book plate
19¾ x 14⅝ - Price £5.5.0 Fixing 5/- 5 10.
A . B A

4.9 Entry in the Powell 'Window Glass Order Book (1906–1909)', dated 23 March 1908, showing the proposed positions of the Wilks and Thorowgood panels

of London' (Figure 4.11).[7] Of particular importance is an additional comment that the 'B cartouch' [*sic*] is to be used. This is the first mention of a cartouche, which tends to confirm that the two cartouche patterns were suggested by Powell & Sons as part of the overall design of the early panels. Yet there is slight doubt about this point, as later in the chapter it will be shown that many subsequent cartouche panels of identical design were supplied by a different company.

In the same book, on 23 March 1908 is an order for an armorial panel for Dr J. C. Thorowgood, the armorial bearings 'to be copied from his own bookplate'.[8] This is accompanied by a drawing of the proposed positioning of the Wilks and Thorowgood panels (Figure 4.9). The letter X in the drawing marks the proposed position of the Thorowgood panel and the letters A and B refer to the two cartouche designs illustrated in Figure 4.3, although, as will be seen later, the blank panel on the right of the trio did not receive its blank cartouche A glazing until much later.

In the event, therefore, the Wilks and Thorowgood panels were indeed installed next to each other in window West 4, the Thorowgood panel being panel 4, a pattern that is confirmed in the 1911 photograph. On 10 April 1908, the payment for each of these panels by their respective donors is recorded, again £5.5.0d for the creation of each panel and 5/- for installing it.[9] In this, as in other instances in the Powell records, the name 'Wilks' is spelt incorrectly as 'Wilkes'. Happily, his name is correctly spelt in his armorial panel.

The six armorial panels that are visible therefore in the 1911 photograph (see Figure 4.10 and Appendix IV pp. 250–1) are as follows:

MASTER	DATE	WINDOW	PANEL
Samuel Clewin Griffith	1897–98	2	6
Clarence Cooper	1903–04	3	4
Albert Bryan Day	1904–05	3	5
James Henry Jeffcoat	1905–06	3	6
John Charles Thorowgood (Warden)	1906–07	4	4
George Wilks	1907–08	4	5

All the other visible panels in all four windows in the 1911 photograph contain clear glass.

The question arises as to when the panels for the three remaining pre-First World War Masters, Thomas Edwin Burton Brown (Master 1901–02), Frederick Gordon Brown (Master 1908–09) and Sir Thomas Boor Crosby (Master 1911–12), were installed, since several panels in window 4 are obscured by the lamp in the middle of the Courtyard in the 1911 photograph. The problem is partially resolved by the 1917 photograph of the

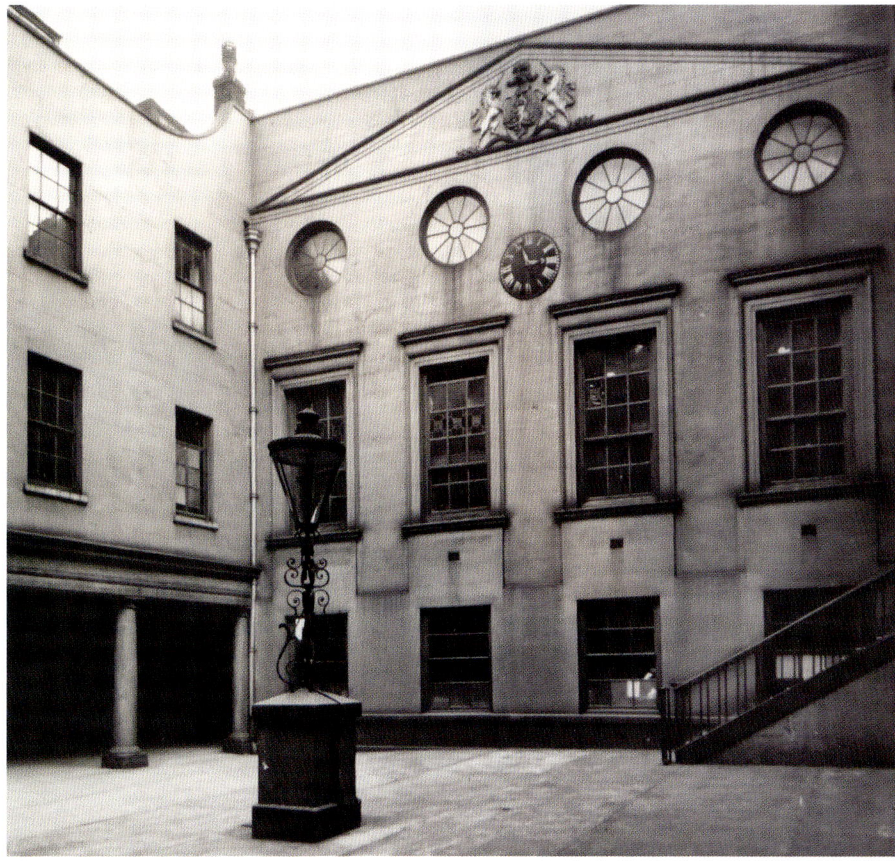

4.10 Photograph of the west side of the Great Hall taken from the Courtyard in 1911

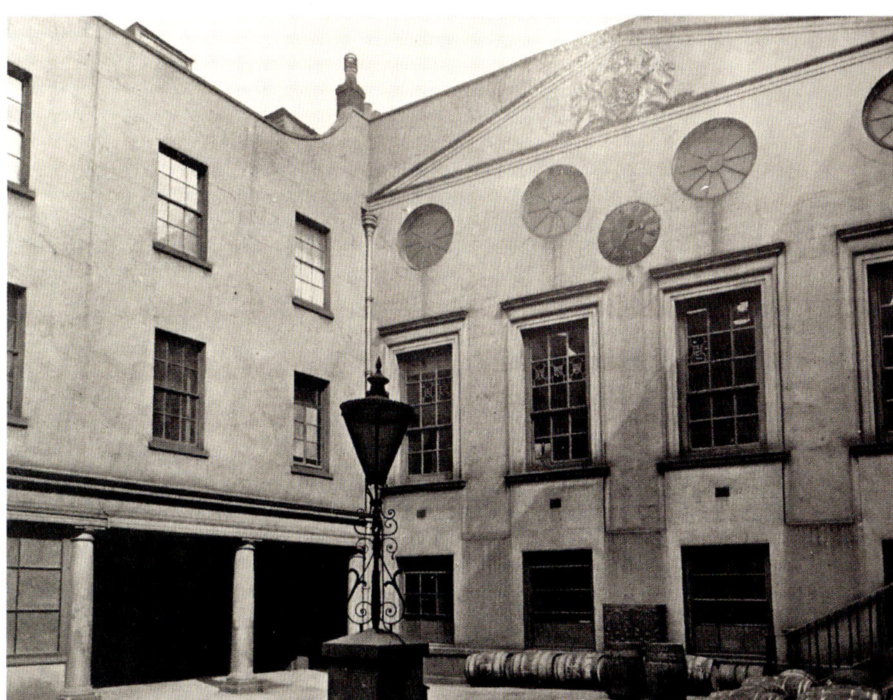

4.11 Photograph of the west side of the Great Hall taken from the Courtyard in 1917

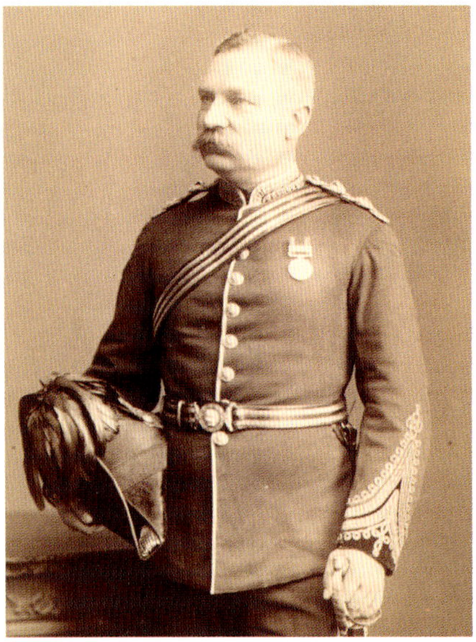

4.12 Dr James Henry Jeffcoat in the uniform of the Army Medical Service; he was the probable initiator of the Great Hall glazing scheme in 1906

Courtyard, which clearly shows that at that date the only stained glass panels in the windows of the Great Hall were the six already described (see Figure 4.11).[10]

Although there is no specific archival evidence to support the claim, it seems reasonable to conclude that it is to James Henry Jeffcoat (Figure 4.12) that credit must be given for the inspirational idea of launching what has turned out to be such an important and attractive asset for the Society.

The Installation of the Next Five Armorial Panels

The next photograph in the archive of the west side of the Great Hall taken from the Courtyard, dated 1922 (Figure 4.13), shows extensive development of the glazing scheme (see Appendix IV pp. 252–3). Eleven armorial panels are seen together with thirty-seven panels, each containing a blank cartouche and along the top row of all four windows twelve panels of clear glass. This scheme was obviously designed in the expectation that future Masters would follow the example of their predecessors, but as will be shown, this was in fact a slow process. It is important to mention here that the folder containing this photograph bears the date 1912. The date on the back of the photograph itself has clearly been altered, the first figure '2' having been changed from a figure '1', converting 1912 to 1922. There is thus some doubt about the accuracy of the 1922 date. However, two of the

PANEL	MASTER	DATE	POSITION
1-3	Plain		
4	Clarence Cooper	1903–04	same as in 1911
5	Albert Bryan Day	1904–05	same as in 1911
6	James Henry Jeffcoat	1905–06	same as in 1911
7	Samuel Clewin Griffith	1897–98	moved from window 2
8	George Wilks	1907–08	moved from window 4
9	John Charles Thorowgood (Warden)	1906–07	moved from window 4
10	Thomas Edwin Burton Brown	1901–02	
11	Frederick Gordon Brown	1908–09	
12	Sir Thomas Boor Crosby	1911–12	
13	Benjamin Bloomfield Connolly	1918–19	
14	Samuel Osborn	1919–20	
15	Blank cartouche (pattern A)		

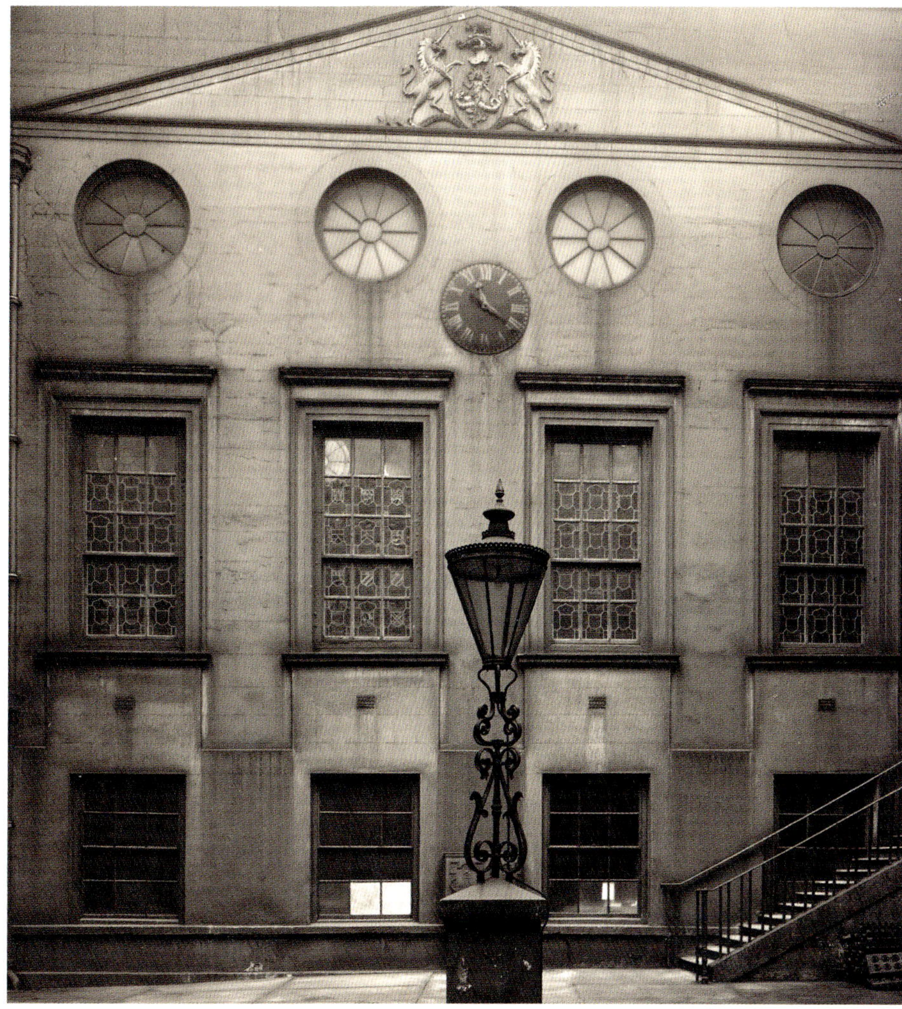

4.13 Photograph of the west side of the Great Hall taken from the Courtyard in 1922

panels in this photograph relate to the Masters in the years 1918–19 and 1919–20, which seems satisfactorily to endorse the 1922 date.

Since the panels of the three further pre-First World War Masters, Thomas Edwin Burton Brown, Frederick Gordon Brown and Sir Thomas Boor Crosby, are absent in the 1917 photograph but present in the 1922 photograph mentioned above, they were obviously installed between those dates, but there is no archival evidence to show when exactly this was done.

In the 1922 photograph, the only window shown to contain armorial glass is window 3. Thus, between 1917 and 1922 panels had been moved from both windows 2 and 4 into window 3, the make-up of which was therefore as listed in the table opposite.

Only four Masters between the years 1911 and 1922 are commemorated in glass. Crosby, Connolly and Osborn are listed above. The fourth, Meredith Townsend (Master 1914–15), now commemorated in window West 2, panel 2 and made by the company of W. B. Simpson & Sons, was probably not installed until 1938 (see below).

There is no record in the Powell archive of orders for that company to make the panels for T. E. Brown, F. G. Brown, Sir Thomas Crosby, B. Connolly or S. Osborn. In view of the later close association of the glass company W. B. Simpson & Sons with the Society, which is described below, it is possible that that company was responsible for making these five panels, but this must remain conjecture, because the Simpson Archive was unfortunately largely destroyed in the Second World War.

Thus in 1922, window 3, comprising eleven armorial bearings all mounted in one or other of two cartouche designs, one blank cartouche panel and three panels of clear glass, viewed from *inside* the Great Hall, would have appeared as shown in Figure 4.14.

Examination of the leading pattern in both the 1911 and 1922 photographs clearly shows the two cartouche designs and that these designs alternate horizontally across all four windows and vertically in each window (Figures 4.13 and 4.14), a pattern long since completely disrupted.

In summary, the panels in the 1922 photograph commemorate ten of the twenty-three Masters between the years 1897–98 and 1919–20. But also commemorated in this period is one Wardenship, that of John Charles Thorowgood (Warden 1905–06). This exception to the general pattern of commemoration requires explanation. The Court Minutes for the year 1905–06 record that on 15 August 1905, the date of the Election Court, Thorowgood was elected as Junior Warden for the year ensuing. The minutes also show that at a meeting of the Private Court on 7 August 1906, he was represented by a deputy. At the Election Court on 14 August of that year, when he should have been elected as Senior Warden, he was again absent and therefore passed over, George Wilks being elected by ballot in his place. It seems that this was due to the ill-health of Thorowgood, for whom an expression of sympathy by the Court was recorded. Although his last attendance at a Court meeting was 18 June 1907, he did not resign from the Court until 1908, his letter of resignation being accepted at the Election Court on 18 August 1908.[11] He was plainly held in very high regard as a colleague and friend by the members of the Court and it seems likely that as a result it was felt that his contribution to the Society should be commemorated by an armorial panel in the Great Hall. Interestingly, he served as Junior Warden in the year 1905–06 but the date on his armorial panel, as indicated in the list above, incorrectly shows his tenure of office as being 1906–07. This panel has also been moved on at least two occasions and is now in window West 1, panel 5.

The Glazing Scheme Loses Momentum

The installation of the thirty-seven blank cartouche panels seen in the 1922 photograph clearly indicates that it was the intention of the Society to continue to decorate the windows of the Great Hall with armorial stained glass, a commitment underlined by the considerable financial outlay for the Society which this entailed. The cost of this development is confirmed by an entry in the Society's 'Ledger 1918–1925', which records the payment of £62.0.0d to the Company of W. B. Simpson & Sons (see Appendix III) on

29 June 1920 for 'New shields to Hall windows'.[12] This presumably refers to the thirty-six blank cartouches in windows West 1, 2 and 4 and possibly the one blank cartouche in window West 3, seen in the 1922 photograph (see Figure 4.13). It is of interest that the Society decided at this point to employ a different company of glaziers to continue its glazing scheme, a decision upon which the Archive is silent. What is not clear is whether the amalgamation of the eleven armorial panels and one blank cartouche into window West 3 was done at the same time, which seems likely, or earlier.

In the Society Archive, there exists a letter dated 10 November 1937 from W. B. Simpson & Sons in which mention is made of a panel which the company 'is executing for Dr Townsend'. This is the Meredith Townsend panel already mentioned. Since Dr Townsend had died in 1918 it is likely that the panel was commissioned by his son Dr Meredith Milton Townsend, who was a member of the Court of Assistants of the Society. Simpsons describe themselves on the letter-head as 'Decorative Art Craftsmen' specialising, amongst other things, in 'Memorial Glass Windows and Leaded Glazing'. The writer of the letter, Graham Colin Simpson, who was a director, also comments that it was his company that had been responsible for 'the original decoration to the windows' at the Hall.[13] While it is not stated, most unfortunately, to what work he refers, it is very likely to have been the installation of the blank cartouches seen in the 1922 photograph. It is a matter of great regret that, because many of the Simpson records were lost in the Second World War, no record of what was done, other than this letter, now exists. Many of the company's pattern books of the period have survived, but none shows designs to match the cartouches. So, there are a number of questions that must remain unanswered. It is clear, however, that the companies of Powell and Simpson were both involved in the early stained glass glazing scheme in the Great Hall.

Before considering the installation of further armorial panels, it is worthwhile considering why at this time the panels in the top row of each window contain only plain glass and not cartouches. One can only guess why this was done. Was it to let more light into the Great Hall, or was it simply a question of expense? A letter in the Society Archive dated 24 January 1938 from James Powell & Sons indicates that both Lord Dawson of Penn's and Lord Nuffield of Nuffield's panels have 'been made for the upper windows in the Great Hall where there is only plain glass at present'.[14] These two panels may indeed have been installed originally in the upper row of panes – although this is unlikely, as will be shown later – and they are not in the top row now, Lord Dawson's being panel 8 in window West 4 and Lord Nuffield's panel 8 in window West 1. But this does indicate, however, that plain panels remained in situ in the top row of each window for many years.

But despite the apparent enthusiasm of the Society to continue with armorial glazing, the whole scheme seems to have come to a virtual standstill in the 1920s and early 1930s. It is likely that between 1922 and 1938 only two panels were installed, those of Algernon Dutton Brenchley (Master 1924–25) and Alfred Hepburn (Master 1926–27). The first of these to be installed was the Hepburn panel, which was made by the well-known stained glass artist Francis Spear. Undoubtedly, Hepburn was stimulated by the decision of the Court in 1931 to commission Spear to make 'The Apothecary' window for the east end of the Great Hall, as described in Chapter 5 (that chapter also describes how both the window and the panel were installed together in 1931). The panel is currently panel 2 in window West 3 and it seems reasonable to presume that that is where it was installed in 1931 as part of the only window at that date to contain armorial glass.

When the above panel and window were installed, a further small panel was also installed by the Francis Spear technicians (also mentioned in Chapter 5). The only Master to have opted for an armorial panel between 1922 and 1931, other than Reginald Whiteside Statham (Master 1927–28) whose panel was not installed until 1938, was Brenchley and so it seems likely that this is the panel in question, particularly as he opted to show only his shield in a cartouche ('a small panel'). It is currently panel 15 in window West 3 and again it seems reasonable to conclude that that is where it was installed in 1931, that being at the time the only remaining blank cartouche panel in that window. Furthermore, the blank cartouche was a type A and Brenchley's Arms are installed in a type A cartouche. What is not clear is whether the Brenchley panel was made by Spear. This is obviously a possibility but is a question that must remain unanswered. The only other candidate for consideration for placement in this position is the panel of Frank Haydon (Secretary 1895–1930), but since his term of office did not end until 1930, it seems reasonable to presume that the making and installation of his panel was later. Incidentally, the Archive is silent regarding any details about the Haydon panel and the current members of his family have no knowledge of these details either.

The W. B. Simpson & Sons panel for Meredith Townsend (Master 1914–15) is of interest (window West 2, panel 2) for he was the first Master in date order to dispense with the cartouche, thus allowing display of his Arms together with crest, mantling and motto. His panel is shown in Figure 4.15. Of more importance, though, is the Hepburn panel for Alfred Hepburn (Master 1926–27) who was the first Master chronologically to adopt this style, a brave decision that seems to have been accepted by the Society without demur. His panel is also shown in Figure 4.15. It is worth noting that of the six Masters commemorated in stained glass between the wars, three dispensed with a cartouche. After the Second World War, the employment of a cartouche has been rare, the last Past Master to use it being Ian McGilchrist Jackson (Master 1977–78) in window West 3, panel 9.

The Glazing Scheme Regains Momentum and Undergoes Major Change: 1938 and the War Years

While the early 1930s was a period of glazing inactivity, it seems that towards the end of 1937 a further decision must have been taken by the Society to expand the scheme. One stimulus for this must have been the fact that by this stage window West 3 contained only two available spaces, both filled with blank panes of glass, so that if more panels were to be accommodated, expansion in due course was inevitable. So, the glazing scheme was given a kick-restart, resulting in the installation of armorial panels in window West 4 and possibly elsewhere.

The principal archival evidence for this kick-restart comes in the form of a round-robin letter written by the Clerk, Group Captain Henry Cooper, some copies dated 13 December and some 14 December 1937, to all Past Masters and Honorary Freemen suggesting that they could, if they so wished, have their armorial bearings displayed in the Great Hall in stained glass.[15] These letters were followed by a personal letter in April the following year, for example to Lady Buchanan, who did not avail herself of the offer on behalf of her husband Sir George Seaton Buchanan (Master 1934–35) and also to Miss Gardiner, the granddaughter of Hugh Worthington Statham (Master 1881–82) and Mrs. N Statham, widow of H. W. Statham's nephew Reginald Whiteside Statham (Master 1927–28), both of whom did.[16] There must have been other similar personal letters sent, but those mentioned here are the only copies with replies to have survived. It may have been this correspondence that stimulated the Townsend family to commemorate their father. It must be presumed, too, that all twelve of the Honorary Freemen were approached, of whom only four accepted the invitation, Sir Buckston Browne, Viscount Dawson of Penn, Sir Arthur MacNalty and Viscount Nuffield of Nuffield.

Further evidence that a major change was envisaged is that the Clerk's letters continue: 'In order to obtain a degree of uniformity it is desirable that the same artist should be employed throughout and the Court recommend [*sic*] that the work be done by James Powell and Sons who were responsible for the most successful of the Arms already installed.' Since detailed examination of the Powell archive shows that the only panels made by that company prior to this date were the first six to be installed, it must be these to which he refers.

A number of stained glass companies were asked by the Society to tender for this work. As the company of James Powell & Sons was included on the list, this would seem to confirm that company had not been employed by the Society or by any of the Past Masters for some years and it is noteworthy, incidentally, that the Powell tendered price was not the cheapest.[17]

Before describing the probable course of events during this period of change, it is helpful to consider all the armorial panels which had to be accommodated between 1922 and 1948. These are set out below in date order of installation. The list clearly demonstrates a flurry of activity in 1938 when there were certainly seven, and probably eight new panels awaiting installation.

These panels are illustrated in Figure 4.15, excluding those of the four Honorary Freemen which are illustrated later in Figure 4.18.

The Powell archive shows that the panels of Sir Hugh Lett, Reginald Hewlett Hayes and Lionel Vernon Cargill were made by that firm in 1943, 1941 and 1948 respectively. Relevant to further discussion below, it is pertinent to record that in the Powell archive the order for the Lett panel includes a note to the effect that the panel is to be delivered to the Hall but not installed until after the war. A note with the Hayes order comments that the Arms are to be inserted in an existing panel, which undoubtedly refers to a cartouche and it is likely that this panel too was not installed until after the war.[18]

It is not unreasonable to suggest that the responses from the Statham family, and from the Honorary Freemen, to the Clerk's letters of December 1937 stimulated the then Master (Sir Hugh Lett) and the Wardens (Reginald Hayes and Vernon

NAME AND DATE OF MASTERSHIP / HONORARY FREEDOM	MAKER	DATE OF INSTALLATION
Alfred Hepburn (Master 1926–27)	Francis Spear	1931
Algernon Dutton Brenchley (Master 1924–25)	Possibly Spear	Probably 1931 with the Hepburn panel
Meredith Townsend (Master 1914–15)	W. B. Simpson & Sons	1938
Hugh Worthington Statham (Master 1881–82)	James Powell & Sons	1938
Reginald Whiteside Statham (Master 1927–28)	James Powell & Sons	1938
The Viscount Dawson (Hon. Freeman 1932)	James Powell & Sonss	1938
Sir Arthur MacNalty (Hon. Freeman 1936)	James Powell & Sons	1938
The Viscount Nuffield (Hon. Freeman 1937)	James Powell & Sons	1938
Sir Buckston Browne (Hon. Freeman 1938)	James Powell & Sons	1938
Frank Haydon (Secretary 1895–1930)	Unknown	Unconfirmed, but likely to have been 1938
Sir Hugh Lett (Master 1937–38)	James Powell & Sons	1946
Reginald Hewlett Hayes (Master 1938–39)	James Powell & Sons	1946
Lionel Vernon Cargill (Master 1939–40)	James Powell & Sons	1948

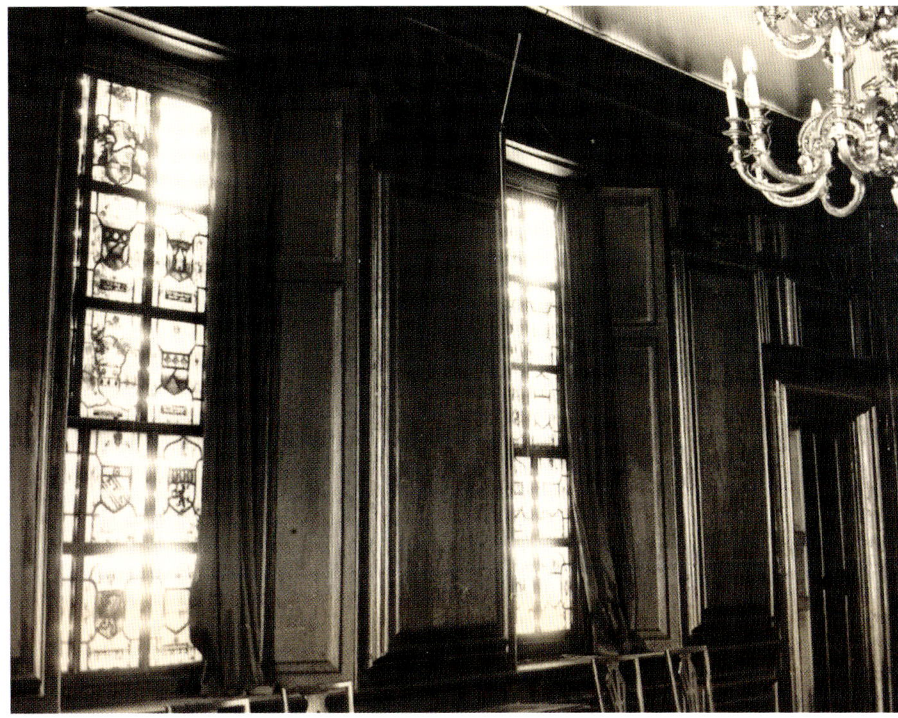

4.16 Detail of a photograph of part of the Great Hall taken in 1941 as part of the 'National Buildings Register' scheme, showing parts of windows West 3 and 4

Cargill) all to have their Arms displayed in the Great Hall windows, a joint venture between the three of them which echoes the initial inspiration for decorative armorial glazing by the Jeffcoat, Day and Cooper trio in 1906, thirty-two years earlier, but not of course realised until well after the end of the war (see opposite).

The only evidence of what installations may have taken place in 1938 is a very blurred and inadequate photograph in the Society Archive of part of the west wall of the Great Hall, taken in 1941 as part of the National Buildings Register scheme (Figure 4.16).

Only part of each of windows West 3 and 4 is visible. In window West 3, the Brenchley panel is installed as panel 15 and the Hepburn panel as panel 2. Panel 8 (Wilks) has been removed and replaced with the panel of Viscount Nuffield. Panel 3 remains as clear glass and, although it cannot be seen, it is likely that for the sake of balance panel 1 remains as clear glass also and that all the other panels remain as seen in the 1922 photograph.

In window 4, the right-hand column of panels can be seen together with only a very narrow sliver of the central column, but enough to identify the panels. It is likely, therefore, that the composition of these two columns is as shown in the list overleaf. The remaining three panels to be accounted for are those of one of the Stathams, Wilks and Sir Buckston Browne. If, as seems reasonable, windows West 1 and 2 remained as shown in the 1922 photograph, with no additions or deletions, these latter three panels must have been installed in the left-hand column of this window. In order to maintain the general cartouche pattern across all four windows, the make-up of window West 4 at this time is therefore likely to have been as follows:

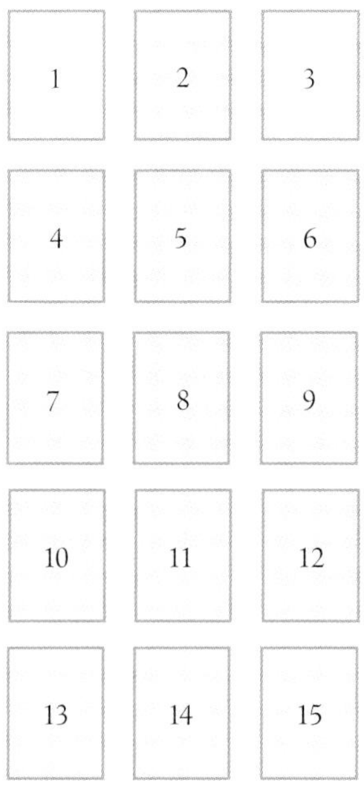

Panel 1 – Clear glass	Panel 2 – Townsend	Panel 3 – Clear glass
Panel 4 – Cartouche A	Panel 5 – MacNalty	Panel 6 – Cartouche A
Panel 7 – Browne (?)	Panel 8 – Dawson	Panel 9 – Cartouche B
Panel 10 – Statham (?)	Panel 11 – Haydon	Panel 12 – Cartouche A
Panel 13 – Wilks (?)	Panel 14 – which Statham?	Panel 15 – Cartouche B

In the Powell & Sons 'Journal Window Department (1934–1939)', a charge of £1.5.0d is recorded on 1 July 1938 for 'removing heraldic panels and fixing in new positions to instructions',[19] a sum which is confirmed in the Society Ledger (1936–43) on 17 August 1938, for 'removing armorial panels in the windows of the Great Hall'.[20] Although this is a comparatively small amount, it is beyond reasonable doubt that these entries refer to the work just described (see Appendix IV p.255).

The war now interrupted the development of the glazing scheme. The remarkable survival of the glass during hostilities, entailing as it did the removal of all the stained glass panels from the west wall windows, is described later in the chapter.

The first post-war evidence of how the glazing scheme continued to develop is a photograph of the west wall of the Great Hall seen from the Courtyard, probably taken early in 1946 (Figure 4.17). Evidently, this was a time when the opportunity to spread the pattern of armorial decoration across the four windows of the west wall of the Great Hall was seized. Although there would have been a desire by all concerned to return all the activities and the fabric of the Society to normal as quickly as possible, it was also an opportunity for detailed aesthetic rethinking.

The exact date of the photograph is not recorded but it is likely to have been taken some time after the date of payment in February 1946 by the Society to James Powell & Sons for undertaking the reinstallation of the glass. Once again, the distinctive leading patterns allow clear identification of most of the panels. This is supported by the fact that in all these cases the panels are still in the same positions today, so that it is very likely that any panel not easily identifiable in the photograph is, in all probability, in the same position in the photograph as that which it occupies in the Hall today. This is illustrated in Appendix IV, p. 257 where these moves can be traced as follows:

> WINDOW WEST 3: The panels of Nuffield, Thorowgood and Griffith have been moved to window West 1; the panels of Cooper, Crosby, T. E. B. Brown and F. C. Brown have been moved to window West 2; the panels of Jeffcoat and Osborn have been moved to window West 4; leaving the panels of Hepburn, Day, Connolly and Brenchley in situ.
>
> New panels for Lett and Hayes have been added.

WINDOW WEST 4: The panels of Wilks, H. W. Statham and R. W. Statham have been moved to window West 1; the panels of Townsend and Browne have been moved to window West 2.

Movements within window West 4 are MacNalty and Haydon, leaving Dawson in situ.

After the 1938 rearrangement and installations, there were twenty-one armorial panels, twenty-nine blank cartouche panels and ten clear panes of glass in the west wall windows. After the reinstallation of all panels in 1946 there were twenty-three armorial panels, thirty-one blank cartouche panels and six clear panes of glass in these windows.

Assuming that the clear panes of glass were not removed during the war, this gives a total of fifty-two panels, fifty from the windows together with the two loose panels of Lett and Hayes which were to be installed after the war. When the panels of Lett and Hayes were installed, the two blank cartouche panels they displaced were installed in the top row of windows West 2 and 3, together with two further blank cartouche panels from the store at Apothecaries' Hall, thus filling the top row of those two windows with stained glass, leaving only six clear panes of glass in the top row of windows West 1 and 4.

The rearrangement of the west wall glass achieved a very satisfactory even spread of armorial glass across all four windows, with a mixture of older and newer panels in each, but sadly this was the time when the symmetrical pattern of cartouches inevitably disappeared.

Although only three Masters and four Honorary Freemen responded positively to the Clerk's offer in 1937 of having their Arms displayed in the Great Hall, the marketing exercise does seem to have been very successful, because after the war it became the rule rather than the exception for Masters to be commemorated in this way.

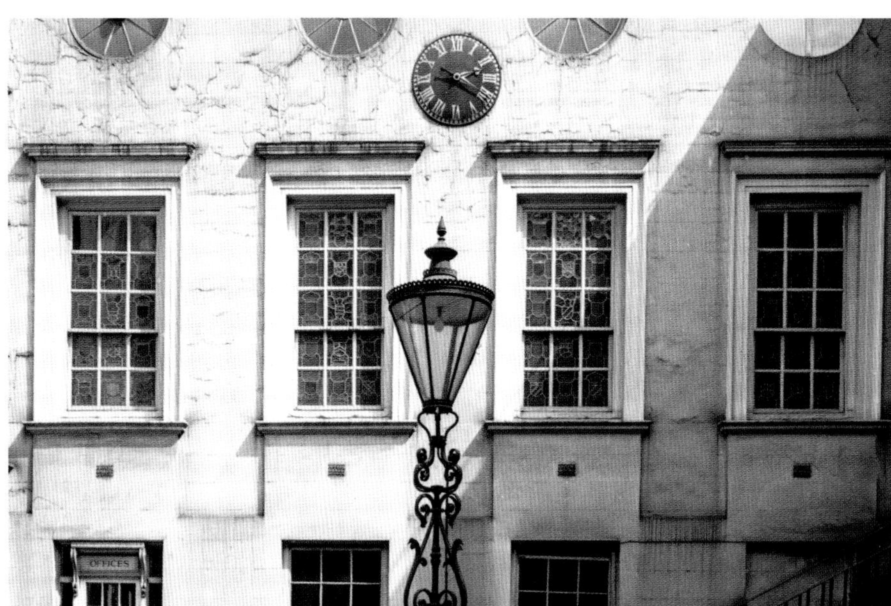

4.17 The west wall of the Great Hall taken from the Courtyard in 1946

Over succeeding years, one by one the panels containing blank cartouches or plain glass have been replaced with armorial glass, so that by 2015 all the panels in the west wall of the Great Hall had been filled with armorial bearings. Of the sixty panels, four commemorate Honorary Freemen, fifty-four commemorate Masters, one commemorates a Wardenship and one commemorates Frank Haydon, who on his panel is simply described as 'Secretary' (Figure 4.15). He was in fact Secretary to the Court of Examiners from 1895 until 1930, a term of office which was plainly regarded as worthy of commemoration in glass. It is of further interest that on his retirement in 1930 his successor's title was changed to 'Registrar' – an appointment that continues to the present day.

The last Master to be commemorated in the west wall windows is Peter John Hocart Tooley (Master 2013–14), window West 1, panel 1, although the glazing scheme was not in fact completed until the installation in 2015 of the panel commemorating the Mastership of Robert George Hankin Bethel (Master 2010–11) window West 2, panel 3.

The Five Honorary Freemen

Five of the Society's Honorary Freemen are commemorated in stained glass (Figure 4.18). Correspondence held in the Archive indicates that four of these panels, all made by James Powell & Sons, were installed in windows on the west side of the Great Hall in 1938.[21] The panel for the fifth Honorary Freeman to be commemorated in stained glass, that of Lord Cohen of Birkenhead, was made by the Carl Edwards Studio in Apothecaries' Hall and was installed on the east side of the Great Hall in 1975.[22] From left to right they are:

The Viscount Dawson of Penn – Honorary Freeman 1932 (window West 4, panel 8)

Sir Arthur MacNalty – Honorary Freeman 1936 (window West 4, panel 11)

The Viscount Nuffield of Nuffield – Honorary Freeman 1937 (window West 1, panel 8)

Sir Buckston Browne – Honorary Freeman 1938 (window West 2, panel 8)

Lord Cohen of Birkenhead – Honorary Freeman 1967 (window East 1, panel 11)

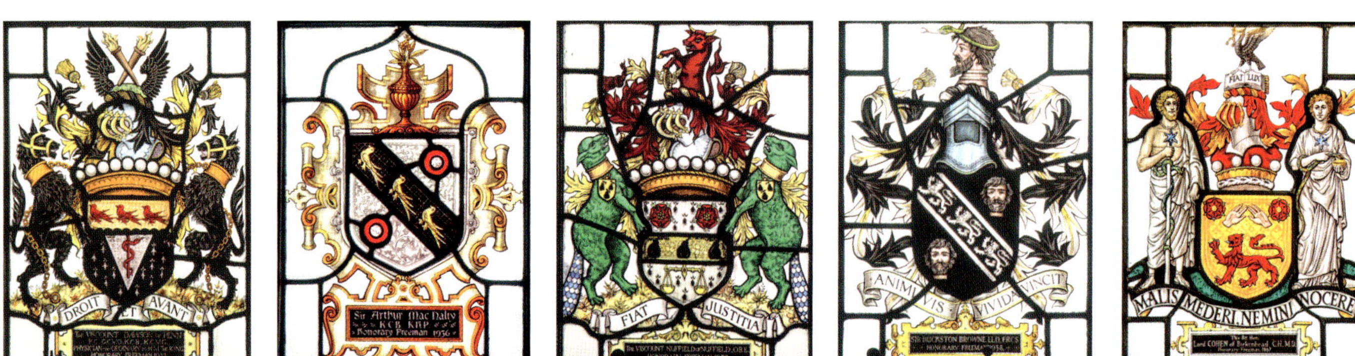

4.18 The armorial bearings of the five Honorary Freemen commemorated in stained glass in order of installation

East Side of the Great Hall

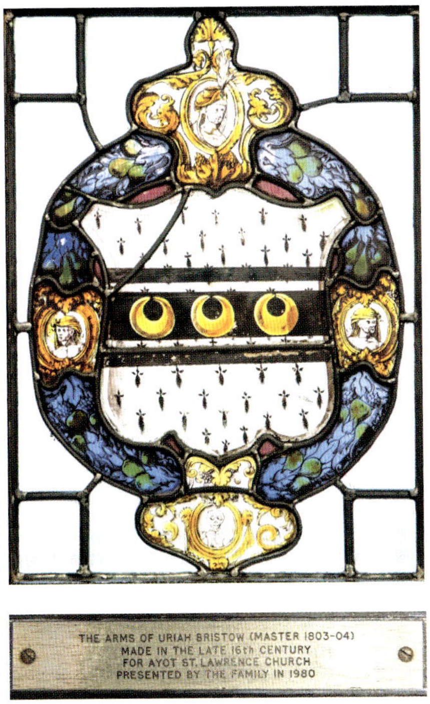
THE ARMS OF URIAH BRISTOW (MASTER 1803-04)
MADE IN THE LATE 16th CENTURY
FOR AYOT ST. LAWRENCE CHURCH
PRESENTED BY THE FAMILY IN 1980

4.19 The armorial bearings of Uriah Bristow (Master 1803–04) and the plaque recording the Bristow family gift to the Society

The glazing scheme for this side of the Great Hall did not start until 1963, when the Arms of Thomas Keith Lyle were installed (window East 2, panel 5). Armorial glazing has continued, and at the date of publication as shown in Figure 4.2, nineteen armorial panels have been installed, seventeen commemorating Masters, one commemorating an Honorary Freeman and one a Registrar and Clerk to the Society.

The oldest glass in Apothecaries' Hall is the Bristow panel (window East 2, panel 14 – Figure 4.19) which dates from the sixteenth century. Chapter 9 is devoted to the history and acquisition of this very interesting and important piece. Suffice to say here that when the panel arrived, it was in poor condition. It was shown to the stained glass expert, Carl Edwards (see Chapter 7), who confirmed that it was indeed likely to be sixteenth century. In a letter dated 2 April 1980 to the Clerk, Major Charles O'Leary, he says:

> *It is a good example of its period. The glass is very thin and fragile and great care must be taken when it is being removed from the frame. I propose to strip off the lead, removing the old cement from each piece of glass and reglaze. The missing pieces to be replaced with glass painted to match and the entire glazing waterproofed. The panel to be squared up by adding white antique glass, matching the glass in the Cartouches panels in the Banqueting Hall [sic], in order that it can be fixed into a window.*[23]

The donors of the panel were both direct descendants of Uriah Bristow (a relationship described in detail in Chapter 9). The donation of this generous gift is recorded on a plaque fixed to the window frame below the panel (Figure 4.19).

Perhaps pertinent to the placing of the Bristow panel is a letter in the Society's Archives, dated 7 May 1980, from the Clerk to Carl Edwards concerning the 'moving of a Coat of Arms in the East side of the Hall from the bottom of one window to the top of the one next to it', which perhaps significantly also accepts Edwards' estimate for doing the conservation work on the Bristow panel.[24] Until 2010, the only panel at the top of either window on the east side of the Great Hall was that recording the Mastership of Dr Elston Grey-Turner (Master 1975–76) in window East 1, panel 2. This must therefore be the panel referred to by the Clerk, because at that time only the central column in each of the two east-side windows contained armorial panels and so it is probable that the Grey-Turner panel was originally at the bottom of the central column in window East 2, panel 14.

The relevance of the move hinges on the debate that must have occurred about where the Bristow panel was to go. Since the panel itself bears no inscription on the glass, an explanatory plaque was obviously required, and this could only be fixed on the adjacent window frame. Since the decision had clearly been taken to install the Bristow panel on the east side of the Great Hall, the only two positions that would allow the explanatory plaque to be easily read, and which would also maintain the symmetry of the glazing,

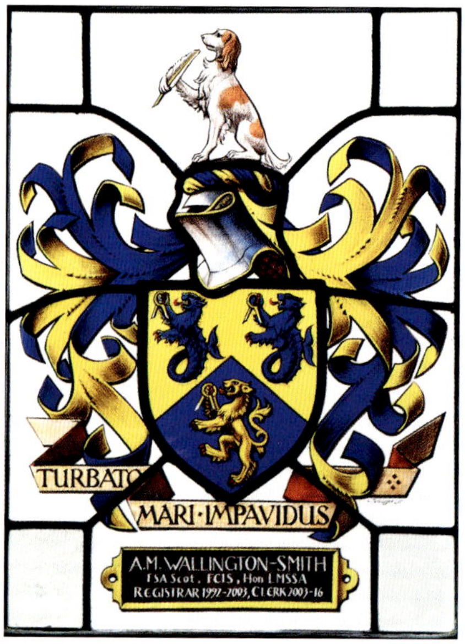

4.20 The armorial bearings of Andrew Wallington-Smith, former Registrar and Clerk to the Society

were the bottom positions of the central column in one or other of the two windows. Window 1, panel 14 records the Mastership of Professor Sir Brian Windeyer (Master 1972–73). Whether he and Dr Grey-Turner were consulted about the proposal to move one of the panels is not known (both were still alive at the time), but it seems reasonable to conclude that the Grey-Turner panel was moved to its present position to make way for the Bristow panel.

On 24 March 2016 Andrew Wallington-Smith retired, having been Registrar to the Society from 1992 until 2003 and Clerk from 2003 until 2016. The Court decided that such a period of service to the Society should be commemorated in stained glass and his armorial bearings were installed in window East 2, panel 1 (Figure 4.20).

Panels 1 and 3 in window East 1 retain blank cartouche panels, design B in panel 1 and design A in panel 3. Hence, a number of panels remain to be filled with armorial bearings. In 2030 or thereabouts, the glazing scheme for the Great Hall will be complete.

The Glass Survives the Second World War

The Court Minutes make no mention of stained glass during the First World War. It is extremely unlikely that it was felt necessary at any time during that war to remove it for safe-keeping. The Court Minutes and other records covering the period of the Second World War do, however, mention the glass in several instances.

The Court Minutes of 13 May 1941 state: 'It was reported that in a recent air-raid the shield of Samuel Clewin Griffith in a window in the Great Hall had been damaged by blast.'[25] Nowhere is it mentioned how this was repaired, but further archival evidence may give a clue. In the James Powell & Sons archive, the 'Journal Window Department (1939–1951)' records on 2 September 1941 the removal of the four (west) windows from the Great Hall, together with the two windows from the Great Staircase and two panels from the Library, at a charge of £25.[26] On 15 October 1941, an entry in the Society 'Ledger (1936–1943)' confirms payment of £25.0.0d to James Powell & Sons for the 'Removal of Cts of Arms from Gt Hall Windows'; as just quoted from their archive, this must include the Staircase windows and the Library panels.[27] Perhaps the damage to the Griffith panel in May of that year was the trigger for all this.

But it was not until 13 April 1943, at a meeting of the Private Court, that 'The Master reported that the Foundling Hospital at Berkhamsted was prepared to accept custody of the Society's pictures and glazed armorial bearings. The Acting Clerk was directed to write to the Secretary of the Hospital accepting their offer and expressing the gratitude of the Court.'[28] The transfer was undertaken by a Southwark removals firm, Samuel Taylor & Son Ltd. of Tooley Street, London SE1, on 22 April 1943. A note in the Archive records that three tea-chests containing respectively twenty-two, sixteen and fourteen panels from the Great Hall were moved, a total of fifty-two panes.[29] It is also noted that a case measuring 5 × 5 feet containing the stained glass windows from the Great Staircase was transferred together with a box containing the two stained glass panels from the Library. There is no mention of the Apothecary window at the southern end of the Great Hall, which presumably remained in situ throughout the war, perhaps because external scaffolding would have been required to remove it. Some rather insubstantial covering of the window nevertheless was undertaken (see Chapter 6).

On 11 May 1943, at a meeting of the Private Court, 'The Master reported that most of the Society's pictures, the glazed Coats of Arms and the painted wood Coat of Arms and an inscription from the Barge had been deposited for safe custody at the Foundling Hospital in Berkhamsted, the glass being stored in the crypt of the Chapel. The Master undertook to consult the Secretary of the Hospital with regard to the inspection of the pictures if the necessity should arise.'[30] Why, one wonders, since the glass was removed from the windows in October 1941 was it not removed from the City until May 1943? A number of items had already been sent to the basement of County Hall but the stained glass windows were not amongst them. The worst bombing of the city was over in 1940 and the first V-1 flying bomb raid was not until 13 June 1944. Perhaps there had been warnings about the imminent doodlebugs.

After the war, the Society's possessions at Berkhamsted were transferred back to the Hall on Friday 17 May 1945 by the removals firm, Messrs. Joseph May of Whitfield Street, London W1.[31] The next relevant entry in the Private Court Minutes is on 12 June 1945:

> *It was reported that the Society's stained glass, silver and most of the Library were returned to the Hall on the 17th May … As it was found that the stained glass belonging to the staircase was cracked, Messrs. James Powell, who had taken it down, were not prepared to re-instate it, or to unpack the glass removed from the Great Hall windows, preferring to leave the whole of the work until they could undertake the repair of the cracked panes.*[32]

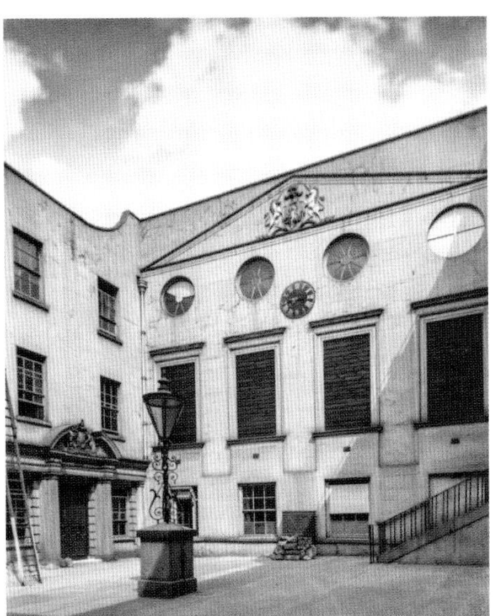

4.21 The windows of the Great Hall still boarded up immediately after the Second World War

In the Powell 'Estimate Book (1937–1948)', an entry for 10 January 1946 refers to the restoration of all the glass that had been removed during the war. Of relevance to the Great Hall, it is recorded that for 'cutting, painting, staining and refitting new pieces of glass to match broken pieces in four of the panels and refixing all the panels in the windows (54 in all)' the charge would be £35.0.0d.[33] This is confirmed in the Powell 'Journal Window Department (1939–1951)' on 30 January.[34] An entry in the Society 'Ledger (1943–1947)' dated 13 February 1946 records a payment of £60.0.0d to James Powell & Sons for 'Repairing and replacing stained glass'.[35] The additional sum of £25 was the estimate for restoring the windows on the Great Staircase (see Chapter 4).

Figure 4.21 shows the west wall of the Great Hall immediately after the war (exact date not recorded), perhaps the nadir of its existence. However, the fabric of the Hall and most of its contents had survived largely unscathed and restoration then began.

In the 1946 photograph of the west side of the Great Hall taken from the Courtyard (Figure 4.17), it is interesting to note that while all the armorial panels have been reinstalled, the circular windows above had not yet been repaired. The full photograph also shows that the two armorial panels in the Landing windows had also not yet been installed (see Chapter 10).

The Society Archive contains many references to the replacement of broken plain glass throughout the whole estate after the war, indicating a considerable degree of blast damage. It is therefore appropriate to emphasise the Society's deep gratitude to the Court for its decision in 1941 which led to the removal of all the heraldic stained glass in the Hall for safekeeping during hostilities.

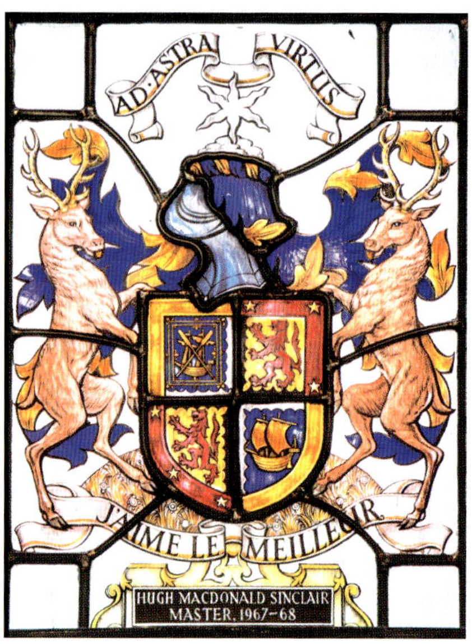

4.22 The armorial bearings of Hugh Macdonald Sinclair (Master 1967–68)

The Sinclair Panel

The Private Court Minutes of 10 March 2009 reveal an intriguing note to the effect that the Clan Sinclair Trust objected to Hugh Macdonald Sinclair's window (window East 2, panel 8) which had been installed in the Great Hall as long ago as 1973! With the permission of the Private Court, the minute can be quoted as follows: 'The Clerk reported that a dispute had broken out with members of the Clan Sinclair Trust following the publication of an image of the late Past Master Dr Hugh Sinclair's stained glass window in the journal of the Heraldry Society of Scotland. It was held by the Trust that he was not entitled to the Arms displayed and the Clerk undertook to research the matter' (Figure 4.22).[36]

These Arms had featured in that journal as an 'heraldic stray' in England and two letters of complaint from Clan Sinclair that these Arms properly belonged to Viscount Thurso were published in the next edition. Hugh Sinclair was the great-grandson of Sir Hugh Sinclair of Ulbster Bt, who had matriculated these Arms with Lord Lyon King of Arms in 1778 and to whom these Arms were re-granted with the baronetcy in 1786. The baronetcy was of Great Britain and therefore registered at the College of Arms. Under English rules, therefore, Dr Sinclair was entitled to assume these Arms in England as a direct legitimate male descendant. The current Viscount Thurso is a second cousin three times removed from Hugh Sinclair and, when approached by the Clerk, was entirely happy that these Arms should be displayed in the Hall.

The entitlement to the supporters is more difficult. Garter King of Arms is restricted to granting supporters mainly to peers by Royal Warrant, but in Scotland it is not uncommon for the minor barons (lairds) and other appropriate armigers to have obtained grants of supporters from Lord Lyon, who exercises the sovereign's whole armorial jurisdiction. The difficulty is that they are hereditary only to the direct heir of the bearer and thus probably should not have been used in this panel.

Marks and Monograms

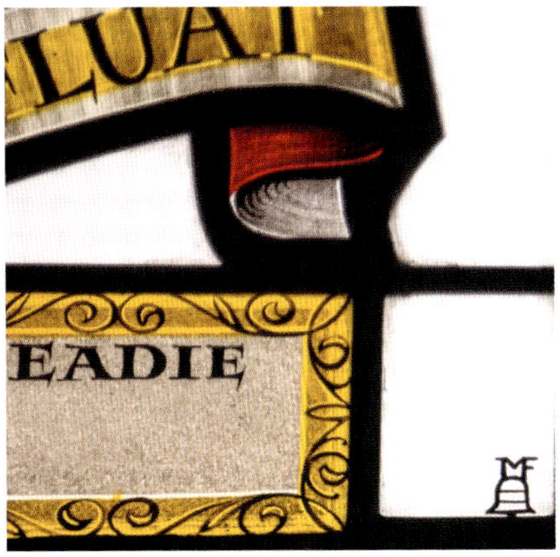

4.23 The mark and monogram of Michael Charles Farrar Bell on the Eadie panel

Many stained glass artists or designers and makers of stained glass 'sign' their windows but sadly many others do not. In the Great Hall only two such marks have been found.

The panel of Douglas George Arnott Eadie (Master 1990–91: window West 3, panel 4) bears the mark of its maker (Figure 4.23), Michael Charles Farrar Bell (1911–1993). He was the great-grandson of Alfred Bell, one of the founders of the Company of Clayton & Bell, one of the largest stained glass firms of the nineteenth and twentieth centuries in Britain (see Appendix III). The company was based in Regent Street in London and boasted that it could make a stained glass church window every day and two on Sunday! The mark is a bell surmounted by the initials MF. Mr Eadie's panel must be one of the last ones that Bell made prior to his death in 1993.

The panels of Sir Peter Tizard (Master 1983–84: window West 4, panel 12) and Professor J. A. Dudgeon (Master 1985–86: window west 4, panel 9) bear the mark of their maker. The initials JG form the monogram of Jane Campbell Gray, née Ross (1933–present) (Figure 4.24).

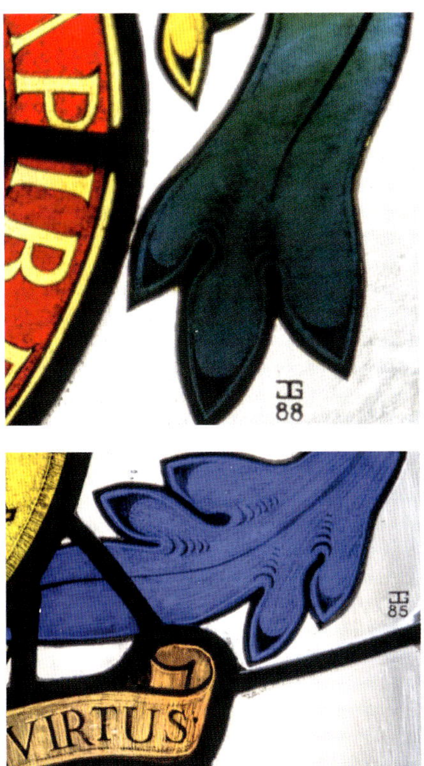

4.24 The monogram of Jane Campbell Gray on the Dudgeon and Tizard panels

Completion

In 1906 an inspirational idea by the Master of the day, Dr James Henry Jeffcoat, persuaded his two predecessors to join him in initiating a highly successful scheme of glazing decoration for the Great Hall. This was echoed by a further trio of Masters in 1937–40.

It is likely that all the panels in the Great Hall will be glazed with armorial panels by 2030 or thereabouts, thus completing a commemorative programme which is unique in the City of London Livery Halls.

Appendix IV, pages 258–60, shows the whole heraldic glazing scheme of the Great Hall as it stands in 2020.

CHAPTER 5

The Great Staircase Windows

Following the destruction of the Hall in the Great Fire of London on Tuesday 4 September 1666, the Society moved quickly to plan its rebuilding. Work began during 1668 and the new Hall was largely complete by the end of 1672.

Amongst the many craftsmen employed was one Thomas Tipping (d.1690), a glazier, who would have been responsible for overseeing the entire glazing of the Hall, mostly with clear glass. In the Society's book of 'Accounts (1669–94)' on 5 September 1670, the

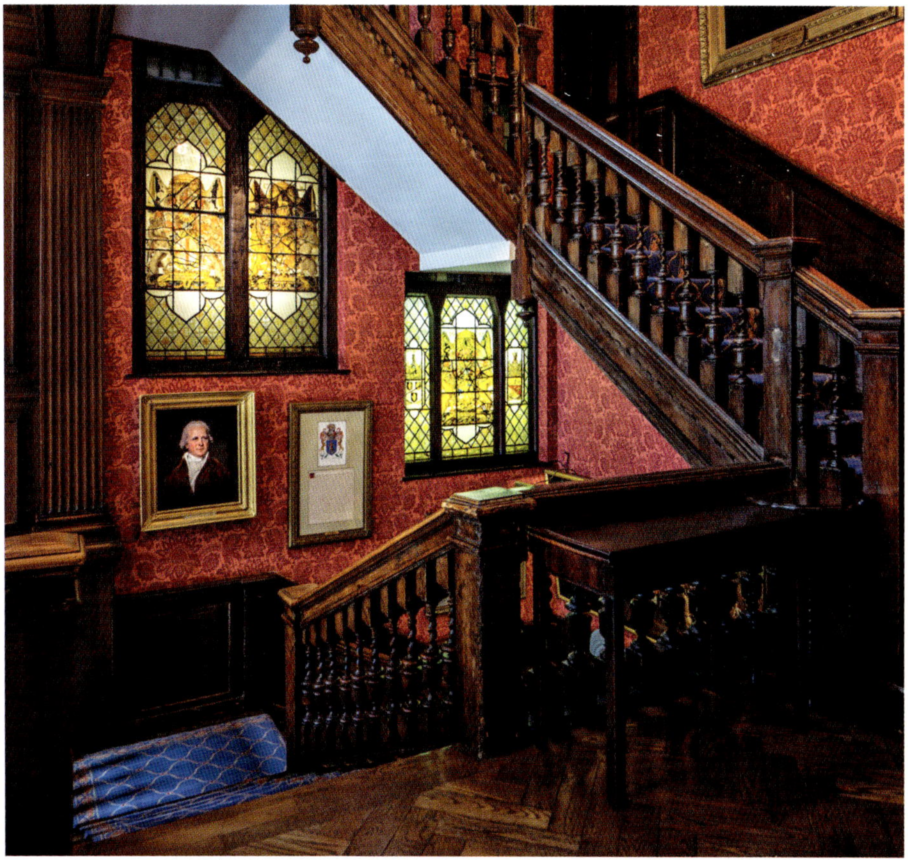

5.1 The windows on the Great Staircase. On the right, the three-light window displays from left to right the Arms of Joannes Lorymer, the Arms of the Society, and the Arms of Jacobus Lowe Wheeler. On the left, the two-light window displays – on the left the Arms of the City of London and on the right the Stuart Arms of King Charles II

5.2 West Wall of the Stairwell
– Overall Window Pattern

A. City Arms

B. Royal Arms

C. Arms of Johannes Lorymer

D. Society Arms

E. Arms of Jacobus Lowe Wheeler

F–O. Contain panes of plain tinted glass

X–Y. Position of the second flight of the staircase (balustrade not shown)

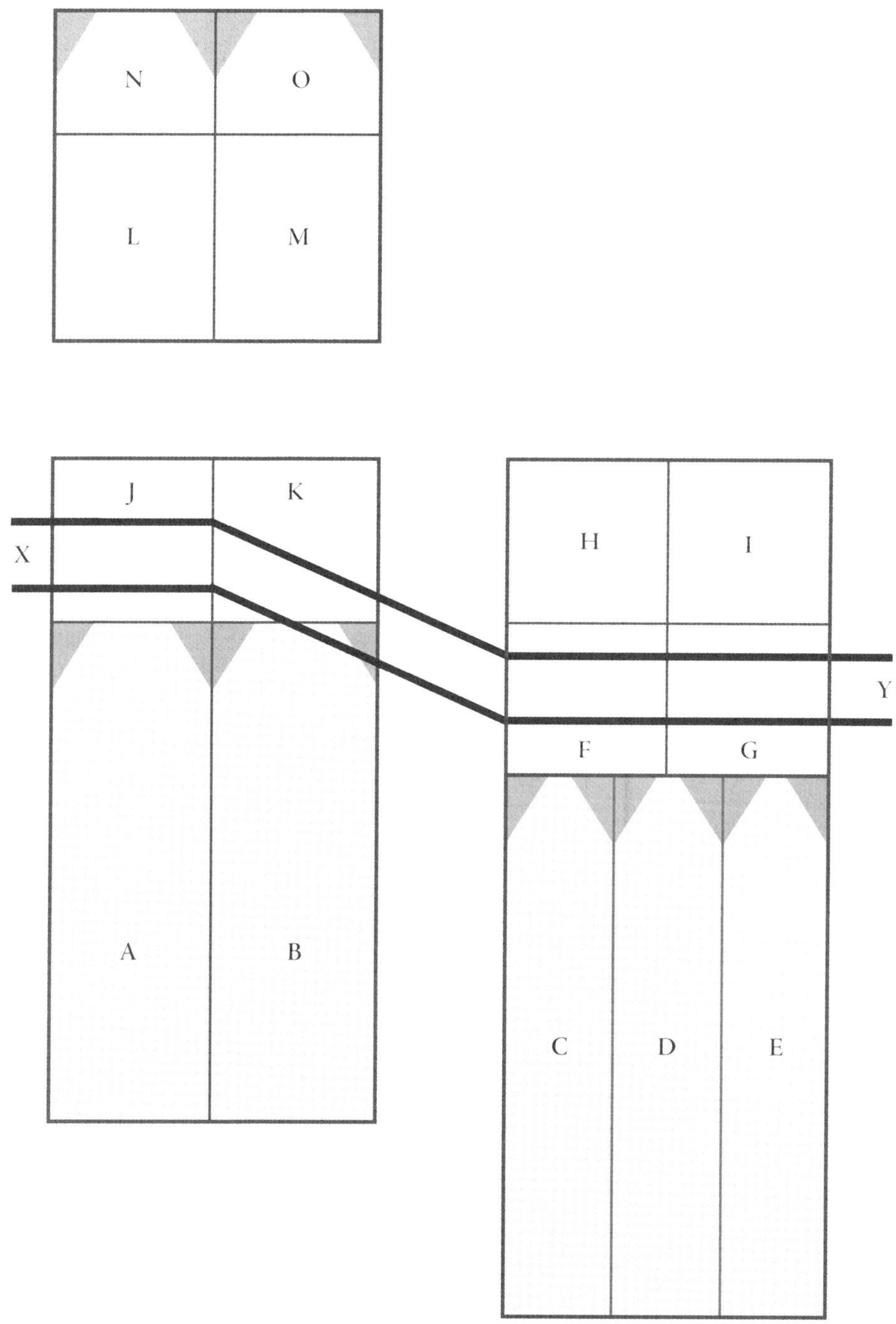

following payment is recorded: 'Mr Tipping the Glazier - £30.0.0d'.[1] This is confirmed by an entry on the same date in the Wardens' book of 'Accounts (1668–91)' which reads 'Paid Mr Tipping the Glazier - £30.0.0d', and in the accounts for the following year in the same book is recorded 'Payd Tipping the Glazier in full and glazing for the Laboratory included – £35.0.0d'.[2] While he would also have been responsible for overseeing the installation of the two stained glass windows on the staircase it is unlikely, however, that Tipping was responsible for the actual painting of any of the panels in these two windows, for reasons which will be discussed below.

The first of the stained glass windows, seen as one ascends from the Entrance Hall, is a three-light window, each light containing heraldic and other glass. The second window, beside the first and at a higher level, is a two-light window also containing heraldic and other glass.

However, on closer inspection it becomes apparent that only part of the whole window is visible in each case. The overall window pattern on this west wall of the stairwell is complex and is illustrated in simplified form in Figure 5.2. Each window is extended upwards by

5.3 'The Staircase' by Barrett 1904

5.4 Appearance of the first flight of the Great Staircase in 2017

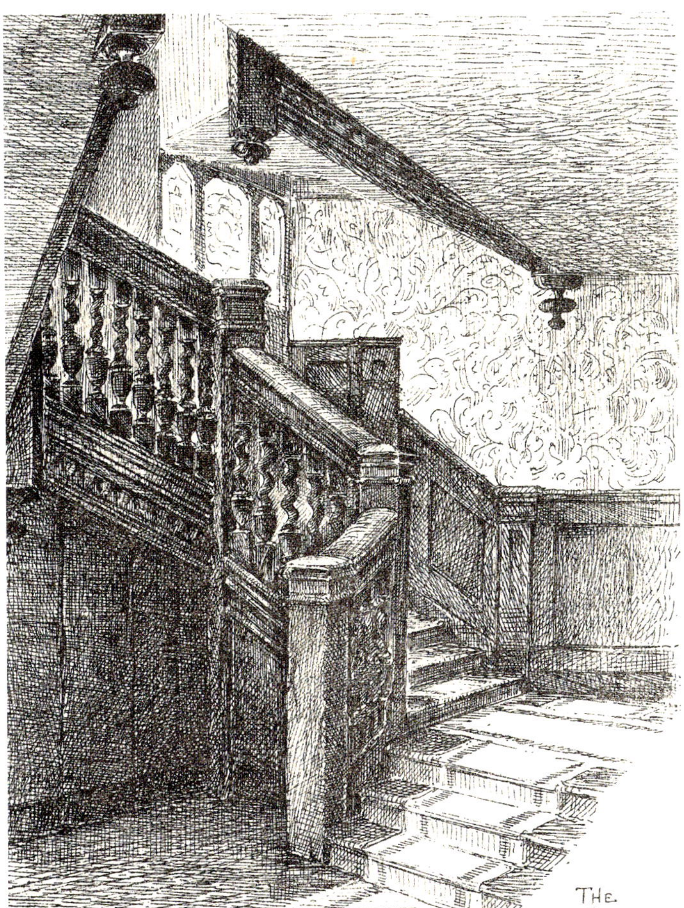

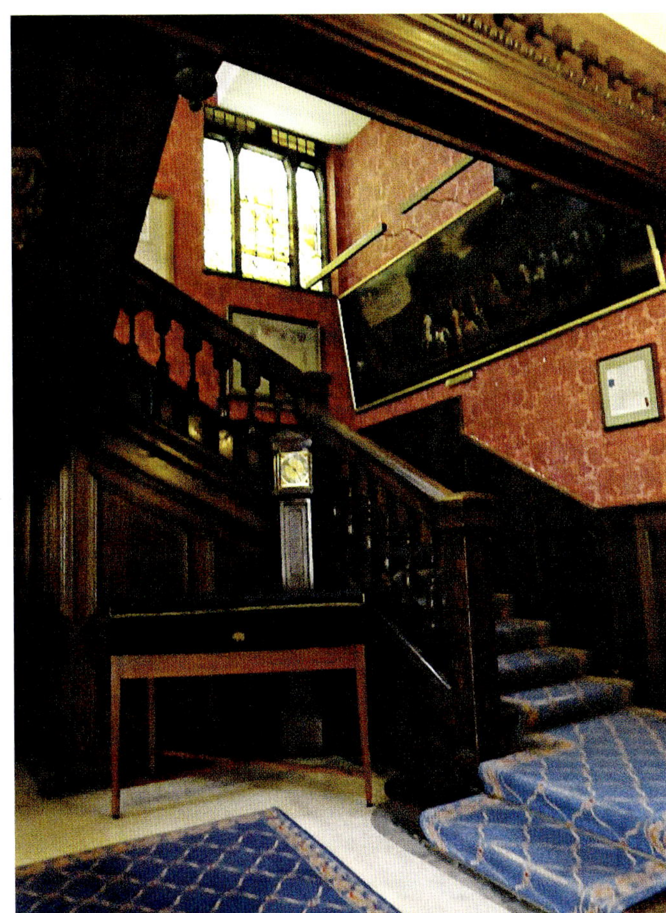

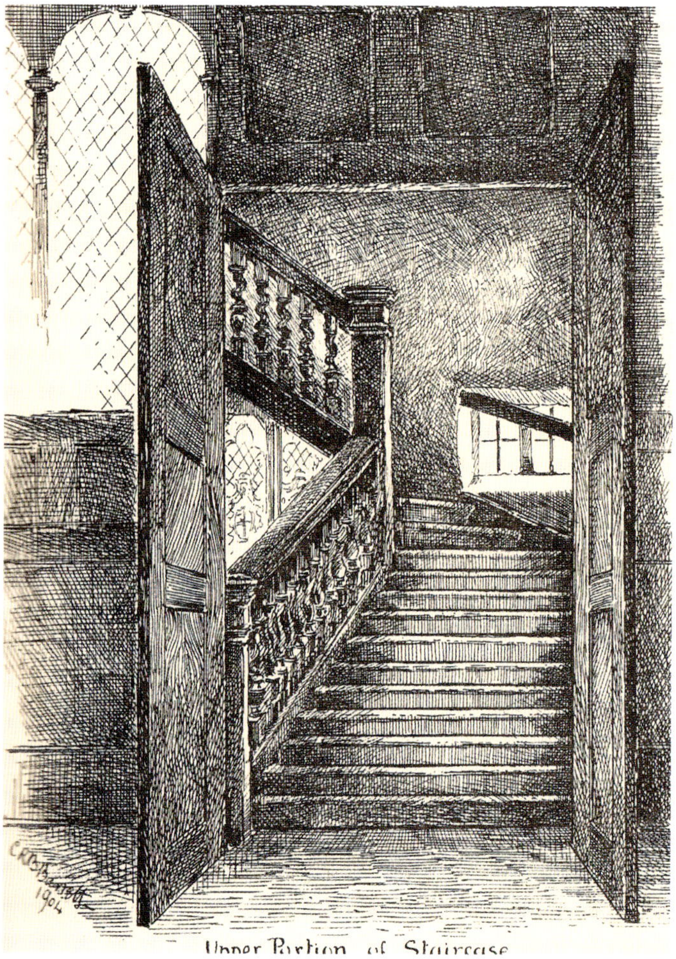

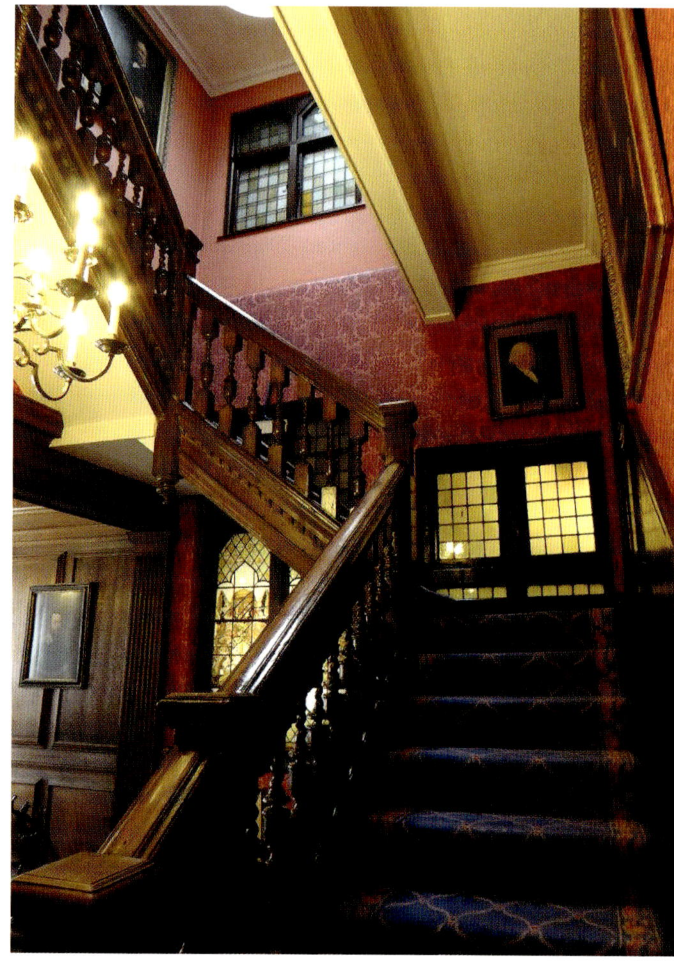

5.5 'Upper Portion of Staircase' by Barrett 1904. Note that the double doors with attached partition and window have long since been removed

5.6 Appearance of the second flight of the Great Staircase in 2017

further panels all of which contain only tinted plain glass. Much of these upward extensions is masked by the rising staircase (X–Y in the figure), from which at upper levels the extensions can be viewed. In addition, there is above the left-hand window at a much higher level a small window which also contains only tinted plain glass and the whole stairwell is capped by a cupola which contains twelve triangular panes of plain clear glass.

Glimpses of the two stained glass windows can be seen in two drawings dated 1904 by C. R. B. Barrett in his book *The History of the Society of Apothecaries*. The drawing of 'The Staircase' (Figure 5.3) shows what can be assumed to be heraldic glass in all three lights of the lower window and the drawing of the 'Upper Portion of Staircase' (Figure 5.5) illustrates more clearly heraldic glass in both lights of the upper window.[3] When these drawings are compared with current photographs of the same views, however, it is clear that some change to the structure of the staircase and to the window embrasures has taken place since 1904 (Figures 5.4 and 5.6). For example, the configuration of the staircase at ground-floor level has been altered and the small window between the first and second floors with its inserted hand-rail has been enlarged, incorporated into the upward extension of the right-hand window, and the hand-rail removed.

It is likely that these alterations were undertaken in 1928–29, when it was discovered that many of the roof timbers and floor joists in the Hall were very badly infested with deathwatch beetle. As a result, it was judged that the building was on the verge of collapse. An extensive programme of restoration was immediately put in place which was supervised by the then Surveyor to the Society Sir William Wells.[4] Unfortunately, no surveyor's reports or records of any details of the work undertaken can be found in the Society's Archive. In view of the extent of the work required, it seems that the opportunity was seized to undertake some reorganisation of adjacent parts of the building.[5]

The Entrance Hall was enlarged by enclosing the pillared portico which was at that time open to the Courtyard. The first-floor landing was enlarged by shortening the east end of the Library, a change which greatly enhanced the lighting of the stairwell. Although not mentioned in the Archive, it is likely that the configuration of the staircase was altered at the same time, together with the addition of the upward extensions of the staircase windows, but it is highly improbable that the main windows and their glazing had to be changed in any significant way.

Additional evidence that this was when the upward extensions of the main windows was undertaken is supplied by a photograph in *The Builder* magazine taken in 1917, which shows no such upward extension at that time (Figure 5.7).[6]

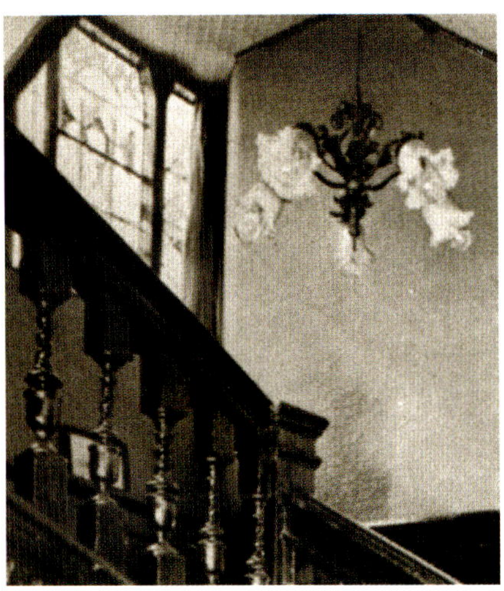

5.7 A photograph taken in 1917 for *The Builder* magazine, which shows no upward extension of the main staircase windows at that date (cf. figures 5.3, 5.4, 5.5 & 5.6)

The 1671 Glass

In the three-light window (Figure 5.8), the central light is dated 1671 and it is the opinion of all the glass experts who have examined the windows that the nine large rectangular heraldic panels in the window can with confidence be ascribed to that date.

Although not dated, the nine rectangular heraldic panels in each of the two lights in the left-hand window are so similar that they too can safely be ascribed to the same period (Figure 5.9). Returning to the right-hand window, Joannes (John) Lorymer (left-hand light) was Master in 1654–55 and Jacobus (James) Lowe Wheeler (right-hand light) was Master in 1864–65. These panels are consistent with these dates, although the similarity between the two is striking. The question therefore arises as to what the whole window looked like before the addition of the Wheeler glass. This and other queries are fully discussed later in this chapter. The remainder of the glass in the windows, that is, the diamond-shaped panes (quarries) and the panes of clear glass, are probably Victorian in date, but could in some cases be more recent, although an intriguing alternative theory will also be discussed below.

In both windows, each of the main heraldic panels is made up of nine rectangular panes. Many of these have additional lead lines which are later additions to secure and cover cracks and are therefore not part of the original design. These could have been

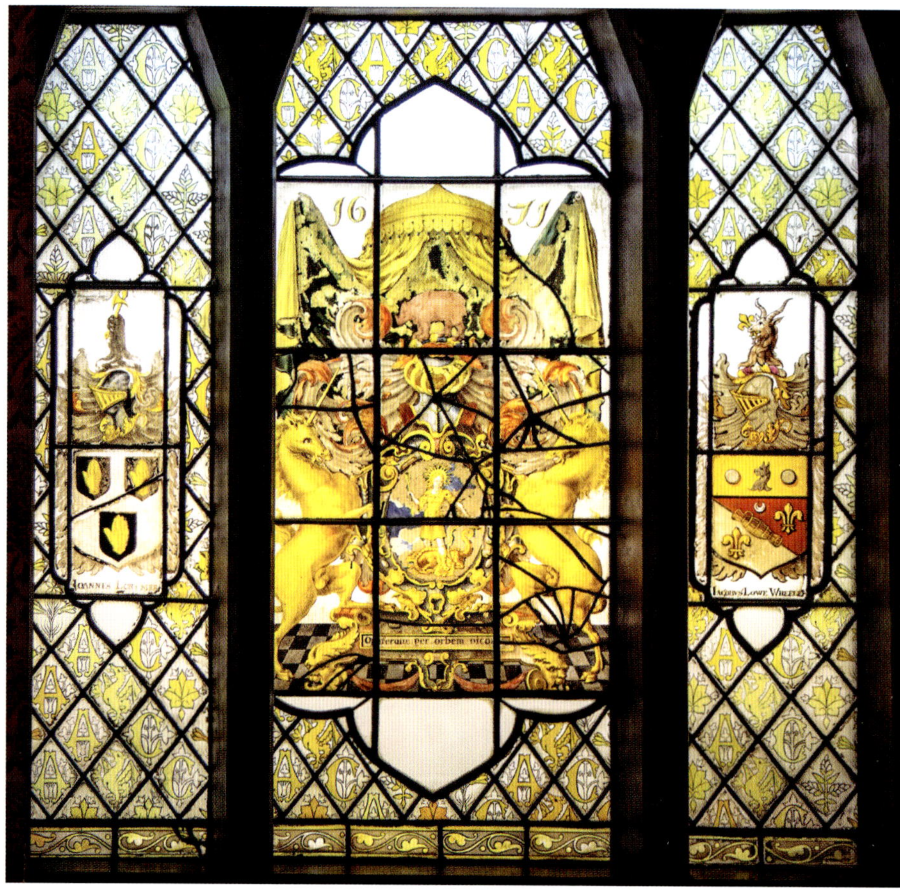

5.8 The three-light window: on the left the Lorymer Arms, in the centre the Society's Arms and on the right the Wheeler Arms

added at any time, but we do know that James Powell & Sons carried out repairs to these windows before their reinstallation after the Second World War in 1946, and some of the extra lead lines may date from that period.[7] Details of the restoration work done after the war are discussed at the end of this chapter.

The twenty-seven panes demonstrate the technique of enamelling on glass in a period when this technique was much in vogue in this country. The much older skill of painting on clear or coloured glass with oxides of iron or copper followed by firing in a kiln in order to anneal the paint permanently to the glass had been practised in northern Europe for many centuries. The earliest glass of this type that still exists in Britain dates from the late twelfth century. A further technique was developed in the early part of the fourteenth century when it was discovered that if oxides of silver were painted onto glass and then fired in a kiln in the same way, these too would seep permanently into the glass, giving various shades of yellow and gold. This was known in the trade as acid or silver staining and is the origin of the term 'stained glass'. All these skills were lost in England after the Dissolution of the Monasteries, when there was obviously no call for stained glass windows.

In the early seventeenth century, however, Archbishop Laud sanctioned the reintroduction of stained glass in churches, but since the skills for making such windows had been lost it was necessary to encourage glaziers from the Low Countries to come over to England – with them came the skill of painting on glass with enamels. In this process, ground glass and other chemicals are mixed to form a paint which is applied to the glass which is again fired in a kiln. This added a large number of colours to the palette of the stained glass artist but was subject to two particular disadvantages – firstly, that the colours created tended to be somewhat less translucent than those seen in glass in which the colour has been produced by the introduction of chemicals at the time of manufacture;

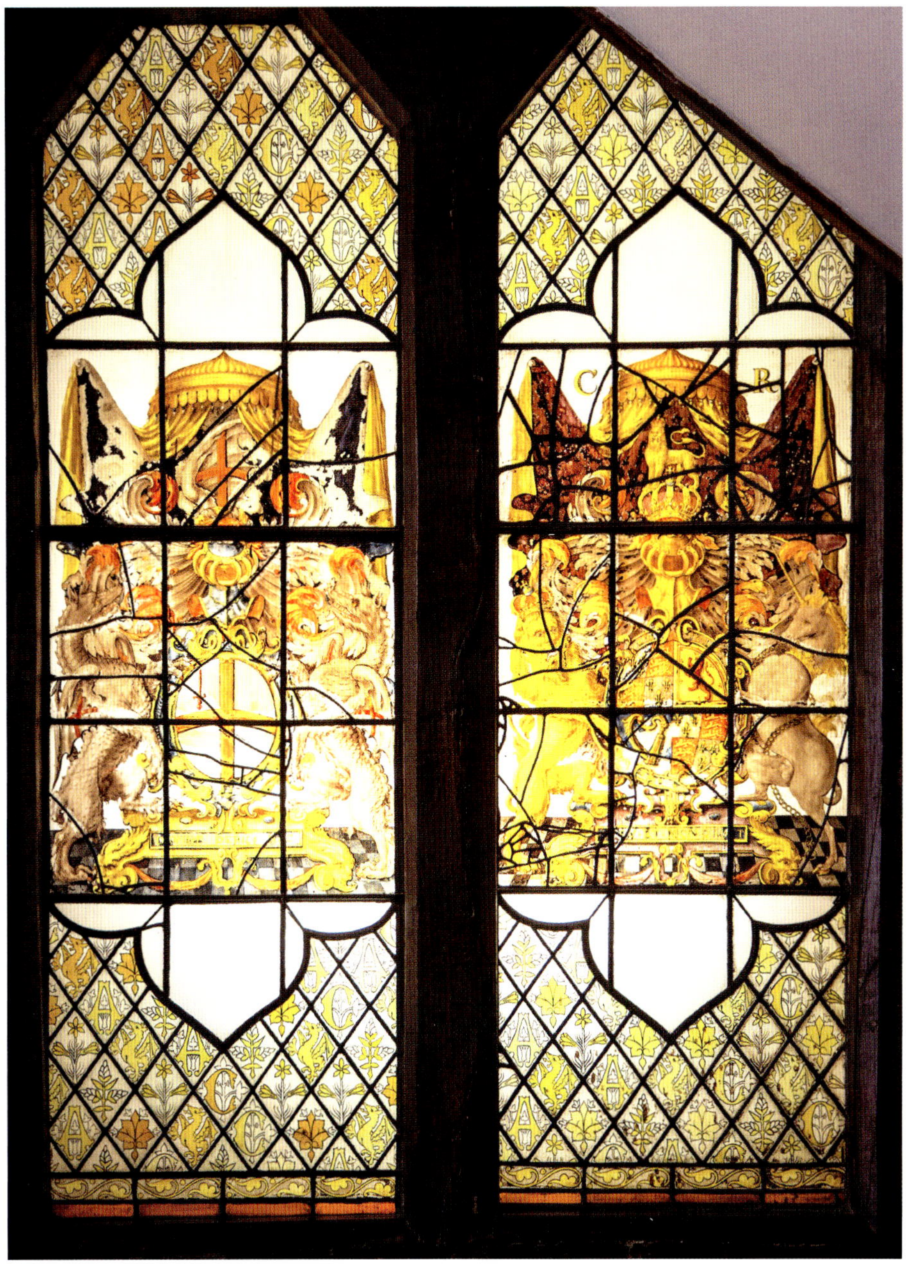

5.9 The two-light window: on the left the City of London Arms and on the right the Stuart Arms of Charles II

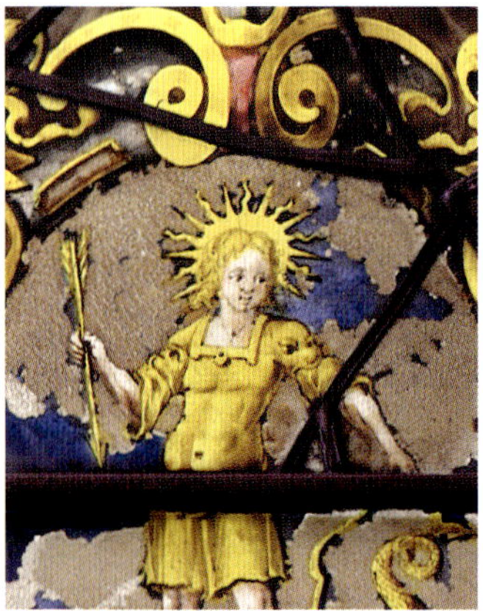

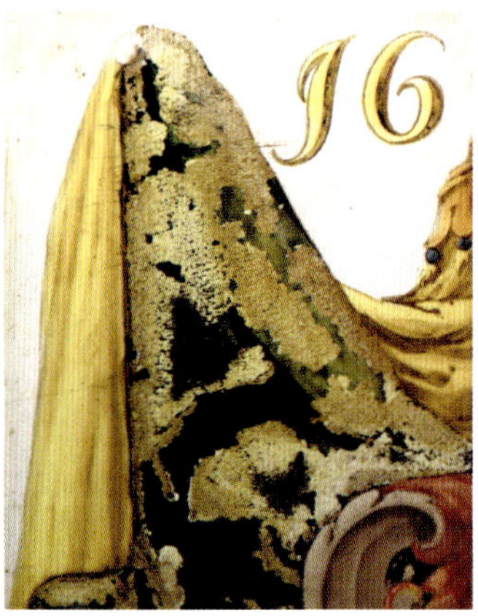

5.10 Flaking of blue enamel from the field around Apollo

5.11 Flaking of grey/black enamel from a canopy

and secondly, and perhaps more importantly, the ground glass and other chemicals from which the enamels are made may not adhere permanently to the glass on which they are painted, so that after a time they tend to flake off, a process that may not occur for many years and which, for reasons unknown, seems to be a failing to which blue enamels are especially prone.

Unfortunately, a considerable amount of flaking has occurred in the Great Staircase windows of Apothecaries' Hall. This is particularly noticeable in the central panel of the right-hand window around the figure of Apollo, which should be surrounded by a uniform field of blue (Figure 5.10) and in the canopies above the Arms in all three windows, which have lost some of their grey-black colouration (Figure 5.11). All three painting techniques, using iron oxide, silver stain and enamels, have been employed on these 1671 panels, enamelling being particularly prominent. Where enamel has flaked off, the underlying glass appears pale brown in colour. This is likely to be a thin layer of glass paint of a light neutral tint applied and fired as a light ground before application of the enamel. The process is described in detail in an article of 1838 in the *Civil Engineer & Architectural Journal*.[8] It may be that the enamels were fired at too low a temperature, so that they did not melt into the paint below and therefore failed to adhere sufficiently to the surface on which they were applied. Hence they began, in due course, to flake off, possibly assisted by condensation.

The Donors

Further examination of the Wardens' book of 'Accounts' for the year 1670–71 gives clues as to who the donors of the panels might have been.[9] In a section listing gifts to the Society the following two entries appear:

> *Received of Arthur Hollingworth for the Company's Arms in glass – £3.0.0d*
>
> *Received of Anthonie Hinton for the King's Arms in glass – £3.0.0d*
>
> On the same page, in a list of payments in the same year, the following entries are recorded:
>
> *Payd for the King's Arms in glass – £3.0.0d*
>
> *Payd for the Company's Arms in glass – £3.0.0d*

It is inconceivable that these four entries do not refer to two of the 1671 panels, and they therefore suggest that they were paid for by private donation by the persons mentioned, both of whom were members of the Society – Arthur Hollingworth being Master in 1670–71 and Anthonie (Anthony) Hinton Master in 1675–76.

No mention is made of the City's Arms, but in the 1671/72 section of the same book the following entry appears: '*Payd to the Glazier - £4.0.0d*'. Could this be payment for the City Arms, presumably paid for by the Society and not by a private donor?[10]

It is extremely unfortunate that no mention is made of the name of the glazier or glaziers to whom these three payments were made. The fact that Tipping is mentioned by name in relation to the overall glazing and not in relation to these entries is one factor which suggests that he was not the glazier responsible for painting these three sets of armorial panels.

So, to whom does the Society owe a debt of gratitude for creating such an inheritance, if not to Thomas Tipping?

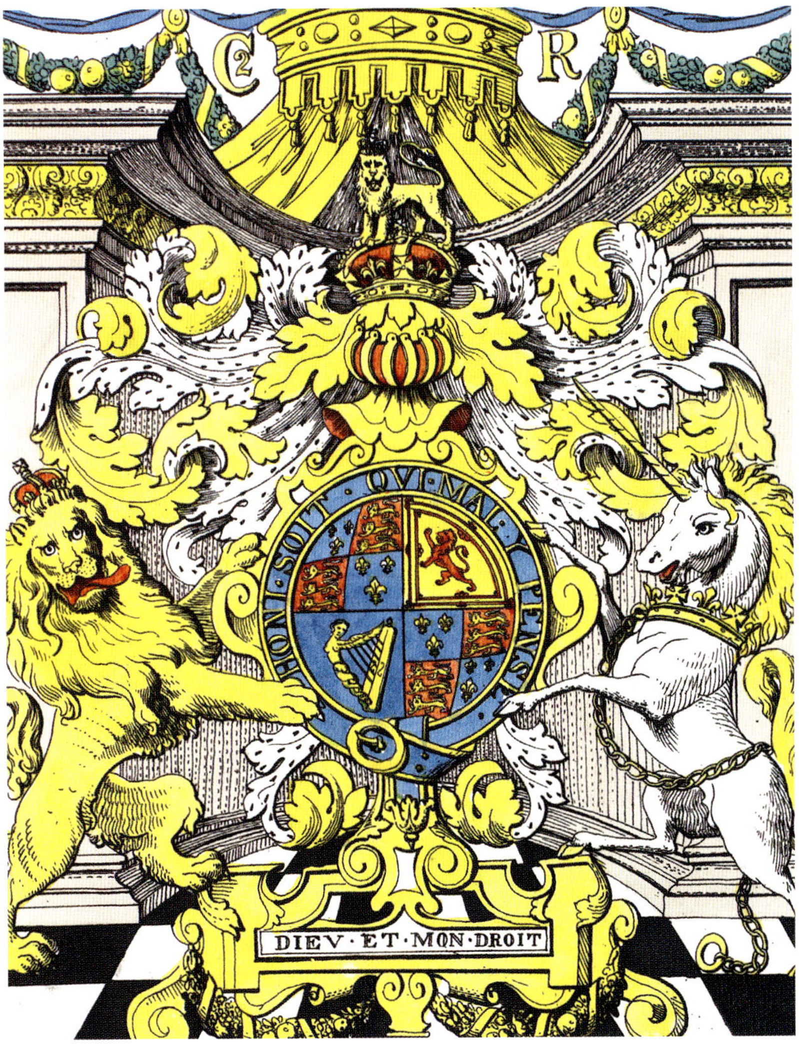

5.12 Coloured drawing of a glass panel by Richard Dutton showing the Stuart Arms, which was at one time in the Church of St Michael's Cornhill, c.1672. This drawing was recorded in 1821 by Thomas Willement, glazier to the Royal family

The Artist

The Society is very grateful to Mr Geoffrey Lane, Librarian to the British Society of Master Glass Painters, who has done a considerable amount of research into the glaziers of this period. He is of the opinion that there seem to be four possible contenders for this work. The two principal glass painters who were active in London at this time were John Oliver (*c.*1616–1702) and Richard Dutton (*c.*1636–1686). Oliver lived in the City in a house rebuilt after the Great Fire, where he also ran a workshop. He was appointed to the post-fire survey of London and was also a member of one of Sir Christopher Wren's teams engaged to rebuild the City churches and St Paul's Cathedral. It is likely, therefore, that he was able to undertake commissions in the City.

Dutton, who lived in Holborn, was the son-in-law of Baptist Sutton (d.1667), one of the most important glass painters in London in earlier years. Dutton inherited his father-in-law's workshop in which he produced panels for the Inns of Court. But he also accepted commissions in the City, painting in 1672, for example, two glass panels, one showing the Royal Arms and another the Draper's Arms for the church of St Michael's, Cornhill (both panels now lost). Figure 5.12 shows an early nineteenth-century coloured drawing by Thomas Willement,[11] glazier to the Royal family, of this Dutton Royal Arms panel which bears a strong resemblance to the Royal Arms panel on the Great Staircase at Apothecaries' Hall – particularly with regard to the unusual canopy and chequerboard flooring.

Another possible contender is John Brace, who was possibly a protégé of John Oliver, about whom much less is known and who died at a young age in 1674. Thomas Tipping himself must be considered a candidate, as he was an eminent glazier, but he is not recognised as a glass painter. Examination of his will in the National Archives does not reveal any mention of glass-painting equipment, which probably rules him out.

On balance therefore, Mr Lane thinks that Richard Dutton is our man.[12] In support of this conclusion is the fact that in the Society's Wardens' Account Book for 1633 a payment to a Mr Sutton, glass painter, on 9 August 1633, for providing two glass dials for the pre-fire Hall is recorded. It is not unreasonable to presume that this is Baptist Sutton, Richard Dutton's father-in-law, which, if correct, makes it likely that Dutton was already well known to the Society.[13]

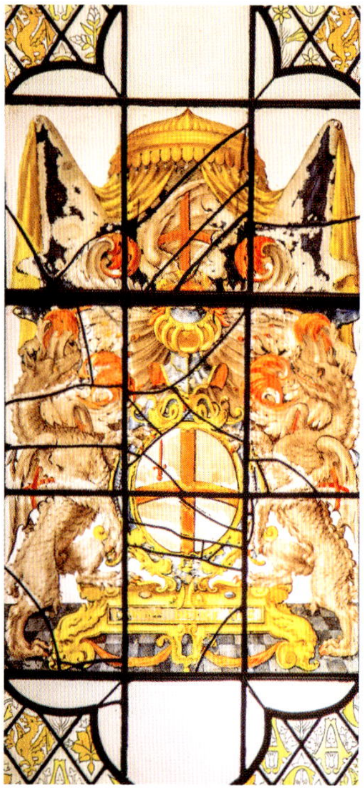

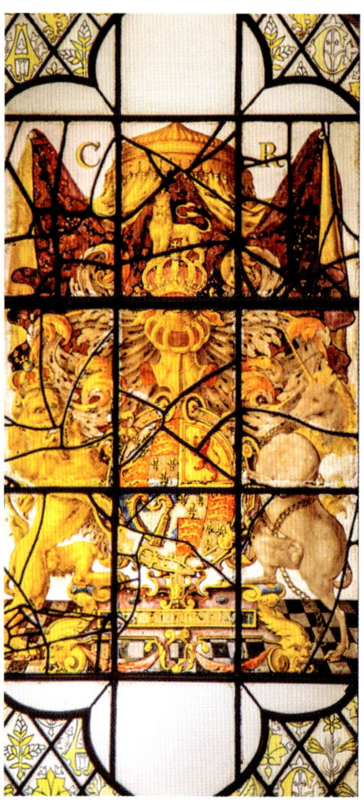

5.13 The City of London Arms

5.14 The Royal Arms

Heraldry

The City Arms

Although the City's Arms (left-hand window, left-hand light – Figure 5.13) are very old, surprisingly they were only granted by the College of Arms on 30 April 1957. This is because the usage preceded the formation of the College in 1494 and the grant of Arms, crest and supporters was confirmed 'as anciently recorded as of right appertaining to them'.[14]

The formal blazon is: *Argent, a Cross Gules, in the first quarter a Sword in pale point upwards of the last; And for a Crest upon a Peer's Helm mantled Argent doubled Gules a Dragon's sinister Wing charged on the underside with a cross throughout Gules; for supporters on each side, a Dragon Argent charged on the undersides of the wings with a Cross throughout Gules*. The motto is *Domine Dirige Nos* (Lord Direct Us).

The representation in the glass is faithful to the blazon but the peeling of some of the colours and the very ornate pavilion over the whole achievement with a black and white chequerboard base below makes the Arms difficult to distinguish, added to which every pane has a leaded repair. The unusual pavilion and chequerboard decoration is a feature of each of the three main Arms on the stairs – another reason for believing that they were all made in 1671.

It is unclear why the City, like the Society, has a peer's helm and also it is incorrectly shown here as affronté with the crest sideways on.

Without a formal grant and description of the City's Arms, various symbols, such as the figure of St Paul, lions, the Swordbearer's hat, the mace and so forth, made their appearance on the Arms in the early years, none of which appears on these Arms. It is sometimes said that the sword in the first quarter represents the dagger used by Lord Mayor William Walworth to end the Peasant's Revolt by killing Wat Tyler, but this cannot be true as the Arms with the sword were in use before 1381, the date of Tyler's death. It is generally accepted that it is in fact the sword of St Paul which has been used as a symbol of the City since at least the early thirteenth century. The earliest illustrations of the dragons and the motto make their appearance at the beginning of the seventeenth century.

The Royal Arms

These are the Stuart Arms of Charles II (left-hand window, right-hand light – Figure 5.14), confirmed both by the date of the window and the initials at the top of the panel. They are identical to his grandfather James' Arms which are fully discussed in Chapter 7. Again there is the problem with the pavilion, the chequerboard and the peeling of the enamels making it even more difficult to distinguish the detail of the Arms. Every pane has a leaded repair.

In this representation the affronté helm is correct but the crown above it and the lion's crown have a distinctly Continental style. The motto *Dieu et Mon Droit* (God and my Right) is shown in the compartment at the base.

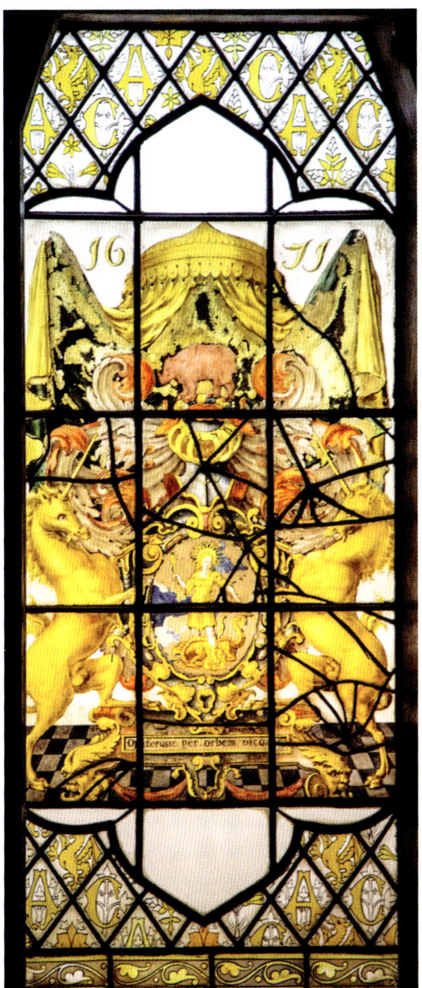

5.15 The Society Arms

The Society Arms

The detail of the window is again very difficult to make out because of the pavilion and chequerboard design and the flaking of the enamels (right-hand window, central light – Figure 5.15). Each pane, apart from those in the top-central and top-left positions, has been repaired, some quite extensively.

The design, which has been discussed comprehensively in Chapter 1, is basically true to Camden's grant, except that the helm has again been turned affronté, the crest remaining in profile. The extensive mantling and the canopy, together with the size of the supporters effectively overwhelm the subject of the glass.

The Joannes Lorymer/Lowman Arms

John Lorymer Senior was Master 1654–55 and at the end of his year, to the surprise and delight of the Court,[15] he paid for the refurbishment of the White or Queen's Room, which is now known as the Parlour. In 1663, shortly before Lorymer's death (*c*.1663–1667) without male issue, his portrait was painted and presented to the Society.[16] This portrait was saved from the Great Fire in 1666, which destroyed the refurbished Parlour.

In 1675 John Lorymer's son-in-law Dr William Croone, Gresham Professor of Rhetoric, offered to redecorate the Parlour in Lorymer's memory to include the placing of the Arms in the window and, indeed, the Court Minutes of 13 April 1675, mention 'the setting of Mr Lorrymer's coate of armes in the glass window'.[17] It is not clear if this recorded an action or an intention but the design and painting of the panels are consistent with this date. Nor indeed is the glass window specified. It could be either the Parlour or the Staircase, and if the four border panels shown were designed as a composite work then the Staircase is probably indicated.

It is likely that this Court Minute refers to only one element of the suggested refurbishment of the Parlour, a project that was in the end never finished by Croone. Amongst other things, the Court was left to pay for the sashing of the window in 1680. It is not clear why Croone failed to live up to his promise as, although he died young aged fifty-one in 1684, he was still active as a Royal College of Physicians Censor in 1679.

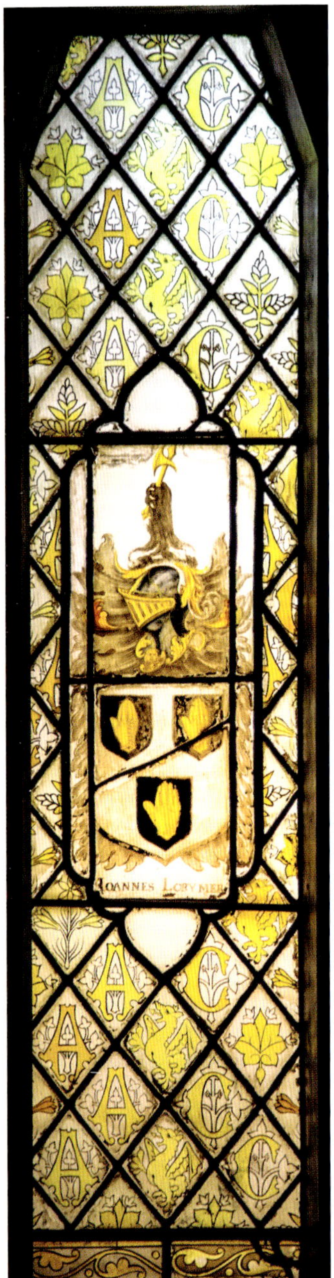

5.16 The Lorymer/Lowman Arms

The Arms in the window (right-hand window, left-hand light – Figure 5.16) are: *Argent, three Escutcheons Sable each charged with a dexter Gauntlet Or, back affronté; and for the Crest upon a Helm mantled, on a Wreath of the colours, a lion's gamb erect and erased Sable holding a battleaxe Or.*

Confusingly, these Arms, granted in 1611, are not the Lorymer Arms but belong to the Devonshire family of Lowman,[18] who have never had any connection whatsoever with the Society. In addition, the Arms are incorrectly shown with a peer's helm.

It is not clear whether John Lorymer actually possessed any Arms, for none are recorded at the College of Arms. When his portrait was returned to hang in the Great Hall in 1675, incidentally a date coinciding with Croone's redecoration proposals, an inscription had been added to it which reads *Joannes Lorymer Armig: 1675*. Yet this is not conclusive as, rather in the way that 'Esquire' was added routinely to twentieth-century post-nominals, it was not uncommon for gentlemen to style themselves as an *Armiger*. On the other hand, John Lorymer was an extremely successful, rich and powerful apothecary, and sometime Alderman of the City, who one might have expected to have been granted Arms.

Any Arms granted to Lorymer would have been transmitted, via his eventual heraldic heiress daughter Mary, to Dr Croone but there is no evidence that he ever used the Lorymer Arms in pretence or that he had any descendants to quarter them. The only other known Lorymer was John *Senior*'s nephew and apprentice, John *Junior*, but nothing is heard of him after his apprenticeship. This, however, does help to date the panel as the Society has had no connection with any Lorymer since the 1670s and there would be no reason to have made glass to commemorate John Lorymer since those years.

Nineteenth-century Arms recorded for English Lorymers are: *Argent, a Chevron Sable between three Spur Rowels Azure; and for a Crest upon a Helm mantled Gules and Argent, an Arm couped at the shoulder in a Maunch embowed and resting on a Wreath.* Scottish Lorimers with different Arms are recorded from 1794.[19]

How the Lowman Arms came to be glazed is a mystery. Seventeenth-century spelling had at least five versions of Lorymer – Lorrimer, Larymer, Lawrymore, Lorrimore. Perhaps the College of Arms, not having any record of Arms for Lorymer, misread Lorymer for Lowman when directing the glazier, with this unfortunate result.

Whether or not Dr Croone knew the Arms to be erroneous cannot be established but, if he did, it may have been the cause of the failure of his refurbishment project. Possibly, the glass was subsequently found in store, the inscription accepted as fact by a later generation, and then installed, although this requires credence that they were stored undamaged for 200 years. There is also the puzzle of what tense – past or future – the Court minute meant by 'the setting', but if the Lowman/Lorymer Arms were actually installed in this window in 1675, then it would have been most unbalanced for 200 years with one blank light.

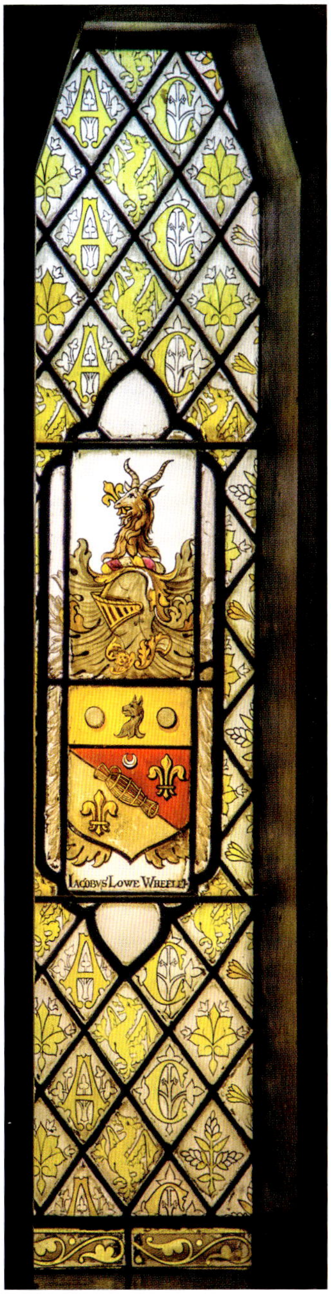

5.17 The Wheeler Arms

The Jacobus Lowe Wheeler Arms

This commemorates James Lowe Wheeler who was Master in 1864–65 (right-hand window, right-hand light – Figure 5.17). So, it is likely that the window dates from this period, although there is no record of this in the Society Archive.

James Lowe Wheeler came from a dynasty of apothecaries (see Figure 5.18). His grandfather Thomas *Senior*, uncle William, and brothers Thomas Lowe and Joseph were Court Assistants over a period of 100 years, whilst his father Thomas *Junior* and brother Charles West were Masters in 1823–24 and 1862–63 respectively. Indeed, he was the Junior Warden when his brother was Master. These relationships are illustrated in Figure 5.18. In 1863 his nephew Thomas Rivington Wheeler presented the portrait of his grandfather Thomas *Junior* which now hangs in the Court Room.

With regards to heraldry, Wheelers or Whelers mostly fall into three groups according to the main charge on their Arms: leopards heads, Catherine wheels or fishwheels. The fishwheel is a most unusual charge and the earliest usage noted dates from 1780 for Worcestershire Wheelers.[20]

The Arms shown in this window, but without the crescent, are ascribed to James Henry Wheeler of Hyde Park Gardens in Burke's General Armory of 1842, but the date of the grant is not given.[21] In the Harleain Society's 1917 list of Grantees of Arms 1687–1898, a grant of 1820 is shown to Wheeler of Piggott's and Gloucester Place.[22] Figure 5.18 shows that James Rivington Wheeler lived in Gloucester Place and that he bought Piggott's Manor from his widowed mother and brothers in 1801. Research at the College of Arms confirms that he is the grantee of these Arms in 1820.[23]

Henry James Wheeler was Thomas Rivington Wheeler's nephew and heir, being the son of his elder brother William. In the General Armory he is described as the representative of the elder branch of the family (see again Figure 5.18).

The blazon of these Arms (see Figure 5.17) is: *Per Bend Azure and Gules, a fishwheel in bend between two fleurs-de-lys Or, on a chief of the last a wolf's head erased Vert between two hurts, in the honour point a Crescent Argent for difference; and for the Crest upon a Helm mantled, on a Wreath of the colours, an Angola goat's head erased Vert, horned or, holding in the mouth a fleur-de-lys gold.*

Most interestingly, the 1820 grant was not just to James Rivington Wheeler but to all the descendants of his father, which include Henry James Wheeler, his nephew and heir, and also, of course, James Lowe Wheeler, whose window this is. It would seem that the crescent was added by his father Thomas *Junior* for his position as a second son. It is unusual and not a little confusing to maintain the cadency mark of the previous generation rather than changing a colour (e.g. making the chief Argent) or changing one of the lesser charges (e.g. replacing the fleurs-de-lys) and establishing a cadet line of Arms. Perhaps the prospect of the College of Arms fees dictated this private scheme!

There is, however, a difficulty with the tinctures, particularly blue and green. The lower part of the field should be blue, as should the two hurts on the chief. Both the wolf's

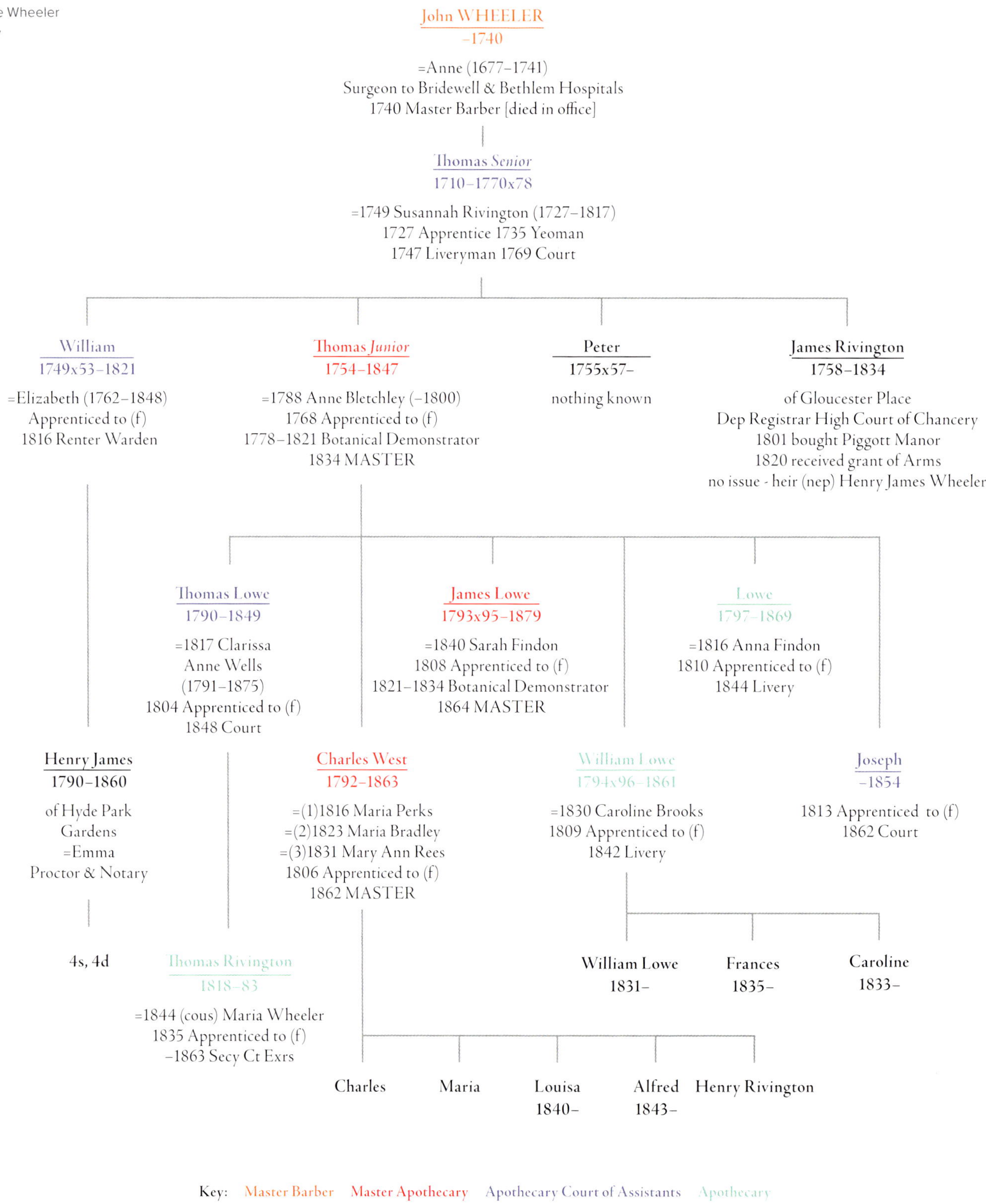

5.18 The Wheeler Dynasty

head on the chief and the goat's head of the crest should be green. It is also likely that the torse above the helm should be tricoloured and that the blue is missing. In all these areas, the glass is a pale brown colour very similar to those areas on the 1671 panels where enamel has clearly flaked off.

In 1983 Past Master Douglas Whittet, in his article on this window in *The Chemist and Druggist*,[24] criticised the glazier as being heraldically ignorant and quoted Carl Edwards' view that the colours had not flaked off. A cursory glance at the Arms might seem to confirm that the glazier has indeed erroneously coloured all these areas Argent (white) but this is not so. Examination of the crescent shows that it is a bright Argent quite different from the colour of the other areas. Furthermore, there is no evidence of any residual colour which, as with the 1671 glass, one might expect if flaking of enamel had occurred. It is likely, then, that the Wheeler panel was designed and painted to match the Lorymer panel in colour as closely as possible in order to achieve a balance across the whole window, deliberately ignoring the ordained heraldic tinctures. In support of this is the fact that the two panels are also strikingly similar in design, so much so that it seems beyond reasonable doubt that the incorrect helm, the overflowing mantling and the entire surround of the Wheeler panel were traced from the Lorymer panel.[25] Analysis of the lettering, that is A, E, J/I, L, O, R, S, seen in both panels, indicates that the glaziers of the panels were different people, which tends to confirm the 200-year gap in the dating of the panels.

The final question to be considered in this section is when the Lorymer/Lowman and Wheeler windows were installed. The Society's Archive is frustratingly silent on this matter. The discussion of the Lorymer/Lowman Arms above suggested that they were not installed in the seventeenth century. This would lead to the amazing conclusion that they were indeed stored for 200 years and inserted together with the Wheeler Arms to form a balanced pair in this window.

One theory discussed by Whittet in his paper postulated that the windows on this wall had to be reconstructed after the major explosion in the laboratory which killed Henry Hennell in 1842.[26] In the Society's pamphlet on its chemical operators, the inquest report states 'but material damage was considerable and the Society was fortunate that the Hall was not destroyed. This was probably because Hennell had taken the precaution of making the preparation in a yard adjoining the Laboratory' and again, 'The glass contained in the whole of the window frames (made of iron) were broken by which at least 1,000 panes were demolished exhibiting a picture of desolation seldom witnessed.'[27] However, there were two thick walls between the Laboratory and the Staircase windows, which perhaps saved the stair glass. There is no recorded damage to any Hall (as distinct from Laboratory) glass but experience shows that archival silence is not conclusive proof.

The main problem with the explosion theory is that James Lowe Wheeler did not become Master until 1864. The supposition must, therefore, be that the two Arms windows were installed together between 1865, the date of James Lowe Wheeler's Mastership, and 1885 when they are described by Corfe.[28]

The Quarries and the Clear-Glass Panes

The quarries, which are typical nineteenth-century copies of mediaeval quarries, exhibit a random display of plants, one dragon-like animal and the letters A and C (Figure 5.19). Most are likely to be no older than nineteenth century and possibly much younger. It is pertinent to note that not one of them is damaged and also that there is considerable colour variation throughout. The lack of damage suggests a reasonably modern date and the colour variation suggests that replacements may have been required on different occasions.

Dr Henry Oakeley, Garden Fellow of the Royal College of Physicians of London, is of the opinion that the plant behind the letters A and C is *Smyrnium olusatrum*, known in English as Alexanders, a plant used for treating bladder pain and strangury.[29] The fact that the same plant is used as background for both letters would seem to tie them nicely together. While the other plants illustrated could, he thinks, be comfrey, asphodel, wheat or cyclamen, it seems likely that they have been chosen at random, with the dragon of disease thrown in for good measure![30]

It is possible that the 1671 panels were reset within the quarry decoration when the Wheeler Arms were installed in late Victorian times, or that this was carried out as part of the 1928–29 refurbishment of the Entrance Hall and Staircase, and it is likely that the

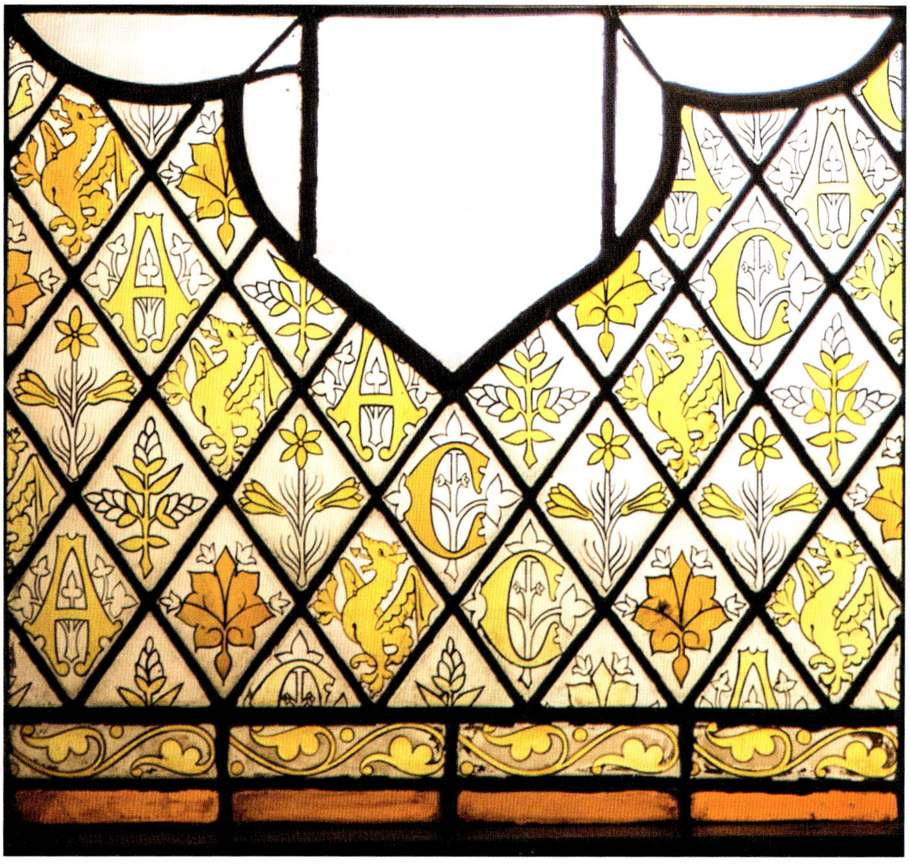

5.19 The quarries

clear-glass panes above and below the 1671 panels were installed at the same time. Unfortunately, no record of any of this work has yet come to light either in the Society's papers or in the Archive of James Powell & Sons who undertook the post-war restoration.

However, it is the opinion of a number of experts that the letters C and A are initials. The only apothecary of note that can be found with these initials is Charles Angibaud. His history is of interest and may therefore be relevant here.

Charles Angibaud, Master 1728–29

Charles Angibaud, a Huguenot, was born in Saintes near Bordeaux in the mid-seventeenth century, the son and grandson of apothecaries from whom he learnt his trade. In due course he became apothecary to Louis XIV, but in 1681 he fled France with his wife and three children to avoid religious persecution and settled in London, where he set up business as an apothecary in St Martin's Lane.

On 6 October 1685, he was admitted as a Freeman of the Society, becoming a Liveryman in 1699, Renter Warden in 1721, Upper Warden in 1726 and finally Master on 22 August 1728. He was appointed Apothecary to King Charles II on 6 January 1684, only three years after his arrival in England and was made Apothecary-General to the Army and Military Hospitals in Ireland under William and Mary in 1689.

Did the Society perhaps feel that such a distinguished career merited commemoration in glass? The Archive is silent on the matter, but plainly Angibaud is a candidate for ownership of the initials.

Wooden Window Frames

While very little detail of the subject matter in each stained glass window is discernible in the 1904 drawings by Barrett (see Figures 5.3 and 5.5), they do clearly show the distinctive shape of the wooden framework around the glass in each case, which matches what was present in 1917 (see Figure 5.7), what was also present immediately after the Second World War (Figure 5.20) and what is still present today (see Figure 5.1).[31]

One further problem arises in trying to ascertain when these windows were installed and whether the current framework dates from 1671, and that is the fact that the window showing the Society's Arms has been narrowed at some point. Accurate measurement of the width of the 1671 panels shows that in the window bearing the Royal and City Arms, all panels are almost exactly the same width. In the Society Arms window, the central panels are the same width as in the other window, but the outer panels on both sides are narrower, especially on the left-hand side. This is clearly corroborated when looking at the painting on the panels. In the Society's Arms window, part of the unicorn on each side is obscured by the wooden frame – a change not echoed in the other window, and which would undoubtedly not have been the intention of the artist.

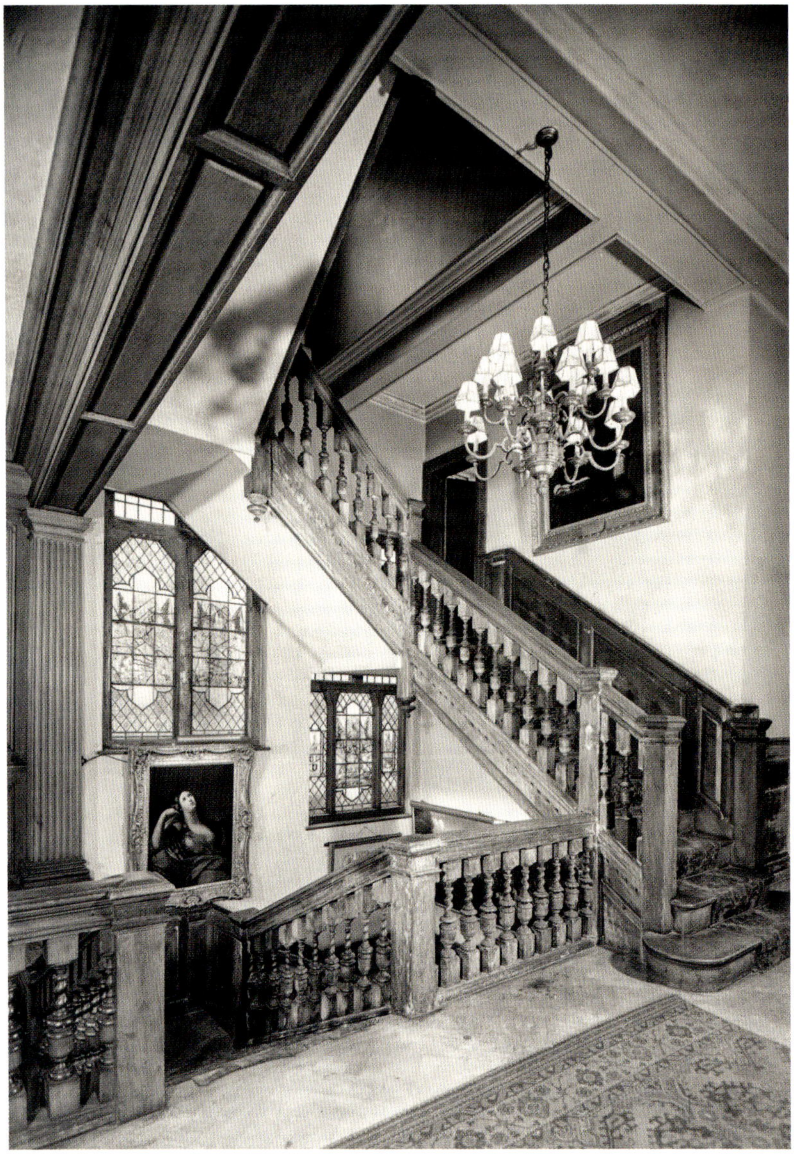

5.20 View of the windows from the landing for an article in *Country Life*, 10 October 1947

This must indicate that the Society's Arms at least are not in their original wooden frame. Close inspection shows that the wooden framework of the lower window is in much better condition than that of the upper window and much lighter in style. It is possible, therefore, that the wooden framework of the upper window is original dating from 1671 and that the newer-looking woodwork around the lower window has been replaced, possibly when the Wheeler window was installed. Furthermore, it is possible that this is when the clear-glass panels and quarries were also added.

Installation and Lighting

When the Hall was built these windows would have been external and probably covered with a protective wire grille. It is likely that they became 'internal' as a result of the major rebuilding programme of 1823, which transformed the west side of the Apothecaries' Hall estate and completed the formation of the Courtyard largely as it is seen today. The work was necessitated by the expansion of the retail activities of the Society, which entailed the provision of larger premises for the shop. As a result of this, the shop now abutted onto the west wall of the great Staircase stairwell, so enclosing and protecting the seventeenth-century windows.[32] The windows were back-lit with artificial lights which were probably installed during the 1928–29 refurbishment.

The 1960–61 Year Book indicates that the Master in that year, Dr Charles White, was instrumental in having all the staircase windows re-lit.[33]

The Glass Survives the Second World War

Together with all the armorial glass in the four west windows in the Great Hall and the two armorial panels in the Library, the Great Staircase windows were removed by James Powell and Sons late in 1941. An entry in the Company's 'Journal Window Department (1939–51)' on 2 September 1941 records that all the glass was removed at a charge of £25.0.0d.[34] This payment is confirmed in the Society's 'Ledger (1936–43)' on

15 October 1941.[35] These windows, together with the Great Hall windows, were taken to the Foundling Hospital at Berkhamsted in April 1943 and returned to the Hall in May 1945.[36]

A further entry in the James Powell & Sons 'Journal Window Department (1939–51)' on 30 January 1946 records the 'repairing and releading where necessary of the three-light window and refixing together with the two-light window' at a charge of £25.0.0d.[37] The detailed material list for this work which is recorded in the 'Estimate Book (1937–48)' includes 'about' 50 feet of lead.[38] This indicates a considerable amount of re-leading, which in turn implies a significant degree of damage to the windows during the whole process of removal and storage. In addition, 'painting' is itemised, which indicates that some glass had to be replaced. This might have been some of the quarries, which could account for the variation in colour of these panes, mentioned above. A payment of £60 to James Powell & Sons on 13 February 1946 is confirmed in the Society's 'Ledger (1943–47)', this being the combination of £35 for the restoration of the Great Hall armorial panels and £25 for the restoration of the Great Staircase windows.[39] Neither of these two latter entries refers to the two Library panels, which although badly scratched received no restoration.

One later instance of damage to a staircase window is recorded. On 10 May 1950, an entry in the James Powell 'Window Glass Order Book (1948–55)' refers to an order relevant to the Society to 'Remove from staircase window a panel 2' 10" x 2' 0" and replace four broken painted pieces. As per estimate 13.4.50 £11.10.0d'.[40] On 11 July 1950, the Powell 'Journal Window Department book' also records 'To repairs to damaged portion of staircase window' at Apothecary Hall at a charge of £11.10.0d,[41] a figure confirmed in the Society's 'Corporation Cash Book (1932–53)' on 11 August 1950.[42] The figure of £11.10.0d is substantial even for 1950 and the damage must have been considerable. Unfortunately, which panels were damaged is not specified in the Company nor in the Society records and measurements of the windows give no clear indication as to which panels these might have been. This may account for further lead lines and possibly new quarries.

In spite of inevitable cracking and some loss of enamel over the years, the 1671 panels on the Great Staircase are very fine examples of their period, and the Society is fortunate indeed that they have survived.

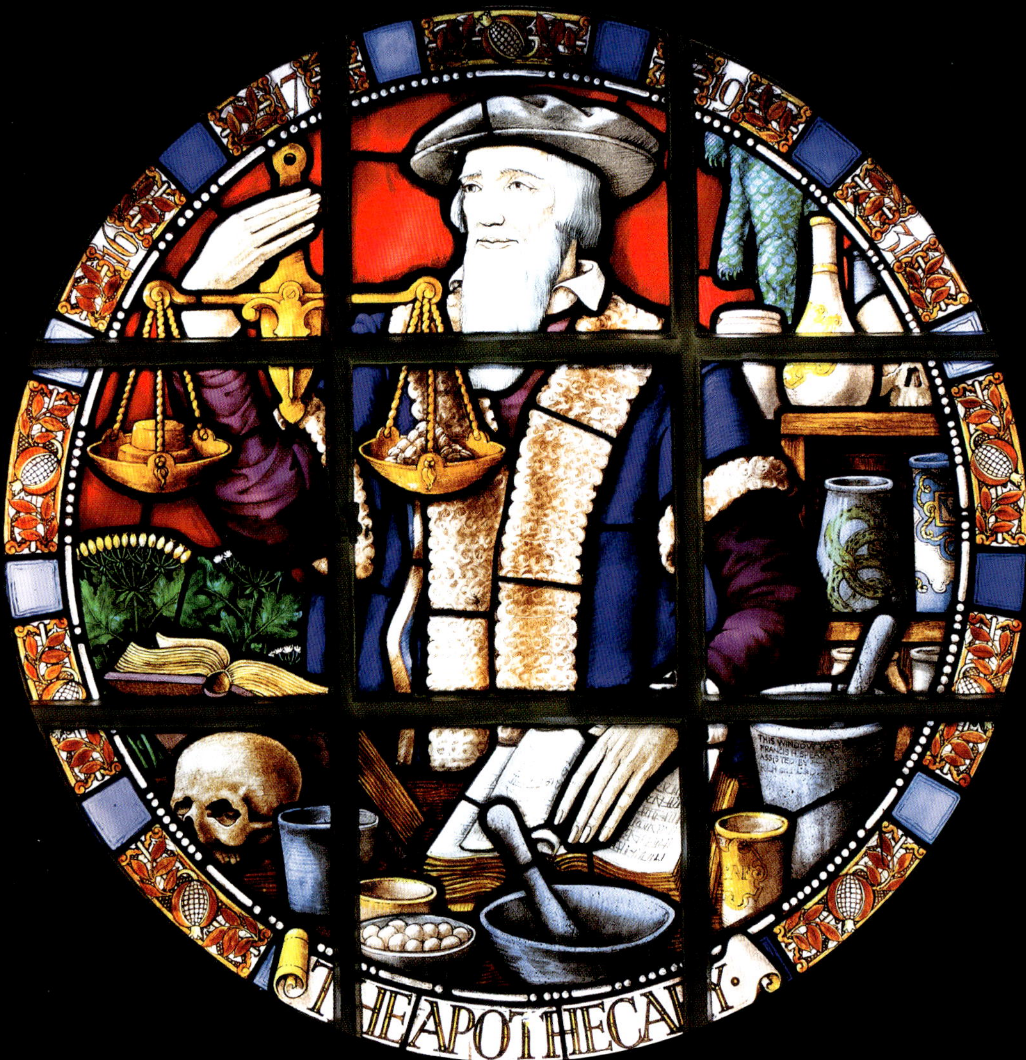

6.1 'The Apothecary' window in the Great Hall

CHAPTER 6

'The Apothecary' Window in the Great Hall

'A circular window in the Hall of the Society of Apothecaries which shows an apothecary of the time of the founding of the Society – 1617 – among his herbs and pots. This window is rich in colour though a good proportion of white glass relieves and at the same time accentuates the richness.'

Francis Spear, 1931[1]

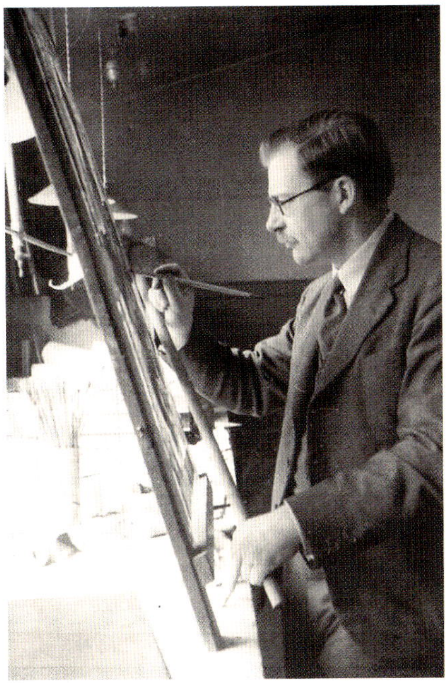

Francis Howard Spear, 1902–79: working in his studio at the London County Council School of Arts and Crafts, Southampton Row, Holborn in London in the mid-1930s

At the southern end of the Great Hall, above the seventeenth-century panelling and old gallery screen, is a window depicting in stained glass an apothecary surrounded by the tools of his profession. This is the only non-heraldic window in Apothecaries' Hall (Figure 6.1). The window has always been known as 'The Apothecary' or as 'Gideon de Laune', the founder of the Society, but until undertaking research for this book everything to do with its provenance was unknown – date, artist, place of manufacture, all forgotten.

The first query to be answered was the date of the window. This was easily established, because as one stands below it, two dates, incorporated into the marginal decoration, can quite clearly be seen with the naked eye, once they have been pointed out. In the margin of the upper-left panel is the date 1617; and in the margin of the upper-right panel is 1931 (Figure 6.2). Examination of the Court Minutes of the Society for 1931 reveals only one relevant entry, namely that at a Court meeting on 10 March 1931: 'It was resolved to instal [sic] a stained glass window depicting "The Apothecary" over the screen in the Great Hall.'[2]

During research into this window, on the occasion of an Open Day on 23 September 2012, a remarkable coincidence occurred. One of the visitors, Mr Alan Brooks, an acknowledged expert on stained glass, not only confirmed that the window had been made in 1931 by the well-known stained glass artist Francis Howard Spear but also had brought with him the original design watercolour painting by Spear himself (Figure 6.3), to compare with the finished window. Mr Brooks also informed us that there are a number of references to the window in the archive of the Company of Lowndes and Drury who, until 1973, were glaziers based in the Glass-House at Fulham.

An entry in the Lowndes and Drury 'Day Book' for 1931 records that on 4 April an order was placed for a 'Circular Window and iron frame for Apothecary Hall – also Small Panel'.[3] This is 'The Apothecary' window, together with the heraldic panel showing the armorial bearings of Alfred Hepburn (Master 1926–27), window West 2, panel 2 (mentioned further in Chapter 4 and described fully in Appendix 1). The details of the order appear in the company's 'Invoices' book on 15 June 1931, namely to glaze and cement a circular window five feet in diameter, total 20 square feet, at 6/- per (sq.) foot, that is £6.0.0d, and to glaze and cement a small heraldic panel 19 × 14 inches, at the same rate, that is 11/-, and so a total of £6.11.0d.[4] A company ledger shows that the order had been completed and paid for by 3 July 1931 for a total charge of £28.7.6d,[5] a figure far in excess of the £6.11.0d just mentioned but which is accounted for by necessary additional work such as supplying an iron frame for the window, painting said frame with two coats of white lead paint, fixing the frame and window at Apothecaries' Hall (together with two small panels, one of which must be the Hepburn panel, the other not being named) and paying a builder's account for supplying scaffolding and carriage of the glass and frame to the Hall. Although the glazing and cementing of the Hepburn panel is included in the total charge, it is likely that the cost of this would have been paid for by Hepburn himself. An intriguing little note in the Ledger on the same date states that Spear was overcharged 10/- for the fixing of the Apothecary window!

It is interesting to note that the word 'Apothecary' in the design painting of the main window is spelt incorrectly as 'Apothecry' (Figure 6.4), but not in any of the Lowndes and Drury records. Happily, this did not transfer into the finished window as we see it today – although in the Lowndes and Drury detailed description of the

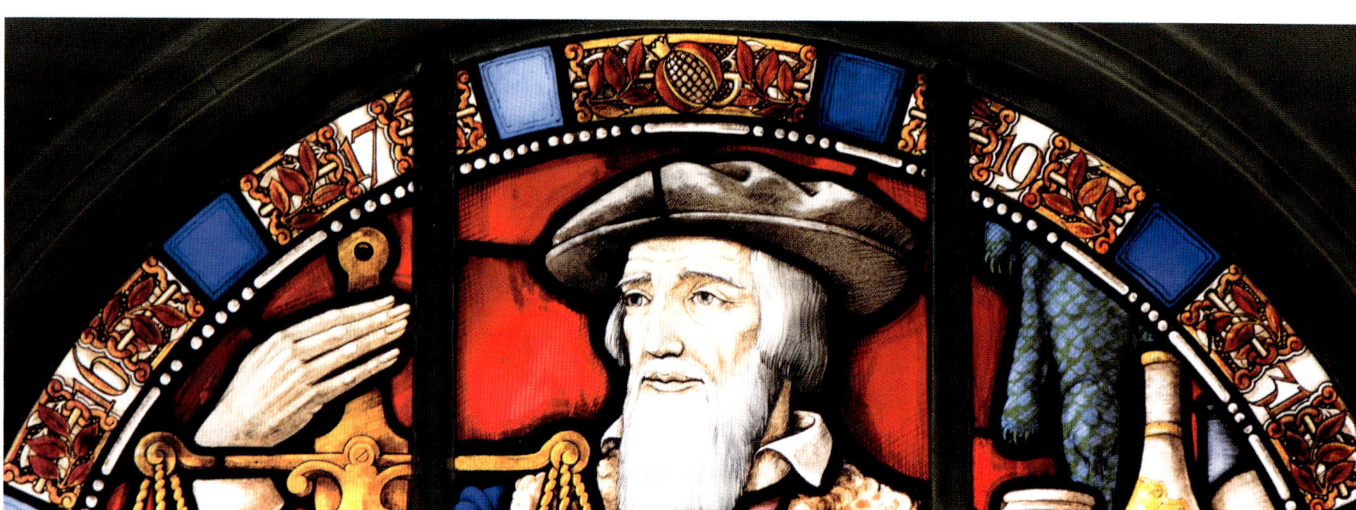

6.2 The dates 1617 and 1931 in the margins of the upper outer panels

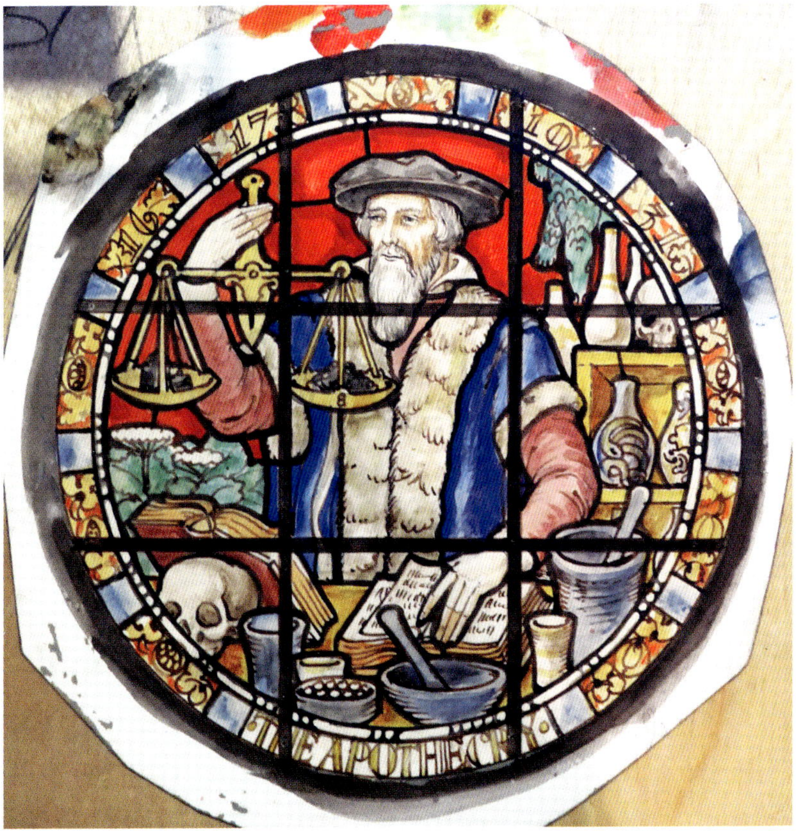

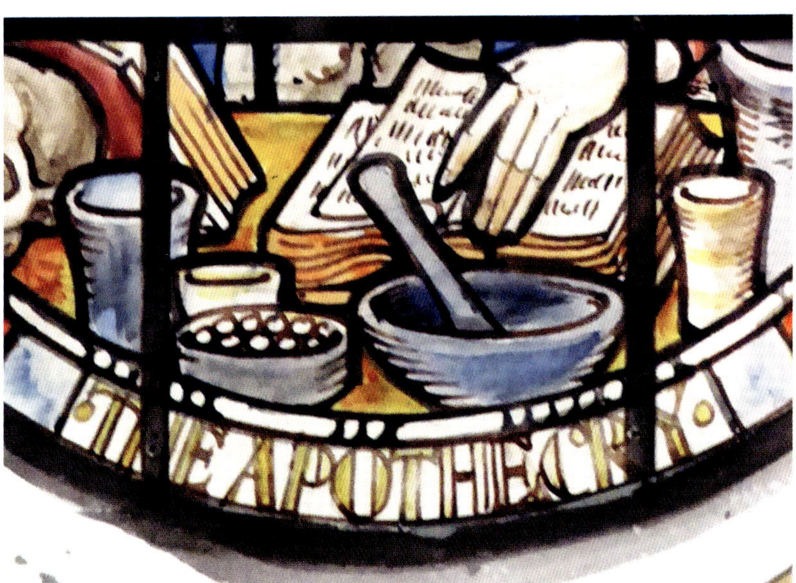

6.3 The original 1931 watercolour painting of 'the Apothecary' window

6.4 The misspelling 'Apothecry' in the design painting

work done, there is one further item which states that a piece of glass had to be removed for lettering to be included, at a charge of 12/6d.[6] It is tempting to surmise that the window was originally installed with the word 'Apothecary' spelt incorrectly and that the lower central panel of the window then had to be removed to allow painting of a new margin with the correct spelling, although there is no reference to this in the Society's Archive.

An entry in the Society 'Ledger for 1928–1935' records a payment of £74.10.0d to Francis Spear on 1 July 1931.[7] This is confirmed by a similar entry the next day in the Society 'Cash Book 1914–1931'.[8] In both books there is an additional comment to the effect that £55.0.0d was payment for the 'Stained window "Apothecary"' and £19.10.0d for 'Lighting'. Today, the window is lit at night from outside by a single halogen lamp on a bracket, a fitting which was last renewed in 2015. It is likely, therefore, that 'Lighting' refers to this outside source of illumination, which would have been installed by an external contractor engaged by Spear.

It was the practice at the time when this window was made for the Society, that the client either engaged an artist of their choice who then used the facilities of the firm in which they worked or vice versa. The fact that the Society paid Spear directly suggests he was the artist specifically chosen and that the former course was adopted. It seems likely that the sum of £74.10.0d paid by the Society to Spear included the £28.7.6d already paid by Spear to Lowndes and Drury in June 1931. After deduction of the cost of the lighting, though, it is not clear whether the balance of £26.12.6d is Spear's fee for designing 'The Apothecary' window alone or whether his fee for designing and making the Hepburn panel is included.

From a medicinal point of view, the pomegranate decoration around the whole margin of the window is obvious (Figure 6.5). Pomegranate has been used since time immemorial to treat many conditions but most

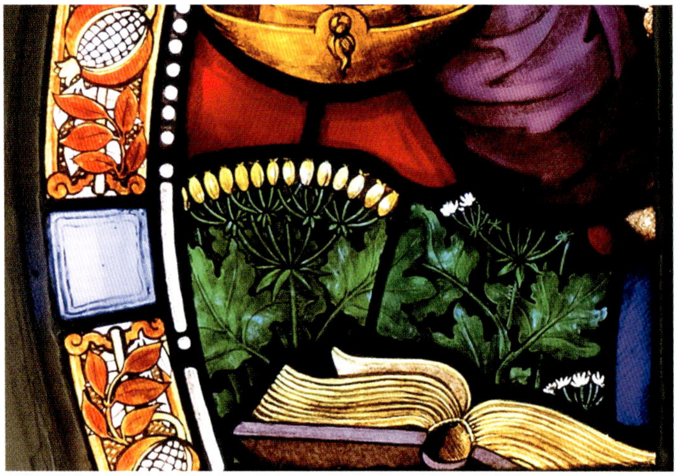

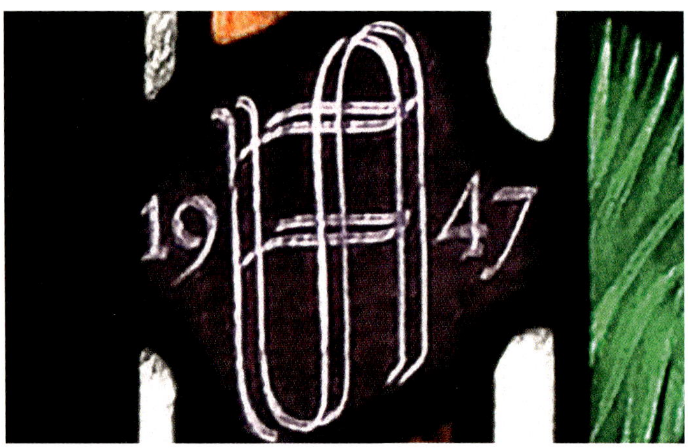

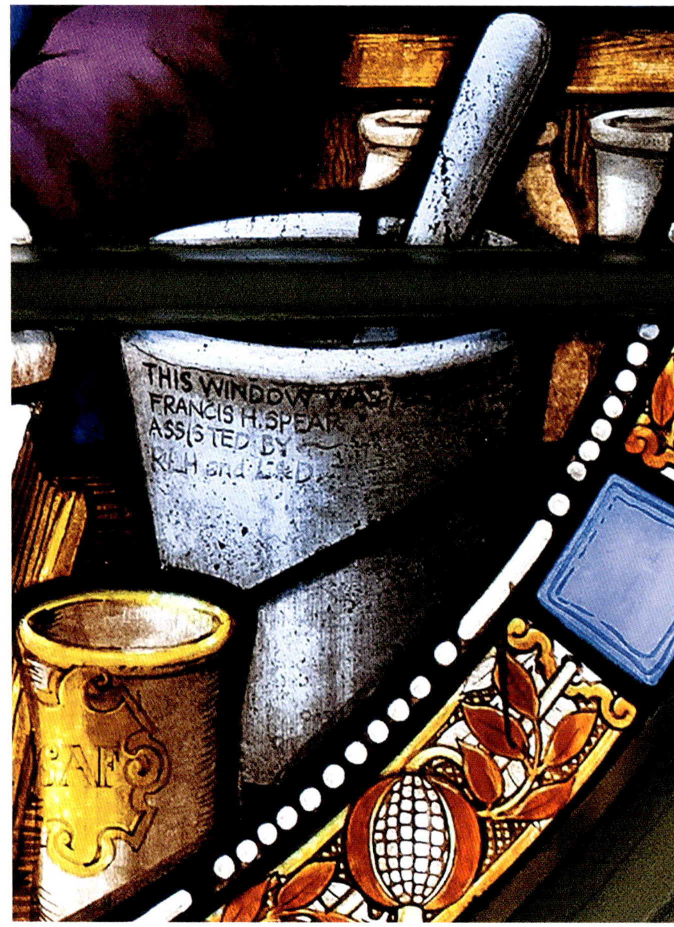

6.5 The plants in 'the Apothecary' window

6.6 The inscriptions on the mortar and the drug jar in the lower-right panel

6.7 Francis Spear's monogram in the Church of St James, Hockwold cum Wilton, Norfolk

particularly tapeworm. Recent studies suggest that it may also have anti-inflammatory and anti-cancer effects.[9] The two plants in the left central panel defy identification.

Close examination of the window through binoculars also reveals two further points of interest. On the mortar in the lower-right panel is an inscription which reads: 'This window was made by Francis H Spear assisted by RLH and L&D' (Figure 6.6). Mr Brooks confirmed that L&D stands for Lowndes and Drury and informed us that RLH refers to Mr Robert Leslie Hendra, who was a student at the Central School of Arts and Crafts in Holborn in London, where Spear was a teacher (1930–1953). Secondly, on the drug jar below the mortar the letters SAF can be seen (again Figure 6.6). It has been suggested by Dr John Ford, Liveryman of the Society, and confirmed by Briony Hudson of the Royal Pharmaceutical Society, that this is probably part of the abbreviation ASSAF for the plant *Ferula assa-foetida*, which was used as a drug to treat constipation.

The fact that the date of the window and the details of its maker and his assistant were plainly there for all to see over the years, underlines the advice given by those who study glass: when viewing stained glass windows, a pair of binoculars should always be

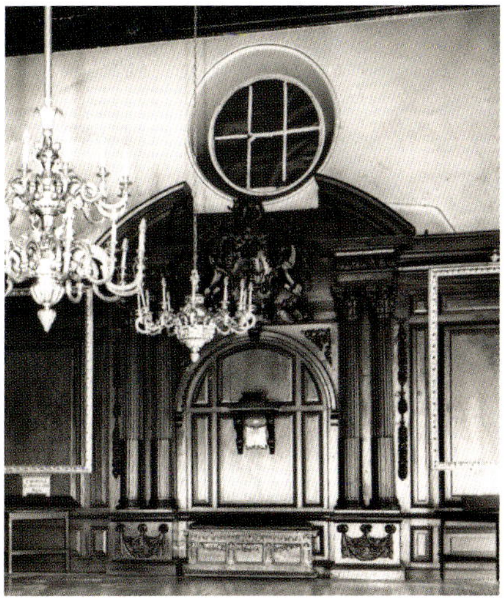

6.8 'The Apothecary' window covered up against blast in 1941

at hand. Spear often 'signed' his work with a very attractive monogram (Figure 6.7), but close examination of 'The Apothecary' window does not reveal such a signature.

There is no record in the Society's Archive that this window was removed to the Foundling Hospital at Berkhamsted for safekeeping during the Second World War, as was all the other stained glass at Apothecaries' Hall. Nor is there any such record in the archive of James Powell and Sons, who were responsible for removing all the other glass. Its removal would have required the erection of quite substantial scaffolding which may have been regarded as a step too far in 1941. However, a photograph of the southern end of the Great Hall, probably taken for the National Buildings Register scheme in 1941 (Figure 6.8), shows that the window was to some extent protected on the inside and this may have been repeated on the outside too.

Mr Brooks and Mr Simon Spear, Francis Spear's son, have very generously given the original design watercolour painting of 'The Apothecary' window to the Society, together with an earlier sketch in ink by Spear (Figure 6.9). It is interesting to note the difference between the original ink sketch and the finished window.

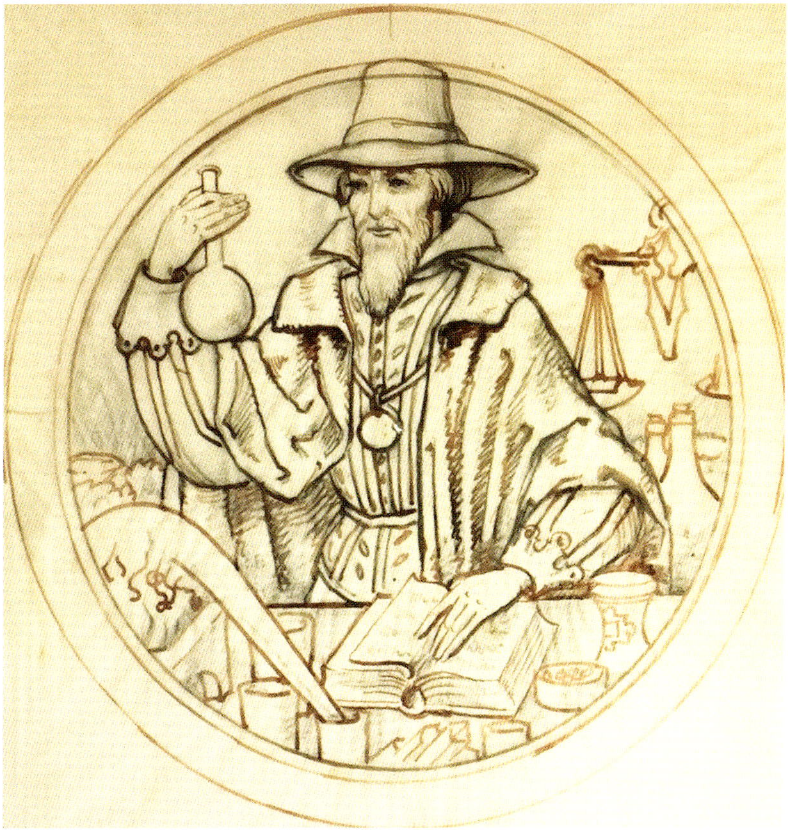

6.9 Francis Spear's early pen and ink design drawing of the window

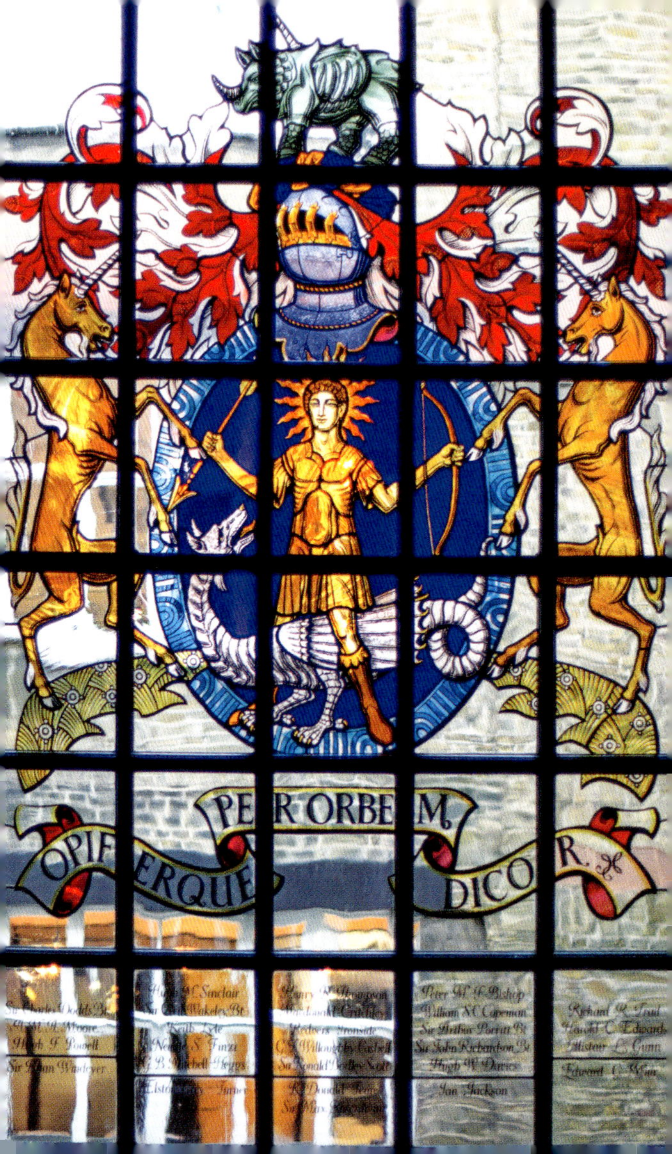
OPIFERQUE PER ORBEM DICOR
Peter M. F. Bishop
William N. C. Copeman
Sir Arthur Porritt Bt
Sir John Richardson Bt
Hugh W. Davies
Ian Jackson
Richard R. Trail
Harold C. Edwards

CHAPTER 7

Whitefriars in Black Friars: Carl Edwards and his legacy at Apothecaries' Hall

The artist has at his command material of incredible beauty. The colours are as rich as jewels, indeed they were once described individually as jewels, ruby for red glass, emerald for green, for instance, and to this day red glass is always described as ruby glass. No other medium has colours that can compare with glass for brilliance and richness.[1]

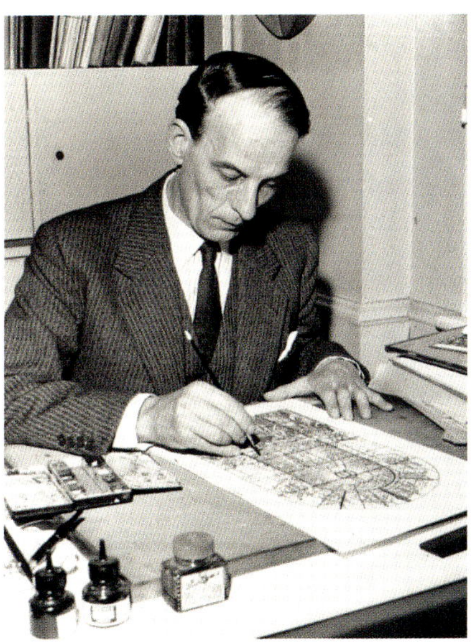

Carl Edwards (1914–1985) working on his design in 1958 for the central East Window for St Clement Danes Church in the Strand, London

In 1952 the internationally renowned stained glass designer Carl Edwards took up a tenancy at Apothecaries' Hall. Over a twenty-year period, the studio he established produced many windows of importance in the United Kingdom and abroad.

The Early Years

Prior to coming to Apothecaries' Hall, Edwards had been working for the glass company James Powell & Sons (Whitefriars) Ltd. This company, originally known as Whitefriars Glass, is said to have been founded in 1680 in Magpie Alley between Bouverie Street and Whitefriars Street south of Fleet Street on the site of a Carmelite Priory, a London house of the White Friars, although written records of the company only date from 1720. In 1834, James Powell, a London wine merchant, purchased the company in order to give his three sons a viable occupation and the name was changed to James Powell & Sons (Whitefriars Glass). The company became very successful, largely as a result of the Gothic Revival and the consequent demand for stained glass windows. Later it produced, in addition, innovative and inspirational ornamental glass and tableware, as well as glass for use in science and industry. In 1923, now known as James Powell & Sons (Whitefriars) Ltd, the company moved to purpose-built premises in Wealdstone near Harrow, but that factory closed in 1980, the 'Whitefriars' trademark being purchased in 1981 by Caithness Glass, which is now part of Dartington Glass.

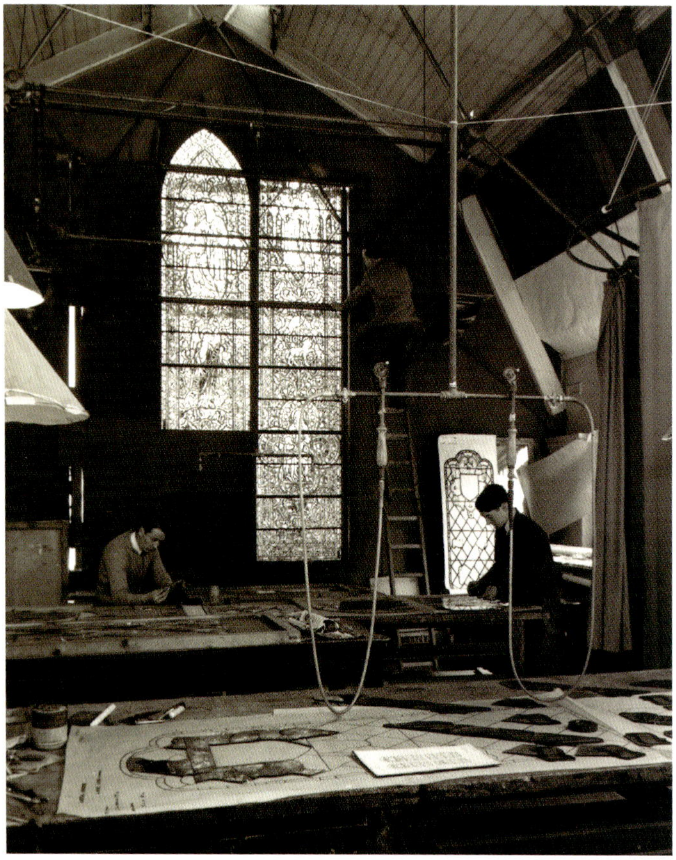

7.1 The Wheeler Room. The east end showing the newly installed window for displaying multiple panels during the creation of a large window, for example for a church. The window on display (in two parts) is the central light of the three-light window on the north side of the east end of the Temple Church in London

In 1928, at the age of fourteen, Carl Johannes Kiviaho (1914–1985) joined the company, working in the office during the day and in the evenings studying architecture at the Regent Street Polytechnic. His parents were Finnish, although Carl himself was born in Marylebone. In due course, he changed his surname to Edwards. By 1936 he had become assistant to James Hogan the head designer at James Powell and Sons, a man who had developed an international reputation for glass design, but his career was interrupted by the Second World War, during which he served in the Royal Engineers.

After the war, Edwards returned to the company and in 1948, when Hogan died, he was appointed to the position of head designer in his place. However, in 1952 he resigned in order to set up his own company and with Hugh Barnaby Powell, who it seems was not related to the founder of Whitefriars Glass, took up a tenancy at Apothecaries' Hall on 1 November of that year, under the name Carl Edwards Studio.

The Apothecaries' Hall Years

The studio that Edwards and Powell and their team established was housed in the Wheeler Room, which was on the top floor of the old Examination Block, a building originally reached by a door now replaced by the left-hand window in the Parlour. The room was named after Thomas Wheeler, one of the twelve members of the first Court of Examiners of the Society appointed on 19 July 1815. He was also Botanical Demonstrator and was elected Master in 1823 (see Chapter 5). In order to make the room suitable for the production of stained glass panels, Edwards installed at his own expense a large window some 14 feet in height at the east end of the room (Figure 7.1).

This photograph, together with a photograph of the west end of the room (Figure 7.2), gives a very good impression of the activity required for the making of stained glass windows.

Figure 7.3 shows a glass painter, Adolphus Augustus Burcombe, working on the cartoon for one of the five lights of a window in the north transept of the Church of St James at Kingston upon Thames. This was the first window to be produced by the company at the Hall.

But in 1956 the Edwards/Powell partnership ceased, Hugh Powell moving elsewhere and Edwards renewing the lease on his own. He was to remain at Apothecaries' Hall until 1972, during which time the output of stained glass windows from the studio was prodigious.

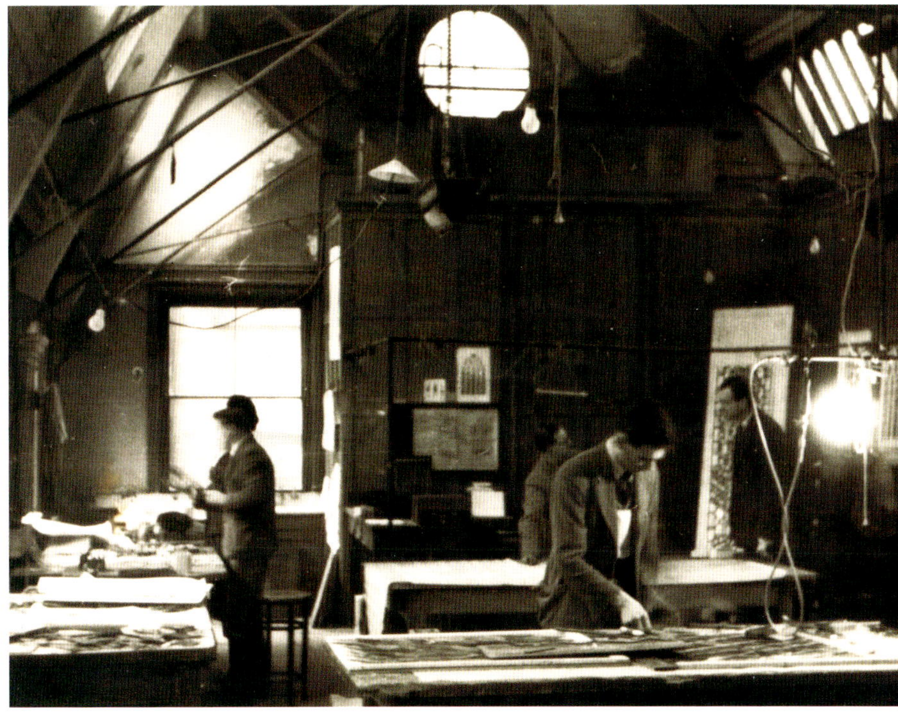

7.2 The Wheeler Room, the west end

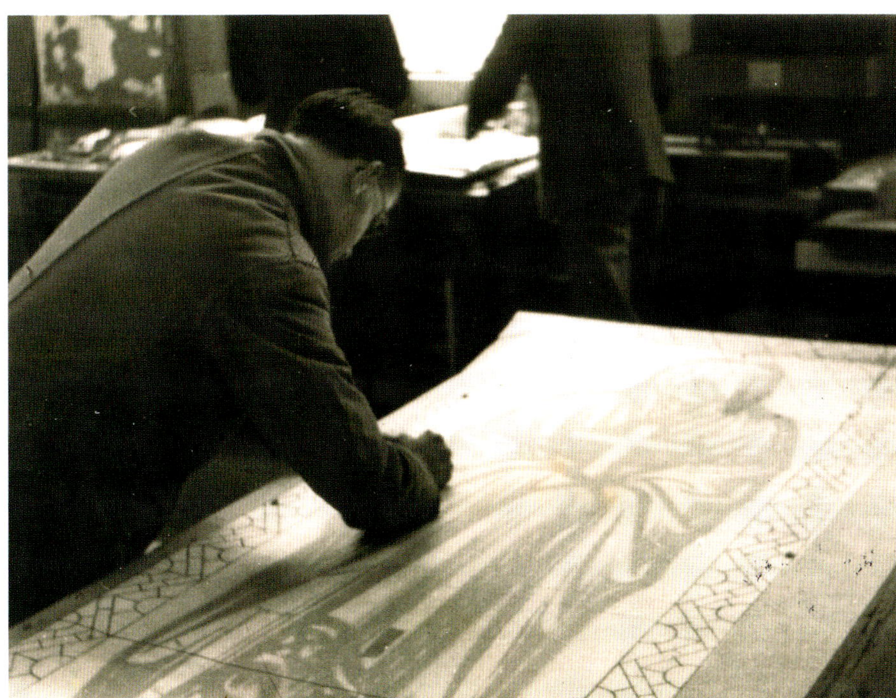

7.3 The first window to be produced by the Carl Edwards studio at Apothecaries' Hall, a five-light window for the north transept of St John's Church, Kingston upon Thames

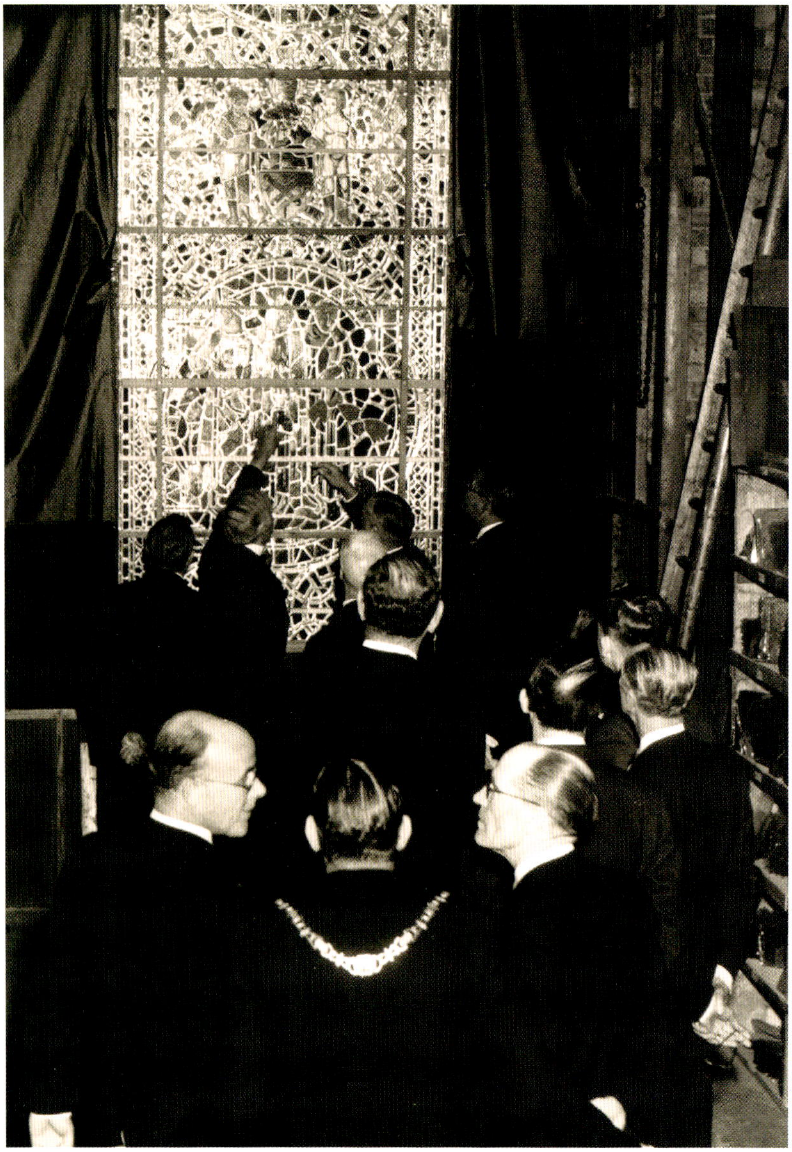

7.4 Society of Apothecaries' soirée in the Carl Edwards studio, 20 July 1954. The window being admired is the lower part of the central light of the central east window of the Temple Church in London. In the foreground, wearing his chain of office, is the Master of the Worshipful Company of Glaziers and Painters of Glass, Sir William Lacon Threlford. Standing to his right in the photograph is the foreman glazier, Edgar Crouch, and on his left is Brian Thomas, a stained glass artist

At the time of his arrival at the Hall, Edwards was working on the three new three-light east windows for the Temple Church in London to replace the windows destroyed in the war. Over his twenty-year period at the Hall, he completed and installed approximately 100 windows in this country and a further fifteen or so in countries as far afield as Australia, New Zealand, South Africa and the United States (see Appendix II). Of particular importance in this country are the seven windows (six of three lights with tracery above and an east window of five lights with tracery) he made for the Chapel at Lambeth Palace in 1955 and the twelve heraldic windows (each of four lights in two tiers with tracery) for the Debating Chamber of the House of Lords in 1956.[2] Again, these were all made to replace windows lost in the war, and in the latter year, he also made six new windows (each of three lights with tracery) for the Prince's Room at the House of Lords, the antechamber between the Royal Gallery and the Debating Chamber. Papers and correspondence relating to these windows can be seen in the Parliamentary Archives. On 20 July 1954 the Master, Dr Henry Morley, with fifty members of the Society and their guests, visited Edwards in his studio and signed his visitor's book during a soirée at the Hall (Figure 7.4).

The Society has benefitted enormously from having as one of its tenants for twenty years an artist of such exceptional talent, a skill he passed on to his daughter Caroline Benyon, now a renowned stained glass artist in her own right, a member of the Worshipful Company of Glaziers and Painters of Glass and, at the time of writing, Chairman of the British Society of Master Glass Painters. Figure 7.5 shows Edwards and his daughter at work in the Wheeler Room on the cartoon for the Great West Window of Liverpool Anglican Cathedral. Caroline recalls that when first drawn, the complete cartoon was so large that it had to be laid out on the floor of the much larger Brande Room below their studio, a room which had previously been used for laboratory work and examinations.

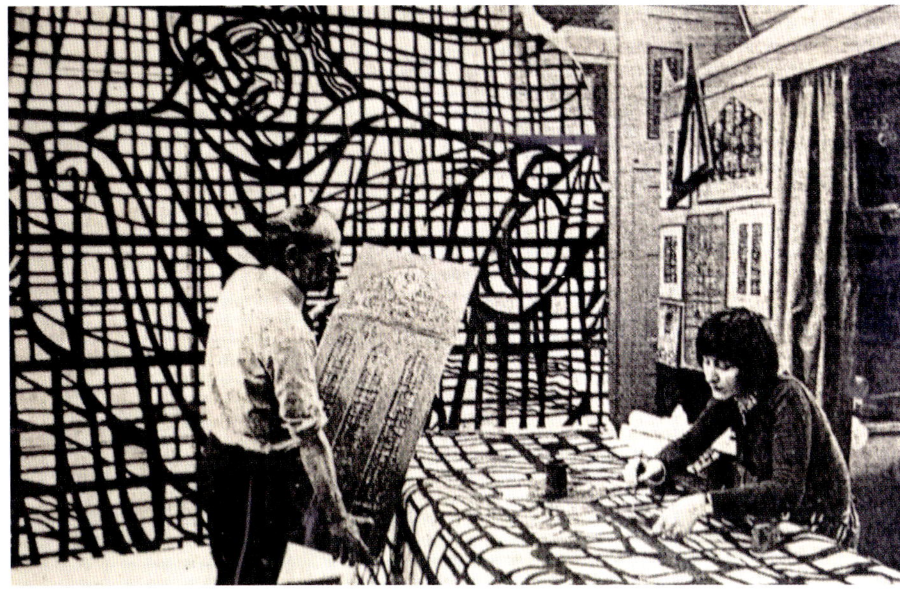

7.5 Carl Edwards and his daughter Caroline at work on the cartoon for the Great West Window of Liverpool Anglican Cathedral

Heraldic Panels by Edwards in Apothecaries' Hall

The Society's Archive shows that Edwards was responsible for the design and execution of ten of the armorial panels in the Great Hall as follows (Figure 7.6):

1. Professor Sir Charles Dodds Bt (Master 1947–48 and 1948–49). Window West 2, panel 14.
2. Henry Morley (Master 1870–71) and his great-grandson Henry Seaward Morley (Master 1953–54) in a combined panel. Window West 1, panel 2.
3. Sir Cecil Wakely Bt (Master 1954–55). Window West 4, panel 1.
4. Thomas Keith Selfe Lyle (Master 1962–63). Window East 2, panel 5.
5. Lord Cohen of Birkenhead (Honorary Freeman 1967). Window East 1, panel 11.
6. Hugh Macdonald Sinclair (Master 1967–68). Window East 2, panel 8.
7. Sir John Richardson (Master 1971–72). Window East 1, panel 8.
8. Sir Brian Windeyer (Master 1972–73). Window East 1, panel 14.
9. Elston Grey Grey-Turner (Master 1975–76). Window East 1, panel 2.
10. Sir Gordon Wolstenholme (Master 1979–80). Window East 1, panel 12.

Caroline Benyon has identified three further panels that are, in her view, undoubtedly by her father. They are (Figure 7.7):

1. Redvers Noel Ironside (Master 1963–64). Window West 3, panel 14.
2. Sir Arthur Porritt Bt (Master 1964–66). Window West 4, panel 14.

3. William Sydney Charles Copeman (Master 1958–59). Window West 4, panel 3.

As a result of close inspection of the quality and style of the painting, she also thinks it very likely that two further panels are by her father (Figure 7.8):

1. Archie Murrell Acheson Moore (Master 1961–62). Window West 3, panel 7.
2. Ian McGilchrist Jackson (Master 1977–78). Window West 3, panel 9.

The Bristow Panel

This panel, from the old church of Ayot St Lawrence in Hertfordshire is sixteenth century in date. It depicts the Arms of Uriah Bristow (Master 1803–04) and comes from a memorial window dedicated to his great-great-great-grandfather Nicholas Bristow, the original armiger. The panel was given to the Society in 1980 and was conserved and mounted by Carl Edwards. It is the oldest stained glass in the Hall and is described fully in Chapter 9.

Turners and Spectacle Makers

In 1944 and 1946 respectively, the Worshipful Companies of Turners and Spectacle Makers became tenants of the Hall. To commemorate this association, Edwards designed and executed in 1962 the Arms of both companies in panels which are now installed in the windows of the Entrance Hall (fully discussed and illustrated in Chapter 11).

The Court Room Windows

Undoubtedly, Edwards's greatest legacy to the Society is the glazing of the two windows in the Court Room in 1967 to commemorate the 350th anniversary of the founding of the Society in 1617 (Figure 7.9). Discussion about how best to mark the anniversary was well underway in 1966. Several options were considered, including a piece of silver, new jewels for the Wardens, a painting and even converting the lamp standard in the courtyard into a fountain which would cascade into the monastery well still in situ below – and of course there were the windows. In a letter from the Clerk to Sir John Richardson, who was Chairman of the Future Activities Committee, dated 12 September 1966, the Clerk mentions that it was he, Ernest Busby, who had suggested the insertion of 'cartouches' in the windows of the Court Room because 'during the day and on summer evenings the outlook is really poor and does, I think, spoil the appearance of the room.'[3] The stained glass project won the day, including, in addition, the repaving of the Courtyard with York stone and the publication of a history of the Society by Dr W. S. C. Copeman (Master 1958–59).

There was much discussion about the cost, and in a letter to the Clerk in August 1966, Edwards suggests glazing only fifteen of the thirty panels in each window. In the event, all thirty panels in both windows were glazed. On 25 October 1966, Sir John

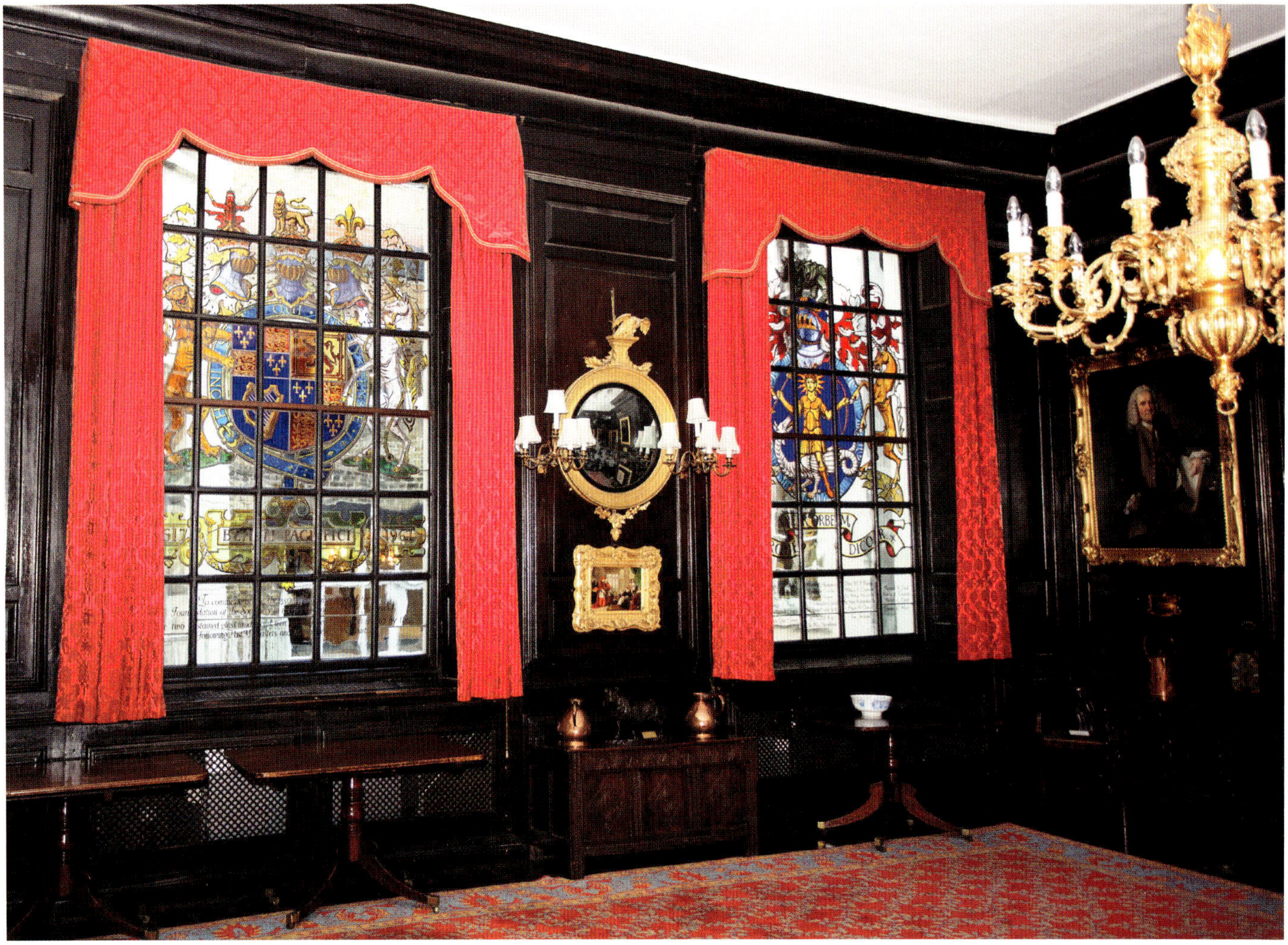

7.9 The Court Room 350th anniversary windows

met Edwards in the Court Room to finalise details. The proposal was for one window to display the Stuart Arms of James I and VI and the other the Arms of the Society. The Archive contains correspondence between Edwards and the Society about possible designs, including a number of early sketches for the windows of which only three survive – two of the Royal Arms and one of the Society's Arms (Figures 7.10 and 7.11).[4]

Edwards was firmly of the opinion that the current glazing bars should not be disturbed and that the upper sash of each window should be advanced to the same plane as the lower sash. Since this would make the windows unopenable, the possibility of providing ventilation by the insertion of grilles in the existing window shutters communicating with channels cut in the outer wall was suggested by Mr Mason, the Maintenance Mechanic, and in due course this was done. Means of artificially lighting the glass were agreed, although why this was considered necessary is not clear. Designs for both windows were also agreed by the Private Court and subsequently accepted by the full Court. At a meeting of the Private Court on 5 June 1967, the wording of the inscription for each window was finally decided (Figures 7.12 and 7.13). All twenty-three members of the Court, together with four retired members, twenty-seven in all, contributed to the cost of the project, and nineteen agreed to have their names recorded in the right-hand window.

These windows are magnificent examples of the traditional techniques of painting on glass, acid etching and silver staining. The only enamelling is on the jewels of the crowns in the Royal Arms window.

The version of the Royal Arms chosen (Figure 7.14) was the full achievement of King James established in 1603 on the union of the Crowns, including the Garter circlet, supporters and, unusually, three crests but without the mottoes.[5] The first and fourth quarters contain the English Royal Arms which had been adopted by Henry IV in 1406. These are quartered to display the three lions passant guardant of England and the three fleur-de-lys of France modern. The fleur-de-lys were first included in the English Royal Arms by Edward III in 1340, as a statement of his claim to the French throne. The old versions of the French Arms showed the fleur-de-lys displayed as semmé-de-lys – in other words, strewn with fleur-de-lys. In 1376 the French King Charles V simplified his Arms to just three fleur-de-lys. Henry IV similarly modernised the Arms in 1406. France was retained in the British Royal Arms until the Union with Ireland in 1801.

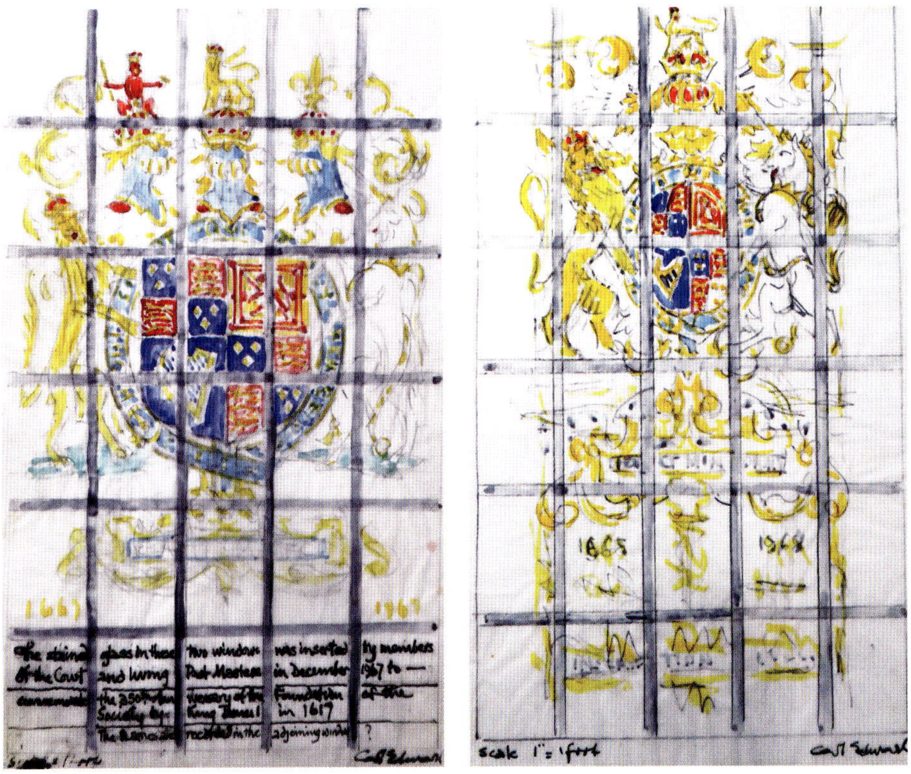

7.10 (below left and middle) Two sketches for the Royal armorial window. The design on the left was the one favoured by the Court

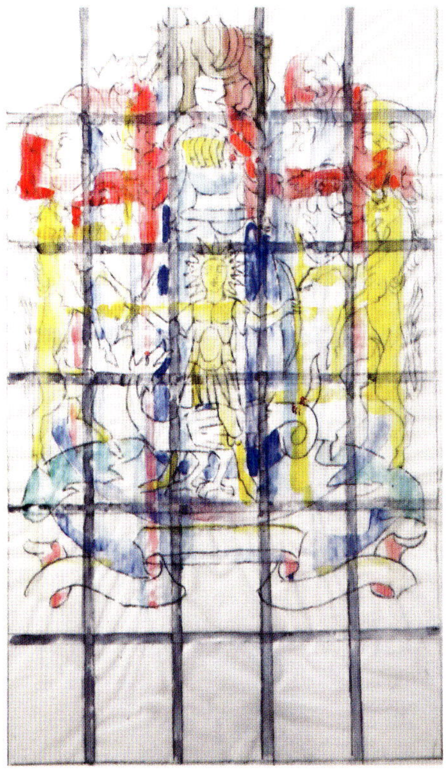

7.11 (far right) The surviving of the two sketches for the Society armorial window. This was the favoured design

The second quarter contains the lion rampant and double tressure of the Scottish Royal Arms, which has been in use since the twelfth century in the reign of King William the Lion (1143–1214). This quarter was introduced into the British Royal Arms on the accession of King James VI to the English throne in 1603.

The third quarter represents the kingdom of Ireland and these Arms were adopted for Ireland by King Henry VIII when he ended the period of lordship (which had existed from 1171 to 1541) and declared Ireland to be a kingdom again. The Arms were integrated into the British Royal Arms on the accession of King James I in 1603 to complete the visual assertion of the unification of the kingdoms of England, Scotland and Ireland.

On King James' accession, a Scottish unicorn supporter replaced the Tudor Welsh dragon although, in doing so, it lost its crown – which, however, continued to be displayed in the Scottish Arms.

The three crests, each on a Royal helm, are, from left-to-right, Scotland, England and France. The Irish Arms do have a crest – *a tower triple-towered Or, from the portal a Hart springing Argent*[6] – which is thought to have been created for King James I's new Royal Arms,[7] but it is very little used.

The traditional Royal mottoes of *Dieu et mon Droit* (God and my right – England), *In Defens* (In my defence God me defend – Scotland) and *Montjoie Saint Denis* (the Oriflamme or banner of St Denis – France) are omitted and *Beati Pacifici* (Blessed are

7.12 The inscription in the window showing the Royal Arms

7.13 The list of donors in the window showing the Society's Arms

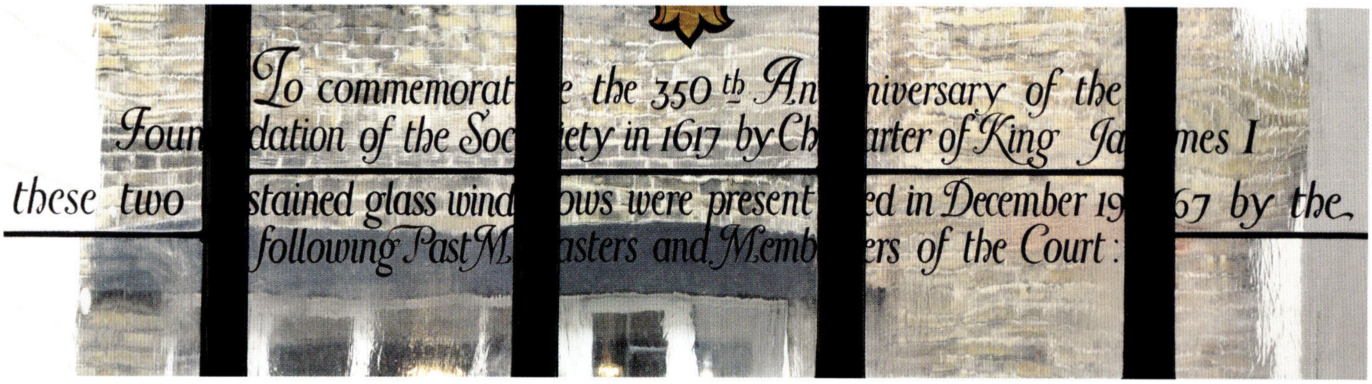
To commemorat e the 350 th An niversary of the
Foun dation of the Soc iety in 1617 by Ch arter of King Ja mes I
these two stained glass wind ows were present ed in December 19 67 by the
following Past M asters and Memb ers of the Court:

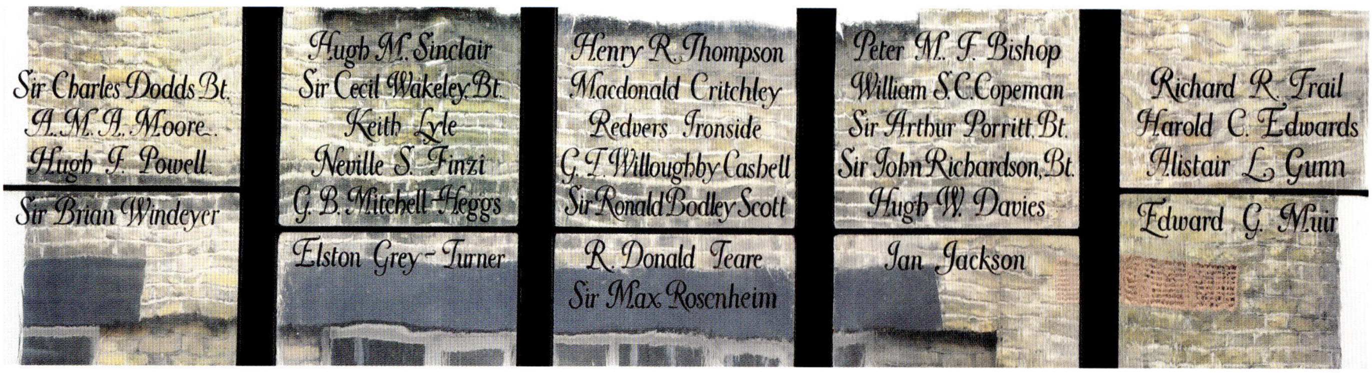
Sir Charles Dodds Bt.
A. M. A. Moore.
Hugh J. Powell.
Sir Brian Windeyer
Hugh M. Sinclair
Sir Cecil Wakeley Bt.
Keith Lyle
Neville S. Finzi
G. B. Mitchell-Heggs
Elston Grey-Turner
Henry R. Thompson
Macdonald Critchley
Redvers Ironside
G. T. Willoughby Casbell
Sir Ronald Bodley Scott
R. Donald Teare
Sir Max Rosenheim
Peter M. F. Bishop
William S. C. Copeman
Sir Arthur Porritt Bt.
Sir John Richardson, Bt.
Hugh W. Davies
Ian Jackson
Richard R. Trail
Harold C. Edwards
Alistair L. Gunn
Edward G. Muir

the Peacemakers) is shown. This was a favourite motto of King James, who saw himself as a peacemaker rather than a warrior and, indeed, his was a reign during which Britain was not at war with itself or with any other country. The Society also sees itself as a peacemaker 'bringing help [peace] to all until time ceases'.

This depiction of the Society's Arms (Figure 7.15) closely follows the Camden original and is one of the best balanced representations in the Hall. All the colours are correct, the helm faces the dexter as it should, the proportions of the rhinoceros, with his dorsal horn proudly erect, and of the unicorns are good and the former is not forced into his usual balancing act. The light blue edging to the shield is artistic licence and Carl Edwards can be forgiven this foible, as it was presumably designed by him to balance the Garter circlet in the Royal Arms.

The 350th anniversary was marked with a week of celebration in December 1967, starting with a Service of Matins at St Paul's Cathedral on Sunday 3 December. On Monday 4 December, there was a soirée at the Hall and on Tuesday a symposium was held at St Bartholomew's Hospital. On Wednesday 6th, the anniversary date of the granting of the Charter, the Court and Livery dined in the Hall in the presence of Her Majesty Queen Elizabeth The Queen Mother, the Lord Mayor and Sheriffs and the Lord Chief Justice. On Thursday 7th, a dinner for the Faculty of the History of Medicine and Pharmacy, as it then was, was held, with the Archbishop of Canterbury, the Most Reverend and Right Honourable Dr Michael Ramsey as the guest of honour. And on Friday 8th, there was a dinner for the Yeomanry. During the week, the windows were 'unveiled' and received with great acclaim.

Until 20 February 2014, the Court Room windows remained artificially lit. On that date the internal lighting and corrugated plastic coverings were removed, allowing these windows to be seen as the magnificent windows they truly are, illuminated, as is almost always ideal for stained glass, with natural daylight.

To have added in the twentieth century two such dominant features to a Stuart Room of 1672 was a courageous decision by all concerned. However, the result is generally agreed to be outstanding and completes the furnishing of the room to perfection.

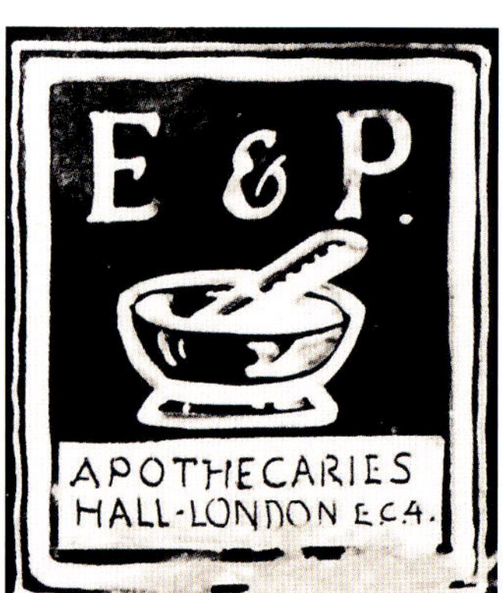

7.16 The Edwards & Powell mark

Signature Mark

During their years together at Apothecaries' Hall, Edwards and Powell used a pestle and mortar mark with their initials and date (Figure 7.16). Unfortunately, glass artists do not always sign their work and there are no examples of this mark on any of the Edwards panels at the Hall.

After the retirement of Powell, Edwards simply marked his more important windows with his name, which can be clearly seen on both windows in the Court Room (Figure 7.17).

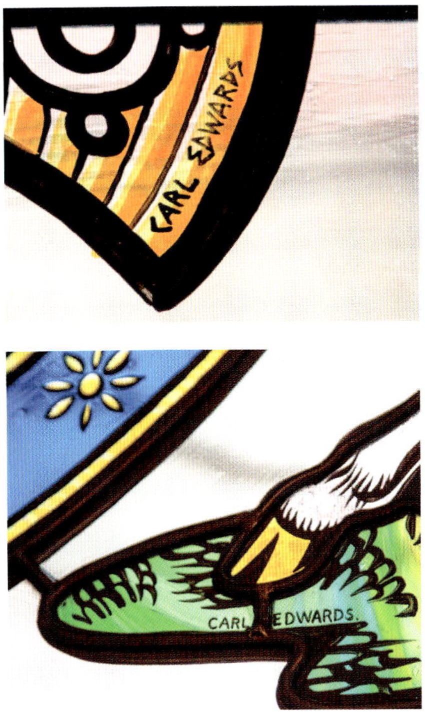

7.17 The Edwards signatures on the two Court Room windows

The Final Years

In the summer of 1972, the Clerk told Edwards that the Society was planning to develop the site upon which his studio stood and that he would have to vacate the premises by Christmas of that year. Edwards is quoted in the *Evening Standard* of 6 June 1972 as saying: 'The Apothecaries Company [*sic*] have told me that they want to build an extra floor on my part of the building. So that means they have to get rid of me. I understand the financial benefit they would achieve as a result of this, and I do not blame them. In fact, they have been very good to me. But it is upsetting.' The article goes on to describe how Edwards would have to convey no fewer than six tons of glass and lead downstairs and out of the building to a new studio, which is exactly what he had to do when he moved to his new studio at the Glass-House in Fulham. The move interrupted work on the Great West Window for the Anglican Cathedral in Liverpool, a commission that was not in fact completed until 1978. In the event, the site at Apothecaries' Hall was not redeveloped until 1980 – becoming what is now let out to tenants as New Cobham House.

Carl Edwards died in 1985, but his name lived on in his daughter's studio which was named after him at the Glass-House in Fulham, until she moved to her own studio in Hampton, Middlesex in 1993.

The windows Edwards produced in the Wheeler Room at Apothecaries' Hall are still much admired around the world. The Society is privileged to possess many examples of his work, none more beautiful than the commemorative windows in the Court Room, all a truly remarkable memorial to a great artist. The Society is hugely indebted to Carl Johannes Edwards.

Appendix II contains a list of the major commissions made in the Carl Edwards studio at Apothecaries' Hall for places other than the Hall itself.

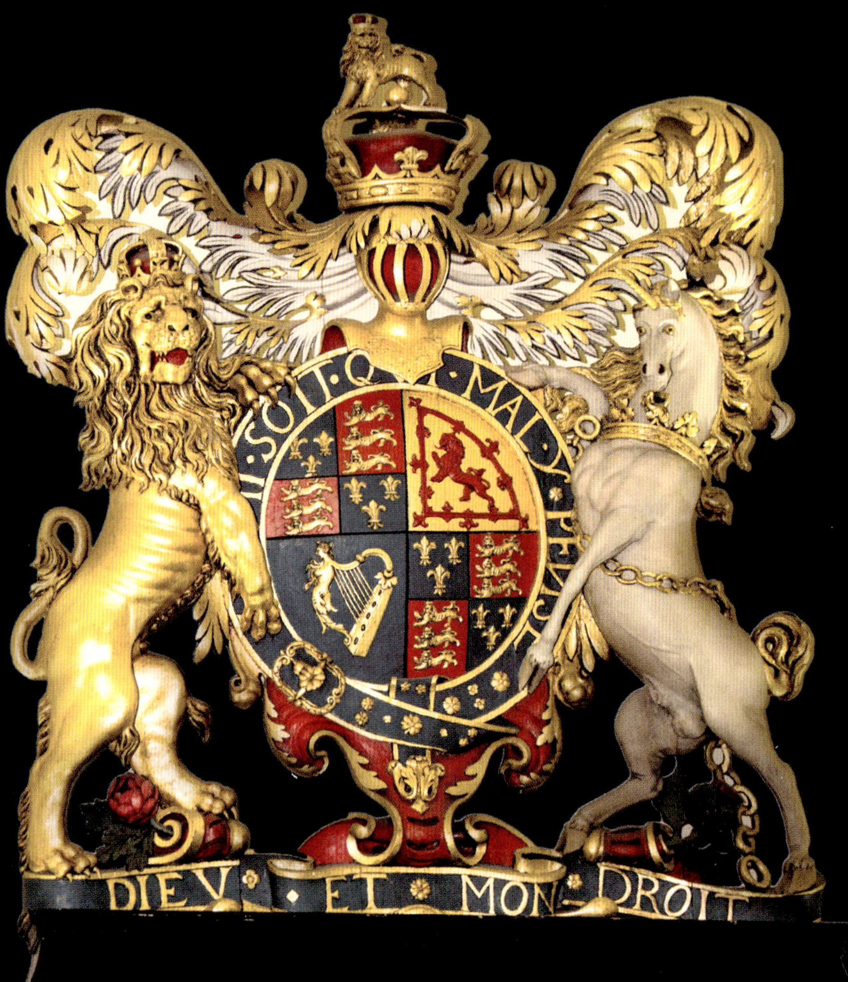

8.3 The Royal Arms in the Great Hall

CHAPTER 8

Royal Heraldry at the Hall

Having been established by Royal Charter, it was natural for the Society to display the Royal Arms and accordingly the Stuart Arms were carved for the pre-1666 Fire Great Hall, but nothing else is known about them. It is possible that they were placed on the north wall, where the current Arms now hang.

There are five representations of the Royal Arms in the Hall today. One on the Great Staircase is described in Chapter 5 and another in the Court Room in Chapter 7.

The City and the Civil Wars

In order to explain how the Society went from being initially a fervently royalist body, particularly after King James' granting of the Charter in 1617 followed by his strong defence of the Society in 1624, to being a supporter of Parliament in only twenty or so years, the twists and turns of the Civil Wars must be charted in some detail.

The philosopher Thomas Hobbes (1588–1679) wrote: 'But for the City the Parliament never could have made the war, nor the Rump ever have murdered the King,'[1] because, he went on to say, the City was the seat of government, the economic powerhouse, and the Tower of London was the country's principal arsenal. The City's adherence to the parliamentarian cause was crucial to the outcome of the First Civil War (1642–47) and its aloofness from the Second Civil War (1648) was no less significant.

After Charles I's accession in 1625, and therefore very shortly after the royal foundation of the Society, the late 1620s saw growing opposition to the forced loans and duties, such as tonnage and poundage, imposed by the King, particularly on the City. During his eleven-year personal rule, Charles also introduced the much-disliked feudal levy of ship money. The Society, under protest, paid £22 in ship money in 1636 and again in 1637 but not apparently thereafter. In 1639 the Crown demanded a loan of £100,000 from the City, of which only a small proportion was raised. A further demand was made in 1640 but this time specifically from the livery companies, of which the Society's share was to be £600, and again this was refused.[2]

Despite these and other impositions, Charles faced bankruptcy in 1640 after the failure of the First Bishops' War in Scotland in 1639. He sought to raise £200,000 from the City but was only offered £50,000. Writs or precepts were again issued by the Lord Mayor to the City Companies and the Society's share was £300, which it met with a loan from a Mrs Monnox at 8 per cent interest. The City refused to extend further loans to the King, so he seized £130,000 of silver bullion held under trust in the Tower. Similarly, the East India Company's stock of pepper and spices was seized. Parliament (the Short Parliament) was also recalled in the King's search for funds in 1640 but was unable to reach a compromise with him and so was dissolved after less than a month. Further warfare with the Scottish Covenanters followed and Parliament (the Long Parliament 1640–60) was recalled that same year, but this too was hostile to the King and intent on reform.

On his return from the Second Bishops' War in Scotland in 1641, Charles was received in London for the first time in his reign and the Lord Mayor wished the entertainment to be sumptuous in spite of previous disagreements. Accordingly, each company had to participate and the Society levied 'Riding Money' of 6/- and 3/- from each liveryman and yeoman respectively. However, support for the King swiftly declined again after this success and public order deteriorated. The City's trained bands were therefore mobilised to contain increased trouble from the London citizenry and apprentices, but nevertheless the situation necessitated the departure of the King to Hampton Court, concerned for the safety of his family. It was at this time that the Society acquired two barrels of gunpowder, four muskets, some swords and three fully accoutred pike men for the defence of the Hall. In Guildhall, the King's supporters were outflanked by the radicals elected in the December 1641 elections and the balance of power shifted away from the Lord Mayor and Aldermen to the Common Councillors.

Following Charles' imprudent and unsuccessful attempt to seize five subversive MPs, who then took refuge in the City, he again fled the capital and Parliament then dominated London. The First Civil War thus began and lasted from 1642 until the King's capture in 1647.

After 1642, demands for loans came from Parliament rather than from the Crown, beginning with an immediate demand for £100,000 from the City for the preservation of the Kingdom of Ireland, the Society's share again being £600. This was provided by individual apothecaries at their own risk. There followed a weekly property tax of £8 on the Hall and further demands for loans totalling some £1,000. In 1643, the Society, facing bankruptcy, let the Hall to a Lady Darcy for a year, meetings then being held in Blackfriars' Church. One of the ways in which the Society attempted to fund these loans was by increasing the livery fine but, as a result, in 1644 for instance, of the sixty-four yeomen called to the livery, only thirteen accepted and paid the fine.

In 1644 the Society was ordered to provide 'able and fit men for Surgeons' to join the New Model Army, but it is not clear that any were sent.[3] The loyalties of individual apothecaries varied with, for instance, Paul de Laune serving as Apothecary to the Parlia-

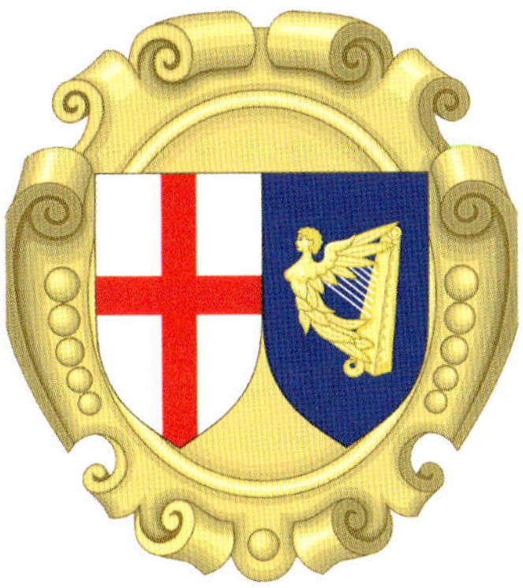

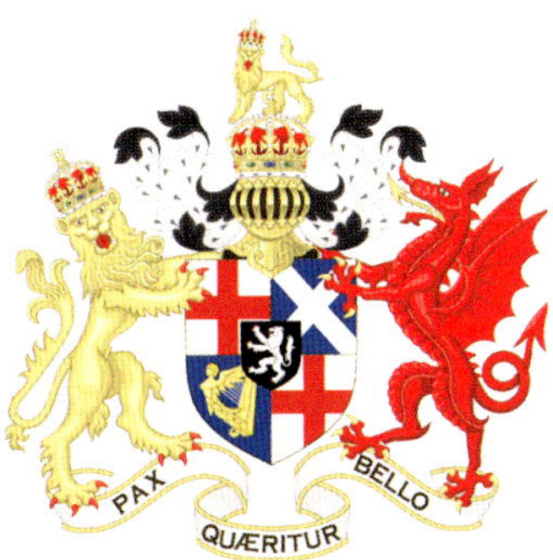

8.1 The Commonwealth Arms 1649–53

8.2 The Arms of the Protectorate 1654–58

mentarian Earl of Essex but Francis Metcalf losing his wagon of goods in the royalist defeat at Naseby.

Whilst the Army and Parliament were divided, Charles escaped from ward in Hampton Court and signed 'the Engagement' with the Scots in 1647 before again being taken into custody, this time in Carisbrooke Castle. The resulting brief Second Civil War in 1648 was a defeat for the Royalist Scots. Disagreements between Parliament and the New Model Army culminated in Pride's purge in 1648, which resulted in the establishment of the Rump Parliament, consisting entirely of MPs who were supporters of the New Model Army and its vision of Commonwealth. The King's trial and execution followed in 1649.

In 1648, some of Lord Fairfax's troops had been billeted in the Hall after his triumphant entry to London and considerable damage was caused to the fabric but not to the valuables, which had already been removed.

On 19 May 1649, the Rump Parliament passed an Act declaring England to be a Commonwealth, with power vested in Parliament and the Council of State, an Army committee replacing the Privy Council. The Rump Parliament passed a number of unpopular laws, such as the ban on theatres and strict observance of Sundays; the uncertainties of the time necessitated economies in the Society such as the abandoning of dinners and the herbarising expeditions. The Rump Parliament lasted until 1653 when it was forcibly dissolved, being replaced by the Army Council and 'Barebone's Parliament' (so called after the City's representative who was named Praise-God Barebone) all of whose members were appointed by the Army.

The Great Hall

In 1650, in response to a precept from the Lord Mayor, the Court paid 12/- for the Royal Arms to be taken down and a further £36.13.0d for a heraldic painter to paint the Arms of the Commonwealth. The first version of these Arms (Figure 8.1) impale St George of England (*Argent a Cross Gules*) with the Harp of Ireland (*Azure a Harp Or*). Note that the red cross symbol of the people has replaced the Royal lions/leopards.[4]

Finding the Commonwealth to be unsatisfactory, Cromwell assumed the role of Lord Protector of a United Commonwealth of England, Scotland and Ireland in 1653 – the Protectorate. Scotland was formally joined to England by an ordinance of 12 April 1654 when it was decreed that new Arms of the Protectorate (Figure 8.2) should be placed on all the public seals, seals of office and seals of bodies civil or corporate as a badge of this Union. The Arms were *Quarterly, 1st and 4th Argent a Cross Gules (for England), 2nd Azure a Saltire Argent (for Scotland), 3rd Azure a Harp Or stringed Argent (for Ireland); on an escutcheon Sable a Lion Rampant Argent (for Cromwell).*

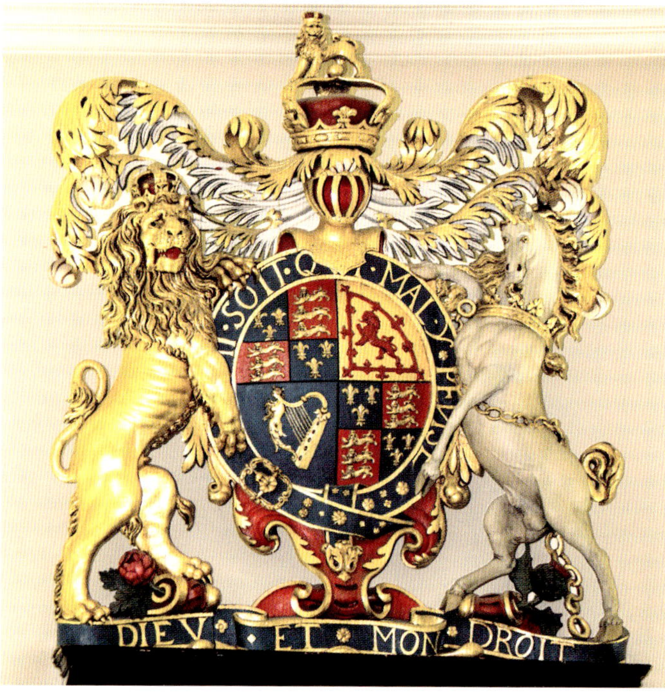

8.3 The Royal Arms in the Great Hall

No representation of the Commonwealth or Protectorate Arms used in the Hall exists and it is therefore not clear which version was painted. Judging by date, it is likely to have been those shown in Figure 8.1 and also likely that they were hung in the position of the previous, and indeed the current, Royal Arms in the Great Hall.

Figure 8.2 shows that the Protectorate Arms retained the Royal helm, crown and crest and for supporters kept the traditional lion but replaced the Stuart unicorn with the previous Welsh dragon. Another variant of these Arms does not use the Cromwellian escutcheon and a second saltire replaces the harp, so possibly these were intended as the Lord Protector's personal Arms. The Society's records do not indicate that a change was made to incorporate any of these new designs.

Cromwell died in 1658 and was succeeded as Lord Protector by his ineffective son Richard. The Rump Parliament was recalled in 1659 and this led to the Restoration of Charles II in 1660.

In 1660 the Society was asked to contribute £72 of £12,000 needed by City companies for the reception of Charles II in the City. The Society also received a precept from the Lord Mayor directing it to remove the Commonwealth Arms and replace them with the King's Arms. At this time, a heraldic painter was paid £3 for the Society Arms and £1 for the King's Arms but these were probably only processional flags for the occasion of the King's reception.

The Society's response to the precept is not clear and the minutes and account books make no mention of any Arms being commissioned. There must have been a queue for carvers to make new Royal Arms after the Restoration and it may be that the processional flags were hung for the time being. However, whatever was in the Hall on 4 September 1666, did not survive the Great Fire.

Barrett records that in 1676 Assistant James Gover paid to gild and paint in heraldic colours the King's Arms in the Great Hall;[5] it seems likely that this action, four years after the completion of the rebuilding, must date the present Arms which hang in the Hall. On 23 May of that year, there was a fire in the wainscoting, caused by the factory chimney overheating but it seems that the Arms were not affected, if indeed they were in place by then, and especially as Dr Gover's offer does not refer to re-gilding.

The Arms (shown in Figure 8.3) are a standard representation of the Stuart Arms with supporters, mantling, motto, helm and single crest showing: *quarterly 1st and 4th; grand quarters 1st and 4th Azure, three fleurs-de-lys Or (France modern) and grand quarters 2nd and 3rd Gules three Lions passant guardant in pale Or, armed and langued Azure (England); 2nd Or a Lion rampant within a double tressure flory-counter-flory Gules (Scotland); 3rd Azure a Harp Or, stringed Argent (Ireland)* (the derivation of the quarters is explained more fully in Chapter 7). This example of the Royal Arms is a magnificent achievement, with the insignificant oddity that the crown has only three arches and looks as if it has been rotated through 45 degrees. It is to be regretted that the carver is unknown.

The Arms were last reconditioned between November 1990 and March 1991, when they were taken down, somewhat perilously, and sent away for four months to be cleaned and re-gilded at a cost of some £4,000.[6] The necessity to refurbish these Arms was first identified by the Sustentation Committee in 1987,[7] with the fascinating additional requirement to correct the detail in the Scottish quartering. There is no further reference to this last action in the records and comparison of the Arms before and after refurbishment reveals no change to the second quarter. Inspection of that quarter shows that the lion cannot be fully rampant but is bent over by the shape of the quarter and the only possible exception a purist could otherwise take is that the tressure is not detailed enough to show it doubled as it should be.

8.4 The carved Royal Arms in the Court Room

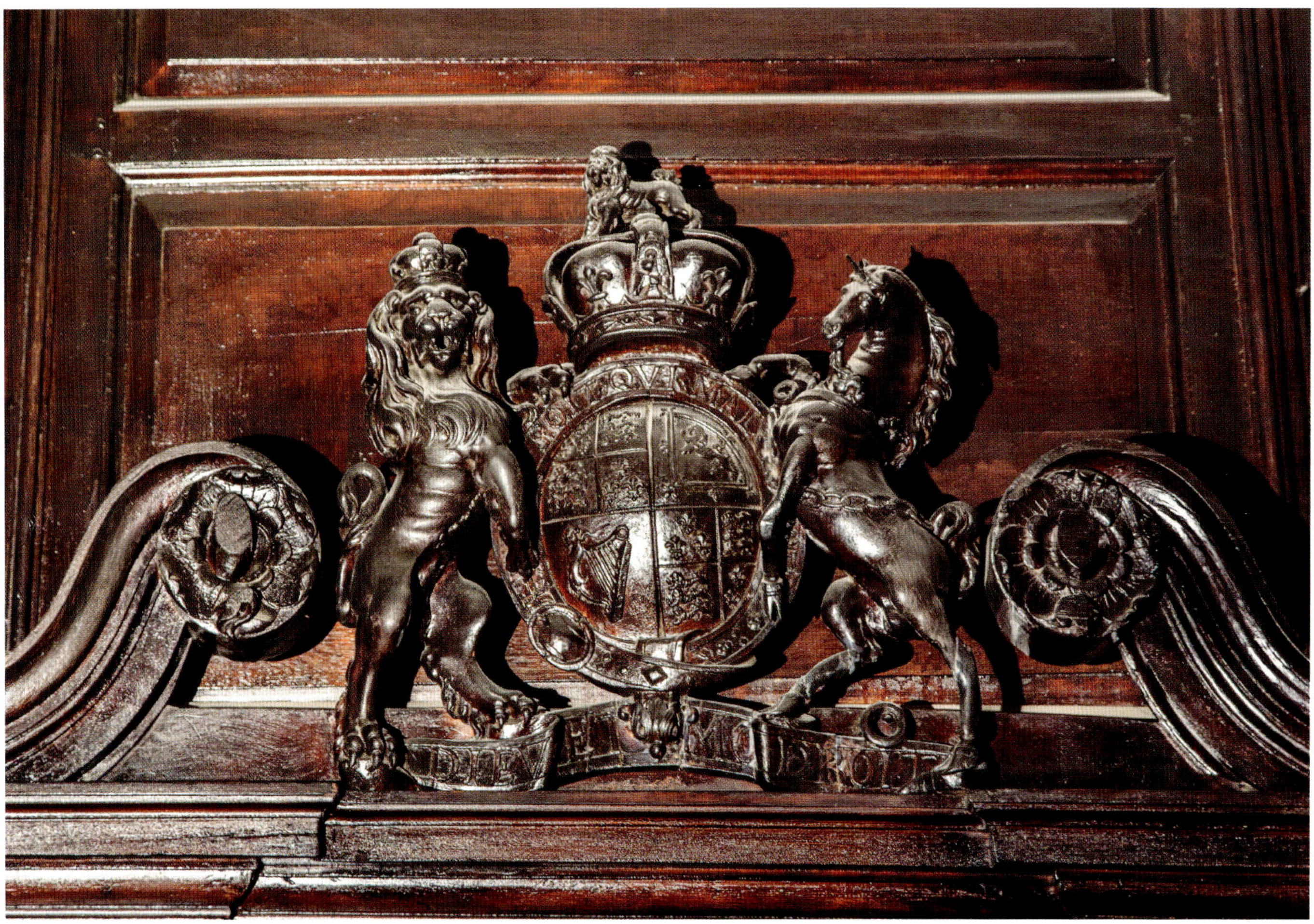

The Court Room

The most obvious Royal Arms in the Court Room are the spectacular stained glass Arms in the window, which were made by Carl Edwards in 1967 to celebrate the 350th anniversary (these are discussed fully in Chapter 7).

Less visible are the oak carved Royal Arms on the north wall of the Court Room (Figure 8.4). At first sight, and bearing in mind that this is the Court Room, with the ornate architrave and lintel it might appear that at one time this formed the backdrop to the Master's Chair at Court meetings. However, the Master not being a Royal official, such as a judge, there would be no reason for him to sit under the Royal Arms.

In fact, this was the original doorway from the Court Room into the Parlour. In due course, this door was closed off and panelling inserted when the Parlour bookcase was installed and a new doorway was formed in the north-west corner of the room. There is no record of when this work was carried out and it must be assumed that the door architrave was retained to highlight the Arms.

This is another example of the Stuart Arms and again the identity of the carver is not known and the date is problematical. Unless it was moved from elsewhere, in which case the earliest possible date is 1603 [accession of James I], it must date from the period 1672 [rebuilding of the Hall] to 1689 [deposition of James II], or possibly it could be as late as 1702–07 when Queen Anne reverted to the plain Stuart Arms before the Act of Union with Scotland.

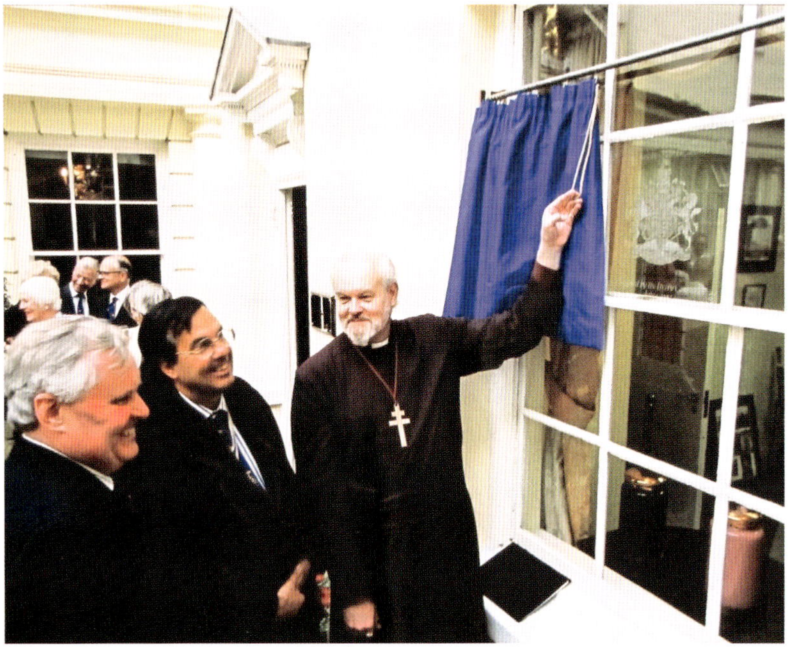

8.5 The Bishop of London unveiling the panel in 2002

One outside possibility, for which there is no evidence except a statement by Barrett that the oak carving is 'of a far more ancient date than the panelling or cornice beneath',[8] is that these Arms may have been produced to comply with the precept of 1660 and were small and portable enough to be saved from the Great Fire. On the other hand, an entry in the Minute Book for 1672 states: 'Subscription towards the wainscoting of the Court Room was £115 + £5 for the King's Arms.' This latter £5 is likely to date the carving of these Arms, as the ones in the Great Hall would have been rather more expensive!

The Arms are in the same form as those in the Hall, that is, quarterly – 1st and 4th England and France modern; 2nd Scotland; 3rd Ireland. Oddly, there is no helm between the shield and the Crown but otherwise they are the Stuart Arms.

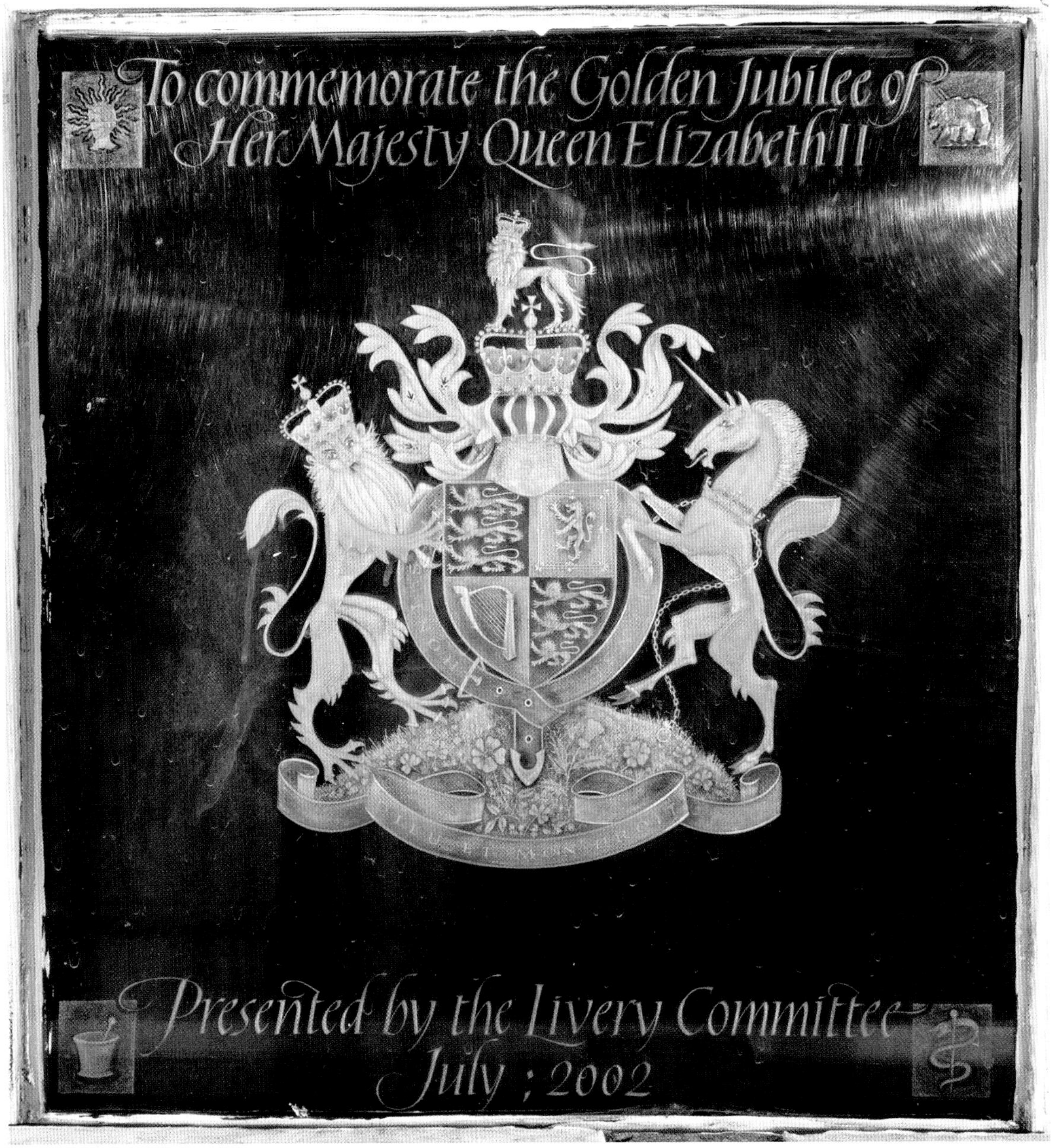
To commemorate the Golden Jubilee of
Her Majesty Queen Elizabeth II
Presented by the Livery Committee
July ; 2002

8.6 Engraved panel showing the armorial bearings of Her Majesty the Queen

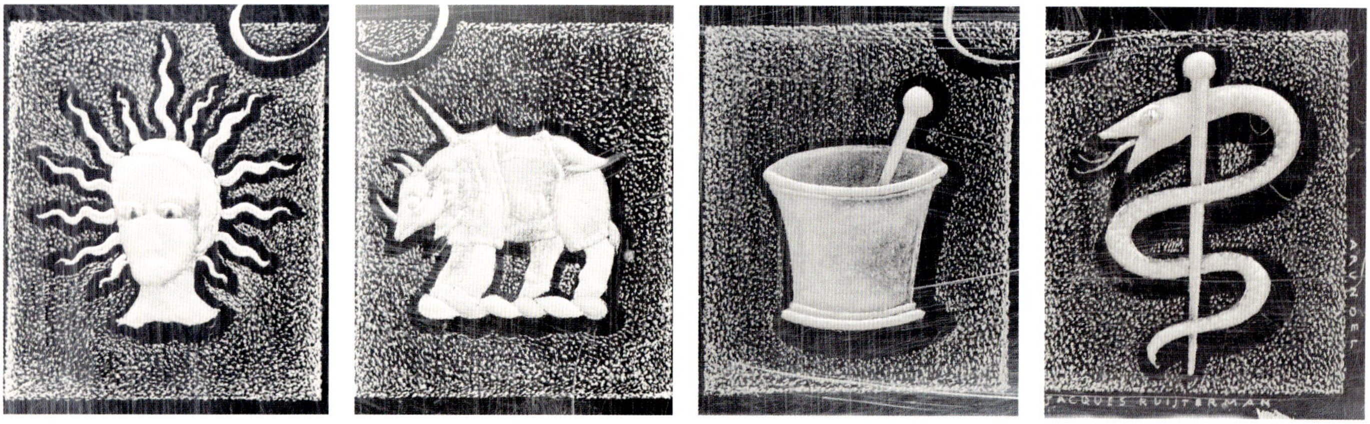

8.7 The four corner engravings: head of Apollo; Dürer's Gomda; pestle and mortar; staff of Asclepius

The Cloakroom

In 2002 the Livery Committee presented to the Society an engraved panel to mark the Golden Jubilee of Her Majesty Queen Elizabeth II (Figure 8.6) and this is placed in the centre of the northern window of the Cloakroom overlooking the Courtyard.[9]

The panel was unveiled by the Right Reverend and Right Honourable Dr Richard Chartres, Bishop of London, on 24 July 2002 (Figure 8.5).[10] Unfortunately, the panel was installed the wrong way round, with the engraved surface on the outside. As all glass should be viewed from inside, the panel was reversed in October of that year.[11] This is also, of course, particularly important for engraved glass, because of the problem of keeping it clean.

The panel depicts Her Majesty's Arms and is the only example in the Hall to depict the current Royal Arms which have been in use since the accession of Queen Victoria in 1837. At each corner of the panel is a small engraving showing details relevant to the Society.

In the top-left corner is the head of Apollo, in the top-right corner a rhinoceros with a splendid dorsal horn, in the bottom-left corner a pestle and mortar and in the bottom-right corner the staff of Asclepius with its snake (Figure 8.7).

The panel was engraved by Mr Jacques Ruijterman using hand-held diamond and carborundum wheel drills. It is 'signed' below the engraving of Asclepius in the bottom right-hand corner and down the right-hand side of the same engraving is the name 'Arundel', the home of the Ruijterman studio. These inscriptions are very difficult to see with the naked eye – a magnifying glass may be required!

Lost Royal Arms

In 1769, as a New Year's gift, Assistant Thomas Basden presented the Society with 'the King's Arms, painted and gilt'.[12] Basden served as Junior Warden 1773–74 and Senior Warden 1774–75 and was to be Master for a few days in 1775 on the death of the incumbent, but he was not re-elected at Election Day in 1775. He died in 1778.[13]

What form these Royal Arms took and where they were displayed in the Hall, if they ever were, is not known as they do no survive but Basden had presented expensively carved Royal Arms to St Dunstan's Church, Cranbrook, in 1756 (Figure 8.8) and the two gifts may have been similar in appearance. Perhaps, if they were similar, he sought to update the Great Hall's Stuart Arms with the then-current Hanoverian version, which impaled England and Scotland in the 1st quarter and replaced the 4th quarter with the Arms of Hanover (*tierced in pale reversed, 1: Gules, two Lions passant guardant Or (Brunswick), 2: Or, semé of Hearts Gules, a Lion rampant Azure (Lüneburg), 3: Gules, a Horse courant Argent (Westfalen); overall an inescutcheon Gules charged with the Crown of Charlemagne*) (shown more clearly in Figure 8.9) – in which case it would appear that the Court may have preferred to retain King James' Arms. Interestingly these St Dunstan's Arms are not quite correct as the lion shown in the Luneburg Arms is Gules rather than the Azure blazoned.

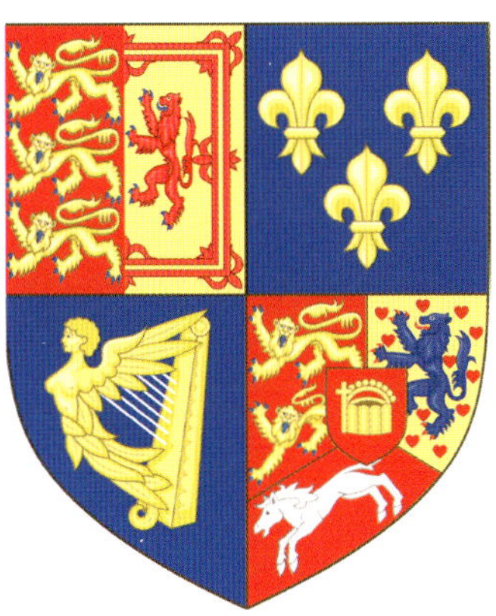

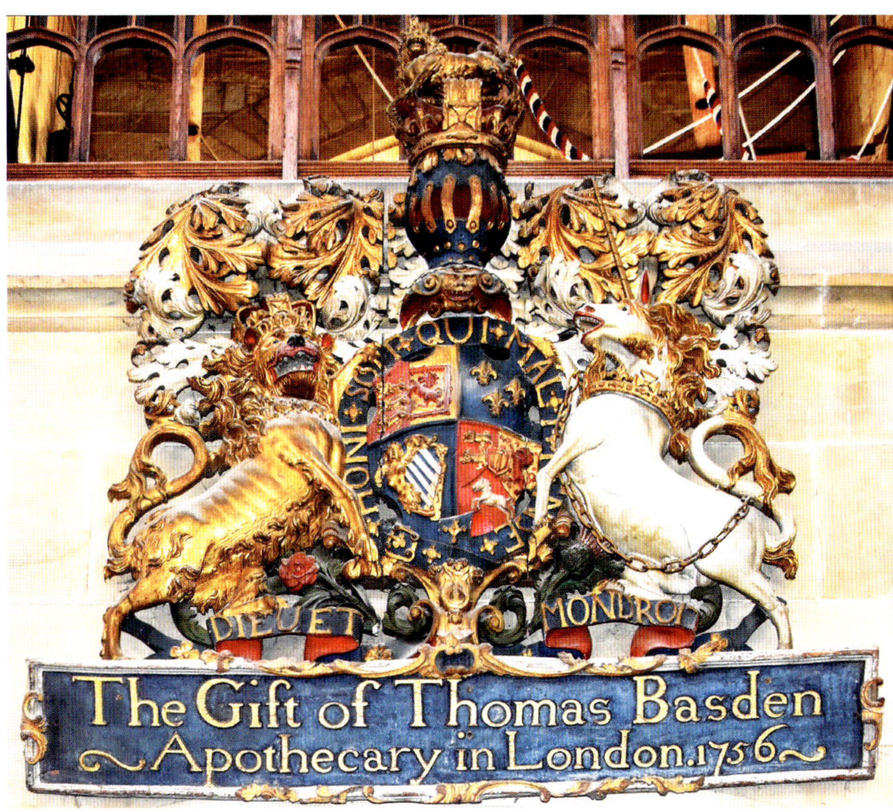
DIEU ET
MON DROIT
The Gift of Thomas Basden
Apothecary in London.1756

8.8 The Hanoverian Royal Arms (1714–1801) in St Dunstan's Church, Cranbrook, the gift of Thomas Basden

8.9 A clearer image of the Hanoverian Royal Arms 1714–1801

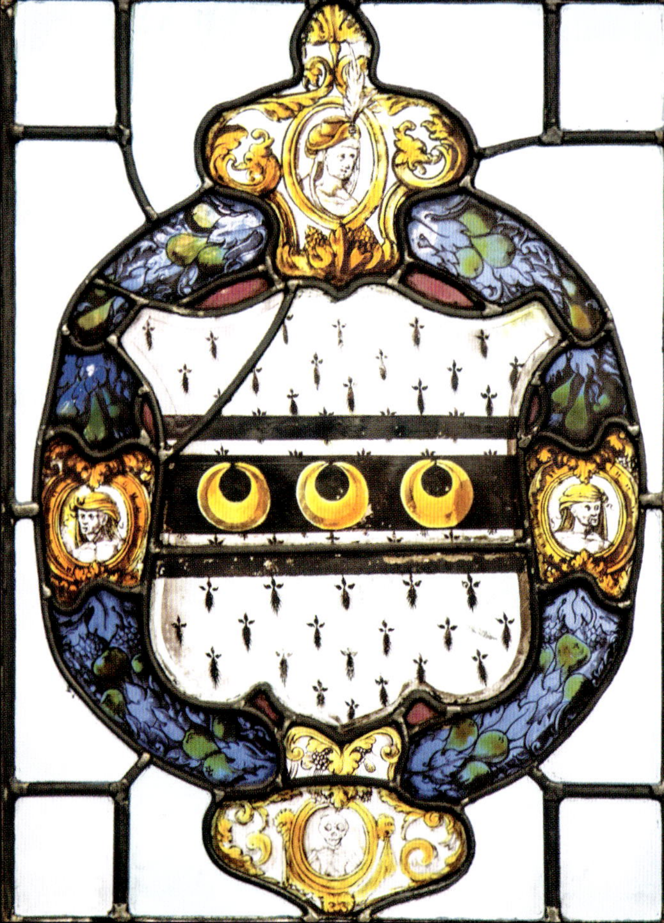

CHAPTER 9

The Bristow Panel in the Great Hall

The Master of the Society in 1803–04 was Dr Uriah Bristow, whose Arms are installed in the Great Hall in Window East 2, panel 14. The glass of the shield within the panel almost certainly dates from the sixteenth century and is therefore amongst the oldest stained glass in London. The history of the Bristow family, its connection with the Society and how this important panel of stained glass came to Apothecaries' Hall has been the subject of much research and is a matter of considerable interest.

In 1544, Nicholas Bristow (1494–1584) of Little Bibbesworth in Hertfordshire, the great-great-great-grandfather of Uriah Bristow, was appointed Clerk of the Jewels to King Henry VIII, a post he held for the remainder of Henry's reign, for the whole of the reigns of Edward VI and Mary I, and into the reign of Elizabeth I, until his retirement in 1561. Bristow accompanied Henry VIII to the siege and capture of Boulogne in 1544 as Clerk of the Wardrobe of Robes and Beds. Following this triumph, the King granted him the right to bear Arms, granted him the Manor of Ayot St Lawrence in Hertfordshire and promoted him to be Clerk of the Jewels.

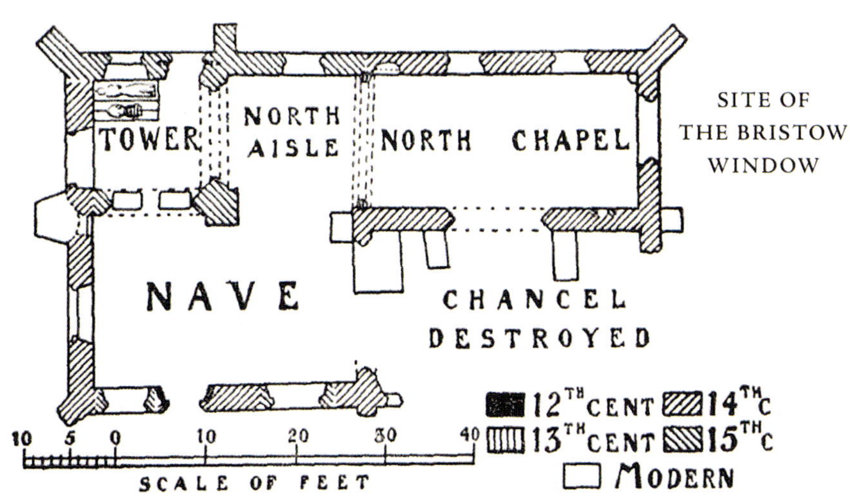

9.2 Plan of the ruin of Ayot St Lawrence Old Church

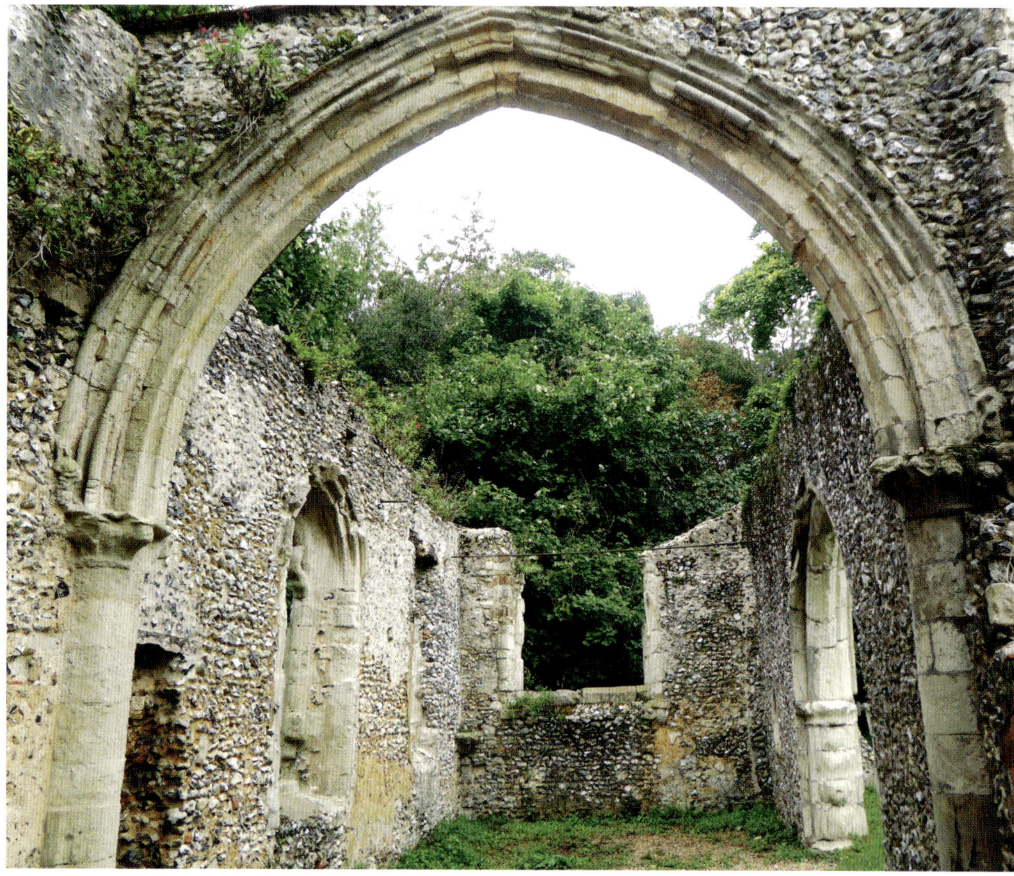

9.3 The Bristow (North) chapel in the ruin of Ayot St Lawrence Old Church, looking towards the former east window where the Bristow memorial window was installed

At the east end of the North Chapel of Ayot St Lawrence Old Church, now a ruin (Figures 9.2 and 9.3), a memorial stained glass window was installed in Bristow's memory, probably after his death in 1584, although, as will be shown below, there is doubt about the exact date of installation, for there is evidence that it may have been some years earlier.[1]

Early Accounts of the Bristow Window

Three early eighteenth-century accounts of the memorials in the church, including the stained glass, give an incomplete and confusing picture of what was actually present in the North Chapel, but a number of salient facts do emerge upon which there is some general agreement. The three antiquaries involved were: Sir Henry Chauncy (1632–1719),[2] Edward Steele (fl.1685–1760),[3] and Nathaniel Salmon (1675–1742).[4]

Chauncy, in 1700, restricts his description of the windows in the church to:

at the East End hereof are two Chancels; the Windows of both have been adorn'd with curious pictures, in stain'd and painted glass, beyond many other Churches; there is a Chapel that belongs to the Bristows, which has a curious wrought Window, in carved

> *Stone, and is adorn'd with painted Glass, wherein are the King's Arms, and the Arms of the Bristows.*

He does not describe the blazons of the Arms. He also mentions, on the south side of the Chapel, the tomb of Nicholas Bristow:

> *Here under lieth the Bodies of Nicholas Bristow, Esq; and Emme his Wife, which served the noble Princes King Henry the Eighth, King Edward, Queen Mary, Queen Elizabeth, and died the – day of – anno 15 - - . The Effigies of Eight Sons Four Daughters in Brass.*

Even in 1700, the engraving on the brass was obviously indistinct.

A collection of loose manuscripts by various writers, compiled and bound into a single volume by the antiquary Steele in *c.*1714, contains one manuscript, otherwise undated, which records the following more detailed description of the stained glass in the window at the east end of the North Chapel:

> *The East Window is curiously Painted and pretty entire but the core part is Wonderful fine wherein the middle light is the Arms and Supporters of Elizabeth. Under is 2 shields* [a description of the heraldry of the Bristow shield and that of his wife follows] … *on the North light is kneeling Nicholas Bristow in Armour and surcoat of Arms, behind him is eight sons. On the South light is his lady with 3 daughters She in her Mantle of Arms. In the middle pane is writt ~~much~~ Nicholas bristow esquire … son of this church and … nicholas served the princes King Henry VIII and ed*[ward] *some* [?] *Anno 1548.*

Again, the inscription was obviously indistinct or in part missing, and one word appears to be crossed out (Figure 9.4).

The mention of a middle, north and south light confirms that this was a three-light window. The description of the Royal Arms as being those of Elizabeth must be an assumption by the writer, since the Royal Arms of all the Tudor monarchs were identical. He may well have assumed that the window had been created after Nicholas Bristow's

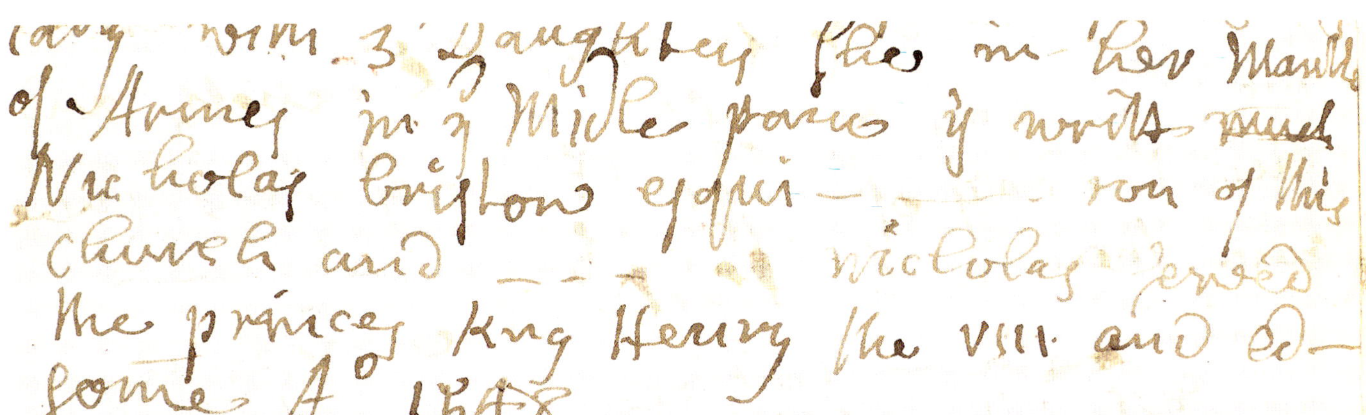
lady with 3 daughters she in her Mantle
of Armes in ye Midle pane is writt ~~much~~
Nicholas bristow esqui — son of this
church and — nicolas served
the princes King Henry the VIII and ed—
some Ao 1548

9.4 Part of the inscription in the middle light, recorded in the Steele manuscript

death, in which case the monarch at the time was indeed Elizabeth. However, although the Royal Arms, the original shield of which may survive (see Figure 9.8), are the Tudor Royal Arms they are differenced with a label of three points for the eldest son of the monarch. As Elizabeth had no direct heir, this raises the first of several questions about the date of the window. The description of eight sons in the north light agrees with the Chauncy description of the brass on the Bristow tomb, but the number of daughters described differs by one. Chauncy does not record the number of kneeling children in the window.

Only Steele's reporter mentions the inscription in the middle pane and plainly he had trouble reading it judging by the two blanks in the line. The inscription will be discussed later in this chapter, but it is not entirely clear what it means nor why it was not recorded by Chauncy in 1700 or by Salmon in 1728. Writing in 1728, Salmon describes the window as follows:

> *In the Chapel Window is fine Painting. The middle pane is the King's Arms. At the bottom those of Bristow; Ermine 3 Crescents Or upon a Fesse Sable. In a Pane to the Right of the King's Arms, a fine Figure of an old Man kneeling, with five Sons kneeling behind him. On the adverse Side the Figure of a Lady kneeling, with three Daughters behind her. On the Man's Habit Arms of Bristow; on the Woman's a Sort of Streamer, Azure 3 Eagles expanded Or. Below, Ermine three Barrulets wavy Or, quartered with this, Gules 3 Barrulets Or, on a Chief a Talbot passant.*

In describing the kneeling man as being in a pane to the right, Salmon must mean heraldic right, that is dexter, and this is confirmed by the Steele manuscript's description of the panel as being the north light. Contrary to the Steele manuscript, he describes the figure in the north light as having five sons kneeling behind him, while his description elsewhere of the brass tomb plate with eight sons agrees with Chauncy. The number of daughters kneeling behind the figure in the south light and on the tomb also tallies with Chauncy. It is of interest that Salmon describes the Royal Arms as the King's Arms. Although he does not mention the writing on the middle light described in the Steele manuscript, one cannot but wonder whether he was influenced by the 1548 date described by the same writer. This point will be discussed later.

It should be noted here that there is also confusion about Nicholas Bristow's wife's name. Chauncy and Salmon record her name on the Bristow tomb as 'Emme', whereas the Steele manuscript records her name on the same tomb as 'Luce'. The Bristow genealogies mostly describe her as Lucy,[5] but it was not uncommon for ladies to be referred to by different names on different memorials.

The Fate of the Bristow Memorial Window

The Manor of Ayot St Lawrence remained in the Bristow family for five generations. William Bristow (1649–1694), Nicholas' great-great-grandson died without a male heir. After his death, his widow Elizabeth sold the Manor to Thomas Lewis in 1714. The Lewis family in turn sold the Manor in 1723 to Cornelius Lyde, and on his death in 1747, it passed to his son-in-law, Sir Lionel Lyde Bt,[6] who allowed the church to fall into ruin and began its demolition. The Bishop of Lincoln, in whose diocese Ayot was then situated, halted the demolition but, with the consecration of a new bishop in 1761, permission was given for Sir Lionel to build a modern Grecian-style church on a nearby site and this was consecrated in 1779,[7] while the old church and its windows were allowed to continue to fall into ruin.

The middle light of the Bristow window, however, was at some stage rescued and moved to the Rectory at Ayot. This would have been between 1747 (when the church was allowed to start to become ruinous) and 1831 (when the window is known to have been in the Rectory – see below). A likely date for the move is *c.*1790, when the Rectory was rebuilt. It is probable that the other two lights were also taken out of the old church and stored at this time.

The much-altered middle light (Figure 9.5) is described by the author Carola Oman in her book *Ayot Rectory* published in 1965. In 1831 the Rector of Ayot, the Reverend John Olive, married a Miss Ellen Brown of Bath. Oman was fortunate to obtain as her principal source of information a manuscript book by Ellen Olive, together with other papers, which formed a memoir of Ellen's mother Mary Sneade. In her book, Oman describes in detail Ellen's first day at the Rectory. An extract from chapter seven follows:

> *As she came down the stairs now she noticed for the first time the brilliant afternoon sunshine glowing through one of the most beautiful windows she had ever seen – fit for a cathedral. Of course when they had arrived last night it would have appeared simply black. It was indeed one of the stained glass windows from the ruined church opposite, no doubt saved and taken across to the Parsonage by the Rector who had built the house in the days of William and Mary. But it was more than a hundred years older than those sovereigns. It displayed three armorial shields, one right royal, with the white and red roses of York and Lancaster, the other two, said John, Arms of a family called Bristow who had held much land hereabouts and were commemorated by a monument in the ruin opposite. There were silver eagles and ermines and talbots, and golden half-moons on crimson. It was impossible to avoid thinking of St Agnes' Eve.*[8]

It should be noted that there is no mention of supporters for the Royal Arms. Instead, the surround of roses (presumably with greenery) is described and there is no mention of an inscription.

This middle light was still in the Rectory in 1910,[9] but is now hung, boxed and backlit, in Ayot St Lawrence New Church. It shows the Royal Arms without supporters and below, the conjoined Bristow and Bristow/Bibbesworth/Barley/Skipwith Arms, each shield surrounded by cameos, roses and greenery, and all mounted in a field of quarries.

It is impossible to determine whether the glass of the three shields is the original sixteenth-century glass, as the window is boxed and sealed and cannot be opened for close inspection. However, in view of the likelihood that the shield from the north light in a panel now in the possession of the Society of Apothecaries is generally agreed to be sixteenth century in date, it is not unreasonable to presume that all four shields are contemporary.

The glass of the surrounds of the lower two shields, together with that of the Apothecaries' Hall shield, may in fact be early seventeenth-century Dutch glass, and the surround of the Royal Arms is thought to be much more recent.[10] It is possible that some or all of this newer glass was added when the window was installed in the rebuilt Rectory in 1790. However, it is also possible that the surrounding quarries may be even more recent and, in addition, the current window is undoubtedly somewhat smaller than the original.

Dr Uriah Bristow, a second cousin twice removed of the last Bristow of Ayot, had no surviving male heir. His youngest daughter married John Hughes (1786–1827). In about 1820, John Hughes visited Ayot St Lawrence and found in the estate yard some pieces of stained glass, amongst which he recognised the Bristow Arms and those of Nicholas' wife Luce/Emme.[11] These he acquired, and with a roundel of his own Arms had them made into a window for his house in Wallasey in Cheshire. The two panels from Ayot must have come from the north and south lights of the original window. The fate of the remainder of those lights, that is the kneeling figures with children, is unknown, despite extensive searches in the Ayot St Lawrence area.

In 1939, three of John Hughes' grandsons, Robert Bristow Hughes (1868–1940), a solicitor, Edward Herbert Hughes (1870–1940) and Leonard John Hughes (1873–1967), an architect, who were living in the Wallasey house, had the stained glass removed, crated and stored in their cellar for the duration of the war. The next year during an air attack on Liverpool, the house was destroyed and the two elder brothers were killed. The glass survived. After the war Leonard lived with his two sisters, Emily Frances Bristow Hughes (1877–1967) and Margaret Bristow Hughes (1879–1965), with the window remaining crated in their garage.

On the death in 1967 of Leonard, the last of the trio of brothers, the crated window came into the possession of his niece Mrs Diana Bousted, a great-great-great-granddaughter of Uriah Bristow. At the suggestion of Liveryman Dr Peter Francis White (1899–1994), who was Mrs Bousted's second cousin and a great-great-great-grandson of Uriah Bristow, the family very generously donated the panel with the Bristow Arms to the Society. The gift was made in 1980, as described in Chapter 4. The correspondence concerning the gift is in the Society's Archive.[12]

The Heraldry of the Surviving Middle Light

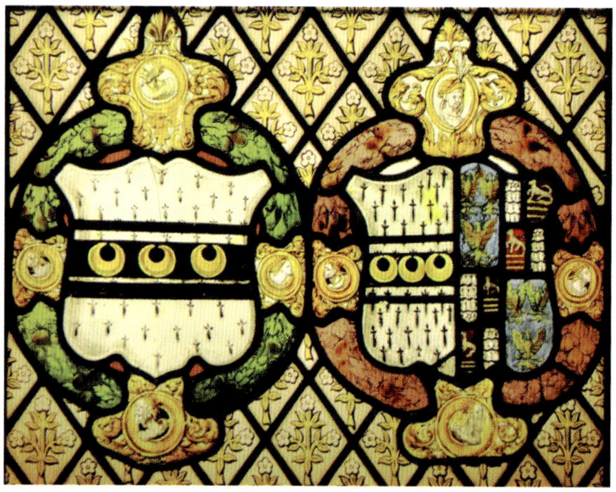

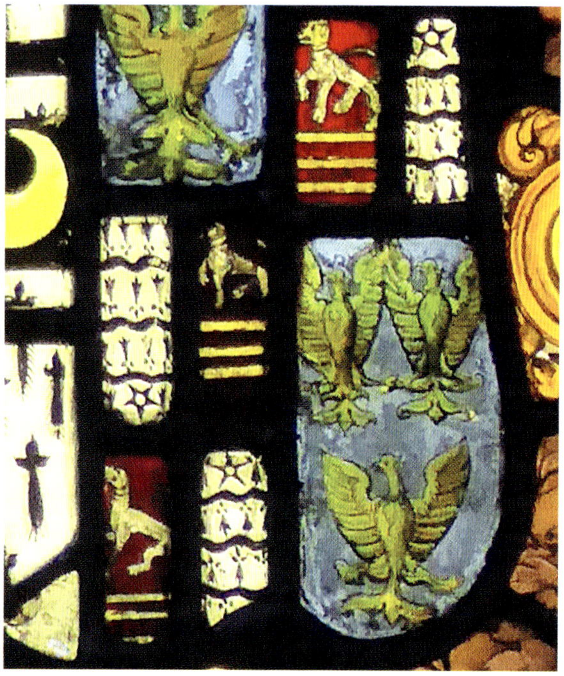

9.6 Detail of the Bristow and Barley family arms in the middle light

9.7 Further detail showing the error in the Barley Arms

The lower left of the three shields (Figure 9.6) is the undifferenced Arms of Bristow and is identical to the shield in Apothecaries' Hall (see Figure 9.1). The surrounding wreath and four cameos are very similar to the Apothecaries' Hall example, except for the colour of the wreath and the details of the cameos.

The lower-right shield is an impaled husband-and-wife grouping (Figure 9.6). The Arms on the dexter side are again those of Bristow but the ones on the sinister side, which should be those of Nicholas Bristow's wife Lucy/Emme Barlye/Barley, display a number of heraldic inconsistencies. They are described in *The Victoria County History* as Bibbesworth quartered with Barley and Skipwith.[13] Lucy Barley was the daughter of Robert Barley of nearby Great Bibbesworth, who married Joan Skipwith of South Ormesby in Lincolnshire.

The Arms of Bibbesworth are *Azure, three eagles displayed Or*; it would seem that the Barleys as lord of the manor of Bibbesworth had appropriated these.[14] The Arms with which they are quartered are described as Barley (1st and 4th) and Skipwith (2nd and 3rd). The Hertfordshire Barleys bore *Ermine three bars wavy Sable*,[15] which is what these Arms are with the addition of a rowel in chief. This must have been an addition for a cadet family of Barleys, possibly a third son using a mullet/spur rowel as a cadency mark. In the 1st grand-quarter of the 3rd quarter, the rowel is shown in base (Figure 9.7), rather than in chief and, in fact, this piece of glass has been installed upside down with the ermine tails standing up rather than hanging down.

The use of the Skipwith Arms is slightly confusing, as Joan Skipwith was not an heraldic heiress, having an elder brother Sir John Skipwith (1454–1518) who continued the Skipwith line and therefore these Arms should not be displayed by the Barleys.[16] The Arms of Skipwith of Ormesby are *Argent, three bars Gules, a Greyhound in full course in chief Sable, collared Or*. A further point of confusion is that the Skipwith Arms in this panel are not the Ormesby colours but a cadet shown as *Gules, three bars, a greyhound in full course in chief Or*.

A possible explanation of Lucy's Arms is that the last male Bibbesworth of Bibbesworth died in 1485 – and possibly young, as the date may connect him with the troubles of Richard III. The Barleys thereafter acquired Bibbesworth, and if it was by marrying the heiress, then they would have quartered the Barley and Bibbesworth Arms. The introduction of Skipwith is perplexing, as discussed above, but this may all have been a status issue. If the spur rowel does indicate a Barley younger son then he may have quartered, however incorrectly, the original family Arms with Skipwith, another important family, to allow his Bibbesworth significance to be stressed by occupying a full quarter rather than the smaller grand-quarter. It was all a question of family prestige, which Arms are very useful to display. All this indicates the difficulties encountered when attempting to interpret the descent of armorial bearings, a problem that has continued through the centuries to the present day, and which has arisen with regard to a number of the armorial panels in the Great Hall (see Appendix I).

The display of the Royal Arms (Figure 9.8) is of particular interest, being extremely rare, as it is differenced with a label of three points for the eldest son of the King. In early heraldry the label could be used to indicate any of the children of an armiger, with different tinctures or additional charges for different sons. The earliest known use of the label was by Saer de Quincy, Earl of Winchester (d.1219), who was a younger son.

During the lifetime of their fathers, the future Edward I (heir 1239–72), Edward II (heir 1284–1307) and Edward III (heir 1312–27) charged their shields with *Azure* labels

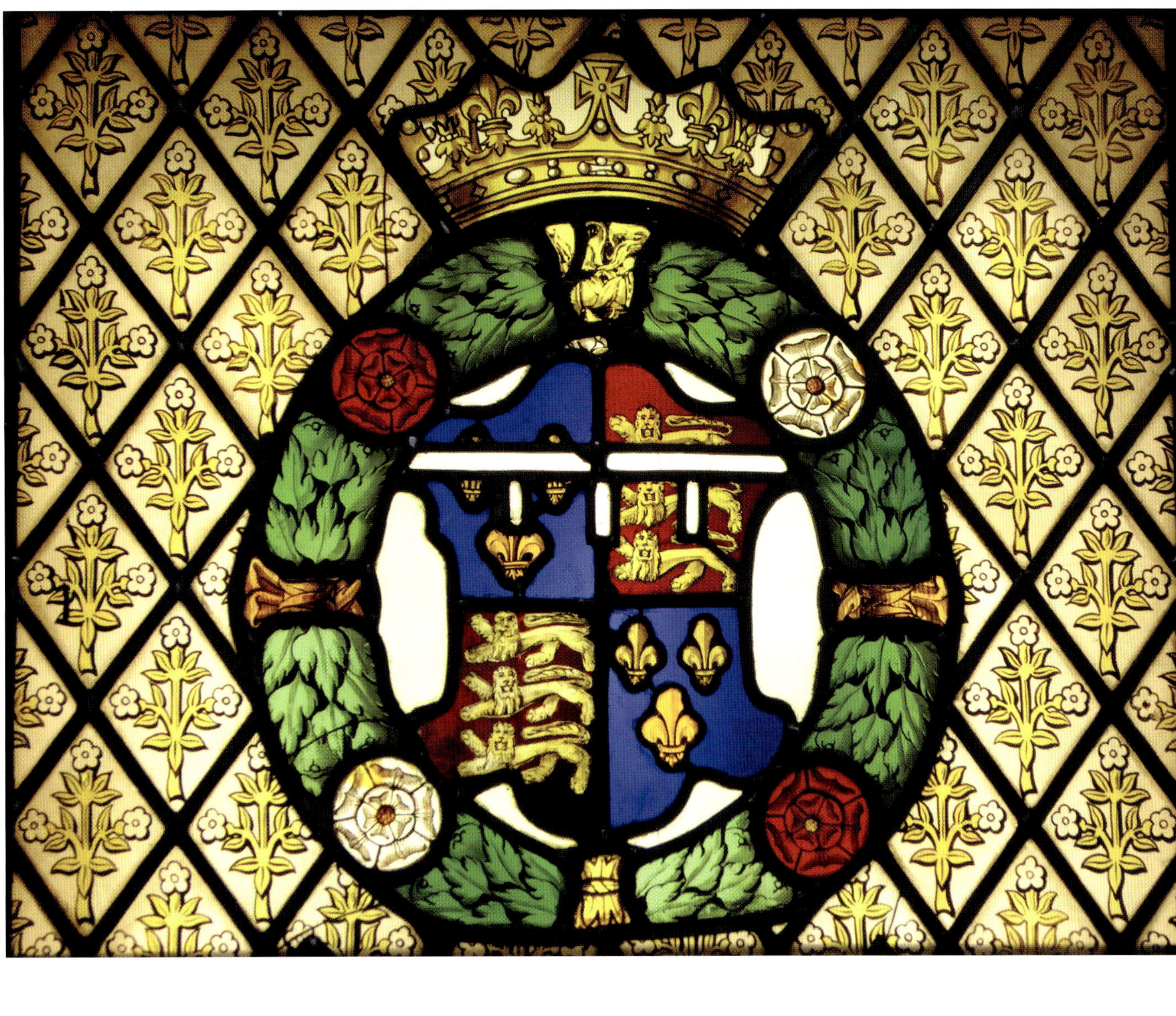

9.8 The Tudor Royal Arms with a Label of three points

of three or five points as the eldest son. It was not until the time of Edward the Black Prince (1330–1376) that the label of the heir became *Argent* of three points. In royal heraldry, younger sons of the king continued to use labels and theirs were differenced by tincture and also by the addition of charges on the points. This practice continues today, although, in non-royal heraldry, the label is used solely by the eldest son in his father's lifetime.[17]

These Royal Arms are those of the Tudor monarchs of England, with the addition of the label. It is thus unique, as the only person to bear these Arms during the period under consideration was Prince Edward in the period 1537–47, before he became Edward VI (1547–53). If this is the original Royal shield, it becomes an important factor in determining the age of all the shield glass. It is worth recording that these Royal Arms could not have been made after 1603, when there would have been a new Stuart Heir Apparent whose Royal Arms would have included a quarter for Scotland, which is absent in this panel.

There is a further perplexing issue to be considered: the surrounds of the three coats of Arms in the centre light. Steele reports that the Royal Arms had supporters, which can only mean that the surround of Tudor roses and greenery was not present when described in the Steele manuscript *c.*1714. This strongly supports the supposition that this surround was added later, perhaps when the window was revived and moved to the Rectory, as discussed above. The impression is that the whole window was in a poor state and that only the significant heraldic glass was recovered.

Assuming that the panels recovered by Hughes in 1820 came from the surcoats of Nicholas Bristow and his wife in the north and south lights, then these elaborate cameo and fruit surrounds are unlikely again to have been in the original composition as they are not part of the family heraldry.

The second shield recovered by Hughes in 1820, of which there is no image extant, is lost, but if it too was surrounded by identical Dutch remnant glass of cameos and fruit, this was presumably all done simply to create a pleasing artistic display. If this occurred at the same time as the addition of the surround to the Royal Arms prior to the transfer to the Rectory, it seems strange that the north and south light shields were similarly decorated just to lie discarded in an estate store. Perhaps there simply was not room for them in the Rectory. This conundrum may never be resolved.

The crown over the Royal Arms is also perplexing. On the face of it, without a cap of maintenance, arches or orb, this is not a king's crown – which reinforces the contention that these are a prince's Arms. It may or may not be original to the original Arms, in that the Arms in 1714 were described as having supporters, which implies also having a crowned helm. Possibly this is the original prince's open circlet, restored when the recoverable parts of the church window were re-used in the Rectory window or a circlet from a separate work added to give the Royal Arms status. The last king to use a crown of this simplicity, without arches, was Henry IV.[18] All depictions of Henry VIII's and subsequent monarchs' crowns have the cap of maintenance and four arches surmounted by an orb.

The Age of the Bristow Shield Glass

It seems reasonable to presume that a memorial, in this case a stained glass window, would not be installed until after the death of the person to be commemorated. Nicholas Bristow died in 1584 and it is therefore strange, to say the least, that the Royal Arms used, if the glass is original, should be those of King Edward VI as Prince of Wales, a position he relinquished on ascending the throne in 1547, thirty-seven years earlier.

As already mentioned, the Steele manuscript describes the middle light as bearing an inscription which includes the date 1548, an inscription which incidentally also seems to refer to Nicholas Bristow as having only served Henry VIII and Edward VI, which was indeed the case in 1548. However, it is certainly not clear to what exactly the date refers. If it refers to the date of installation, then it is perhaps not unreasonable to postulate that the glassmaker may simply have assumed that the Arms used by the Heir Apparent would continue to be used when he became king. This was after all only one year after Edward's succession to the throne.

However, Steele is the one source which calls the Royal Arms the Queen's Arms, which may, of course, simply indicate that the writer writing about 120 years later was aware that Bristow had died in the reign of Elizabeth, the window having nevertheless been installed at an earlier date.

If this window was made in 1548, during Bristow's lifetime, what reason was there to make it? It was not a significant year nationally nor, it seems, in Bristow's career. Bristow was a powerful royal official close to the old king, but this was no reason to install a memorial window for himself. The gaps in the inscription might have told the story, perhaps a generous endowment to the church from Bristow as the Patron of the Living? There is simply not enough evidence to draw any firm conclusion. If it does date from 1548, this might explain the varying number of sons and daughters recorded on window and tomb, as some failed to survive childhood and others were born after this date.

Leonard Hughes, who died in 1967, sent a photograph of the window in his house at Wallasey to the Victoria and Albert Museum. In a paper dated July 1980, the year in which the family gave the Bristow panel to the Society, his descendent, Liveryman Dr Peter White, records this and quotes the reply from the museum as follows:

> *I should say the uppermost shield [Bristow] was made about mid-16th century. In style it very closely resembles some heraldic glass at Chequers, Bucks, known to date from 1540. It is possible that the fragments with fruit flanking the shield may come from a Dutch enamel painted window of the beginning of the 17th century. There is another similar window in existence. This, probably formed from the centre light of the Ayot church window, is now in the possession of Lord Brocket, the present owner of Ayot. The Hughes window would have come from the two outer lights.*[19]

Enquiries at Chequers in 2019 failed to corroborate the above statement. Enquiries in Ayot St Lawrence suggest that the connection with Lord Brocket is likely simply to refer to the fact that the window was somewhere on the Brocket estate. It seems beyond reasonable doubt, therefore, that the window described as being in the possession of Lord Brocket is the window which was in the Rectory and which is now in Ayot St Lawrence New Church. The dates when it was removed from the Rectory and subsequently installed in the New Church are not known.

When the Bristow panel arrived at Apothecaries' Hall in 1980 it was shown to Carl Edwards, who reported that:

> *there seems to be no doubt that the Coat of Arms is 16th century. It is typical work of that period and it is possible that the Society of Antiquaries might even know where it was made and give a fairly accurate date. As a point of interest Southwark Cathedral were given a 16th century Coat of Arms and were claiming to have the oldest piece of stained glass in London.*[20]

The suggestion that the Society of Antiquaries should be approached was followed up by the current authors, but no further information was discovered.

Conclusion

It is likely that the five armorial shields (the Centre light Royal Arms, Bristow and impaled Arms (see Figure 9.5)) plus the North light Bristow Arms (see Figure 9.1) and the missing South light Bibbesworth/Barley/Skipworth Arms without their surrounds are sixteenth century and contemporaneous. The exact date of this stained glass must remain uncertain. Nicholas Bristow entered royal employment in 1542, was granted Ayot St Lawrence in 1544 and died in 1584, so it is virtually certain that the Bristow Arms shield is mid- to late sixteenth century in date.

The pointers that tend to support a late sixteenth-century date (post-1584) for the Bristow shield glass are:

- A memorial window almost invariably post-dates the death of the individual commemorated.
- The kneeling figures in the north and south lights, together with their children and the later addition of the skeleton in the bottom cameo, suggest that this was a *post-mortem* memorial window, although, if of an earlier date, the skeleton could simply be a *memento mori*.
- In 1728, Nathaniel Salmon described the north light as showing 'a fine figure of an <u>old</u> man'.

– The Royal Arms are described by an observer in about 1714 as 'the Arms and Supporters of Elizabeth'.

– In the key inscription on the window, mentioned in the Steele manuscript, a transcription error by the painter of the glass or the antiquarian may have occurred, simply recording 1584 as 1548.

The clues that might indicate an earlier mid-sixteenth century date (1548) are:

– the assessment of the date of the shields by the Victoria and Albert Museum.

– the specific date of 1548 recorded by Steele.

– the Royal Arms of Prince Edward with the label of three points and Prince's circlet.

– the Royal Arms are described by Nathaniel Salmon in 1728 as 'the King's Arms'.

– the lack of any mention of Queen Mary or Queen Elizabeth in the Steele inscription, possibly indicating that the glass was made before their reigns.

While we are unlikely ever to know the exact date of the Bristow panel, it is undoubtedly the oldest glass in Apothecaries' Hall and one of the oldest panels in the City of London.

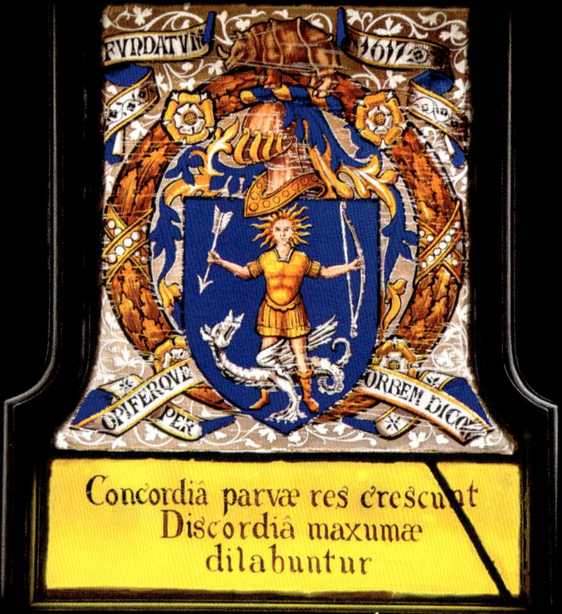

FVNDATVM
1617
OPIFERQVE
PER
ORBEM DICOR
Concordiâ parvæ res crescunt
Discordiâ maxumæ
dilabuntur

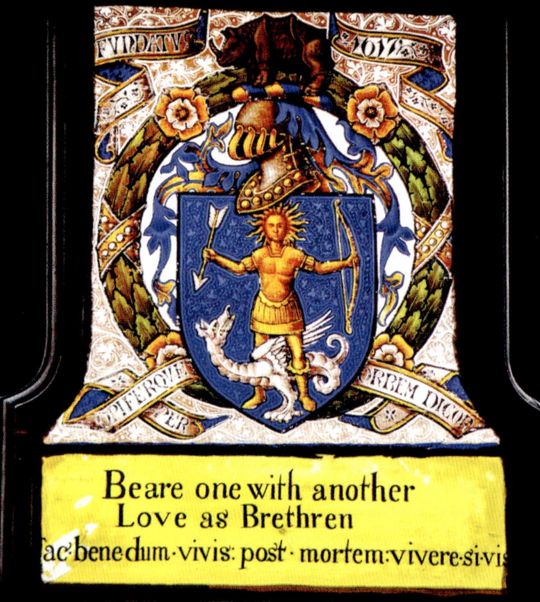

1617
OPIFERQVE
PER
ORBEM DICOR
Beare one with another
Love as Brethren
ac·bene dum·vivis: post· mortem:vivere·si·vis

CHAPTER 10

The Landing and Library Windows and the Missing Panel

The First Floor Landing

At the time of writing, nothing is known of the provenance of the two stained glass panels in the Landing windows (Figure 10.1).

In his book *The History of the Society of Apothecaries*, C. R. B. Barrett describes the panels as being in the Library in 1905.[1] Until the major refurbishment of 1928, described in Chapter 4, the Library was a longer room, extending eastwards towards the doors of the Great Hall and incorporating what is now the right hand of the two windows on the Landing as viewed from inside. A photograph taken from the Courtyard in a paper in the Society's Archive dated 7 December 1917 shows only the two most easterly windows of the Library before it was shortened, but the unusual shape of one of the panels can be clearly seen in the left-hand window, although which of the two it is impossible to identify (Figure 10.2).[2]

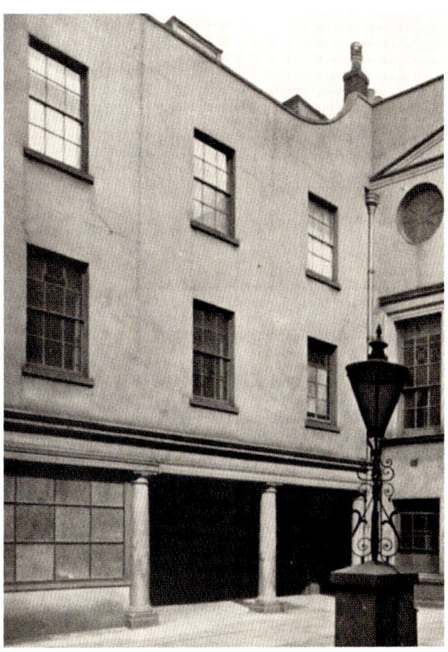

10.2 A 1917 photograph, showing on the first floor, the two easterly windows of the Library, one with a stained glass panel, and the then single Landing window

Together with other stained glass from the Hall, these panels were removed to the crypt of the Foundling Hospital at Berkhamsted for safe-keeping during the Second World War. The estimate by James Powell and Sons for removing the stained glass from the Hall windows, dated 2 September 1941, includes the removal of 'two small windows from the *Library*', an entry which must refer to these two panels.[3] After the panels were returned from Berkhamsted after the war, it is not clear when they were installed in their present position. An undated photograph, likely to have been taken in early 1946, shows the west wall of the Great Hall with all its armorial glass reinstalled (by James Powell and Sons), but with the circular windows above still unrepaired and the Landing windows with no armorial glass. A photograph of the Courtyard in 1980 does, however, clearly show the distinctive shape of the two panels installed in the Landing windows (Figure 10.3). On balance, therefore, and in the absence of any archival evidence to the contrary, the likelihood is that they were in due course installed in their present position by James Powell.

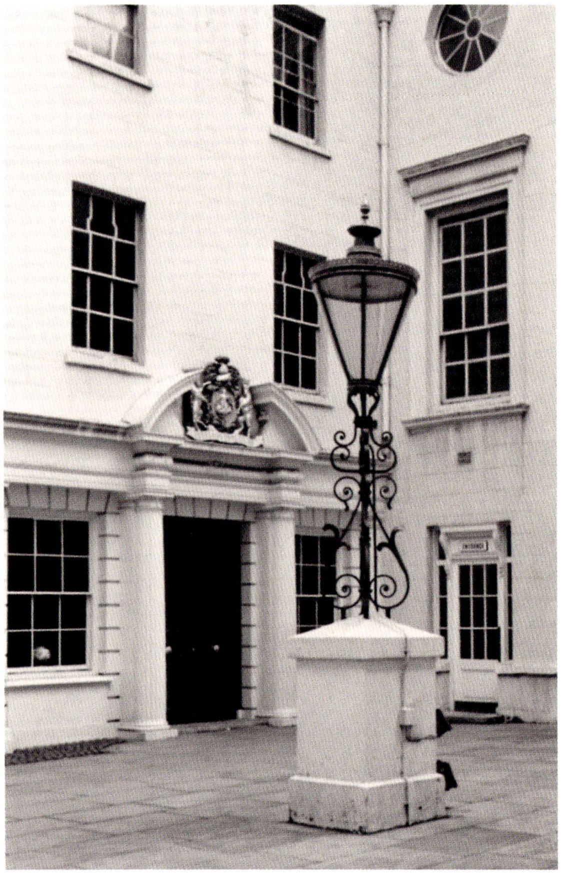

10.3 The Courtyard in 1980, showing the distinctive shape of the two stained glass panels in the Landing windows

The Panels

In each of the two Landing windows the upper-middle pane is a panel of stained glass of very distinctive shape, featuring in both cases the armorial bearings of the Society (Figures 10.1 and 10.3). The two panels are similar in that they both depict Apollo astride the dragon, with the rhinoceros crest above, the motto below, but without supporters and each headed 'Fundatum 1617'. The Arms sit within an unusual wreath, one green, the other gold and both decorated with four roses. Erroneously, the mantling is shown in the Society colours, *Azure doubled Or*, rather than the prescribed *Gules doubled Argent*.

The panel on the left shows Apollo on a clear field of blue flashed glass. The quotation beneath is painted in black on clear yellow glass. The whole panel is very badly scratched, damage which may have occurred at the time of storage during the war. It is the opinion of Dr Jasmine Allen, Curator of the Stained Glass Museum at Ely Cathedral, that the panel is probably eighteenth century in date.[4]

The panel on the right is more delicately painted which, in Allen's opinion, may indicate a more recent date, probably nineteenth century. The quotation beneath is painted in black on a panel which has been stained yellow on its outer surface with silver stain, the sheen of which can be clearly seen from the Courtyard. The patterned decoration around Apollo is mediaeval in design but the whole panel is Victorian in style. A few scratches are present.

Allen is also of the opinion that the script beneath the left-hand panel looks more recent than that beneath the right-hand panel, and she therefore wonders whether the inscriptions may have been switched at some stage.

No explanation for the curious shape of the panels has been found. The first letter of the third line of the inscription on the right-hand panel, a capital F, is obscured by the woodwork of the frame, which may indicate that the panel was originally made for a larger frame. The wording, translation and source of each inscription is as follows:

Left panel

Concordia parvae res crescent Discordia maxumae dilabuntur, which translates as 'With harmony small things grow, while with discord the mightiest are ruined.' This is taken from 'Bellum Jugurthinum' Chapter 10,[5] by the Republican Roman writer Gaius Sallustius Crispus (86–*c.*35 BCE), commonly known as Sallust.

Right panel

'Beare one with another Love as Brethren.' This comes from the first epistle of St Peter 3:8.

Fac bene dum vivis : post mortem : vivere si vis. This an anonymous mediaeval Latin proverb.[6] The full couplet is:

> *O dives, dives non vives omni tempore*
>
> *Fac bene dum vivis, post mortem vivere si vis*
>
> *O rich man, rich man, you will not live for ever!*
>
> *Do good while you live, if you want to live after death.*

The Library

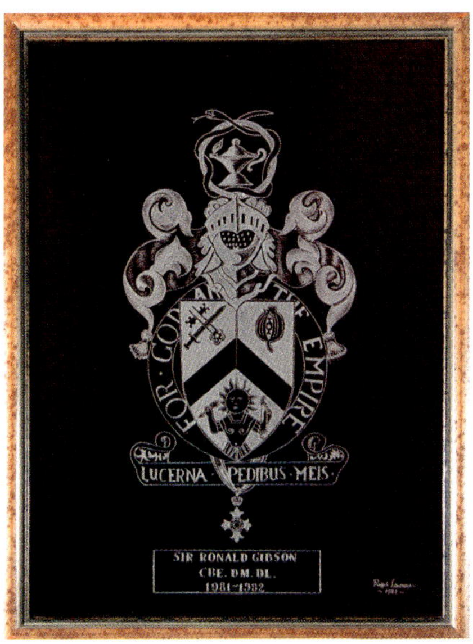

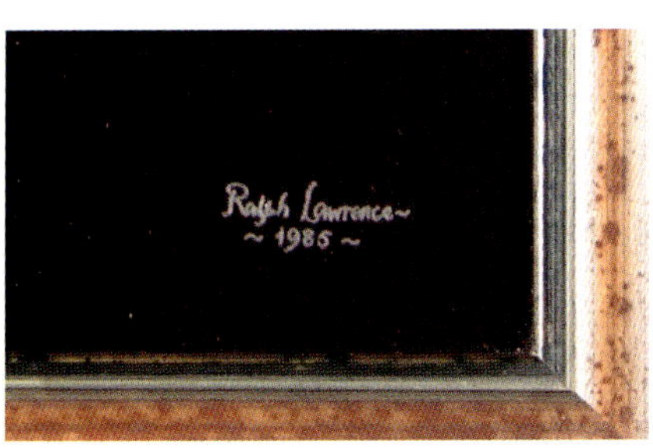

10.4 The Arms of Sir Ronald Gibson

10.5 Signature of Ralph Lawrence

In the Library hangs the only modern panel displaying the armorial bearings of a Master which are not in the Great Hall. These are the Arms of Sir Ronald Gibson (Master 1981–82). They are engraved on plain clear glass and set in a frame with a burgundy velvet background (Figure 10.4). The panel was designed and executed by Ralph Lawrence in 1985 and is signed and dated (Figure 10.5). The Arms are blazoned thus:

> *Per pale Sable and Argent, a Chevron counterchanged between in chief two Keys endorsed in bend, bows interlaced, the upper Or, the nether Argent, with a Sword interposed in bend sinister also Argent, hilt and pommel Or, and a Pomegranate Proper, in base issuant a representation of Apollo with bow and arrow also Or; And for the Crest upon a Knight's helm, mantled Sable doubled Argent, an ancient Lamp Or, enflamed proper, within an Annulet also Or entwined by a Serpent Vert.*

The motto comes from Psalm 119, '***Lucerna pedibus meis*** *verbum tuum et lumen semitis meis*' (Thy word is a lamp unto my feet and a light unto my path) and alludes to the crest, which also appears in the Arms of the Royal College of General Practitioners (RCGP). The field and chevron are from the Arms of St Bartholomew's Hospital, where Sir Ronald trained and also from the RCGP Arms; the interlaced keys and sword are from the Arms of the Bishopric of Winchester; the pomegranate is a symbol of fertility and appears in the Arms of three medical Royal Colleges and the British Medical Association; Apollo is from the Society's Arms.

The disadvantage of displaying the Arms in this way is that the colours are lost and they do not lend themselves to the conventional hatching for two-tone heraldry (see Glossary). As a result, the artist has an impossible task. The shield is wrong, as the counterchanged field and chevron cannot be displayed correctly. The left-hand side of the field should be dark with a light chevron, which would make it difficult to display the

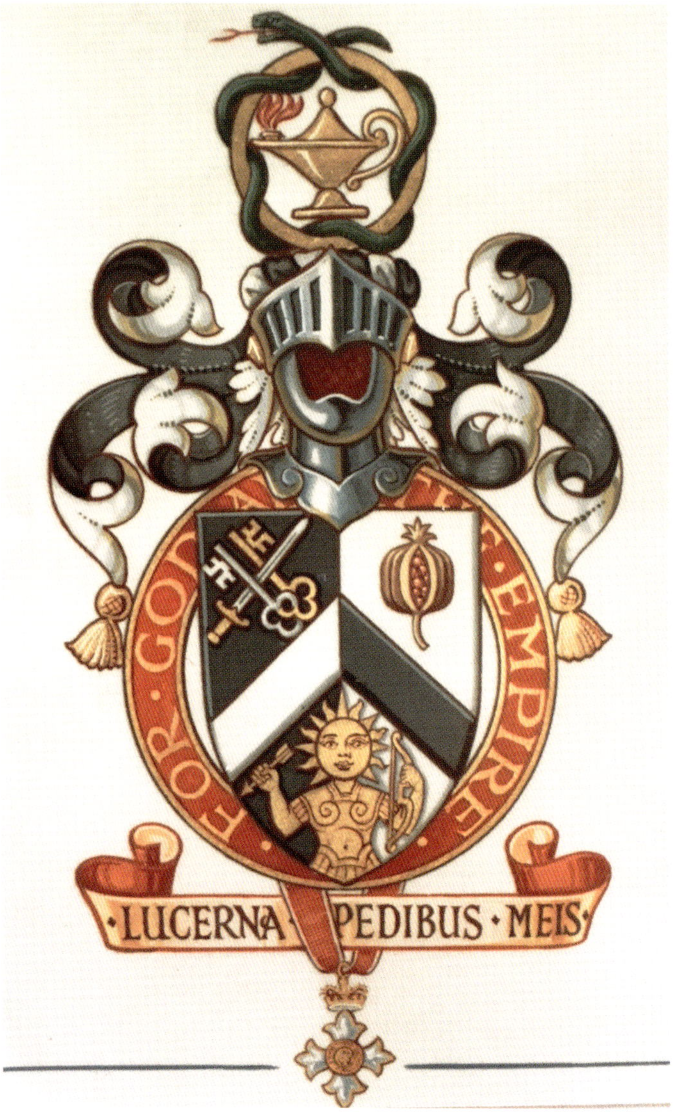

10.6 The Gibson Arms in colour

keys and sword, and a third colour would be needed for Apollo as he should not be two tone. The correctly coloured version of the Arms is shown in Figure 10.6.

The technique employed was hand-held diamond and carborundum wheel engraving, as for the Ruijterman panel in the Cloakroom.

Although it was plainly the choice of Sir Ronald Gibson himself that his Arms should be engraved rather than displayed in stained glass, his decision engendered a considerable amount of discussion in various committees. At one point, it was suggested that all armorial bearings should be displayed only in stained glass,[7] but it may have been the intention that this should apply only to the Great Hall. The possibility of back-lighting the panel was also discussed but finally a black, non-lit background was agreed upon. In the event, a burgundy-coloured background was used – and to good artistic, if not heraldic, effect.

The Missing Panel

In the same chapter in which Barrett mentions the two panels on the Landing, he also describes the first-floor landing – or 'main corridor' as he calls it – as being 'long and lofty; lighted at one end by a window in which … appear the Arms of the Society'.[8] Photographs of this window in 1910, 1911 and again in 1917 taken from the Courtyard show that at those dates the glazing was very different to that in the window to its left, which was still within the Library at that time (Figure 10.7).

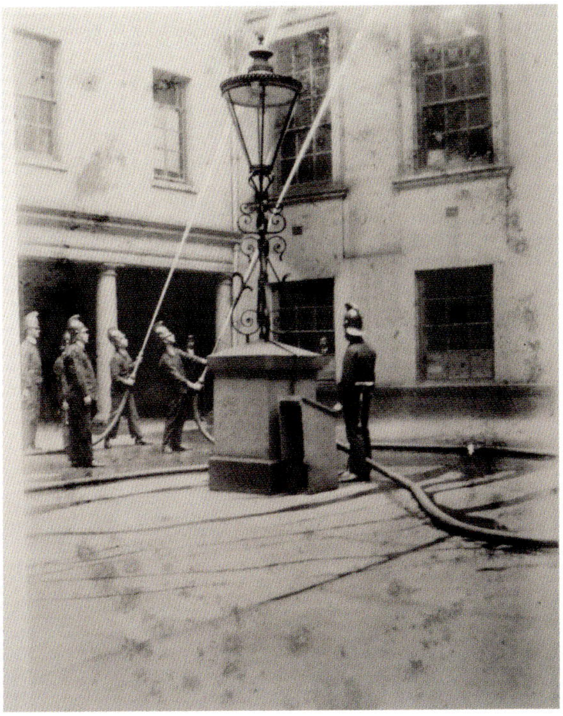

1910

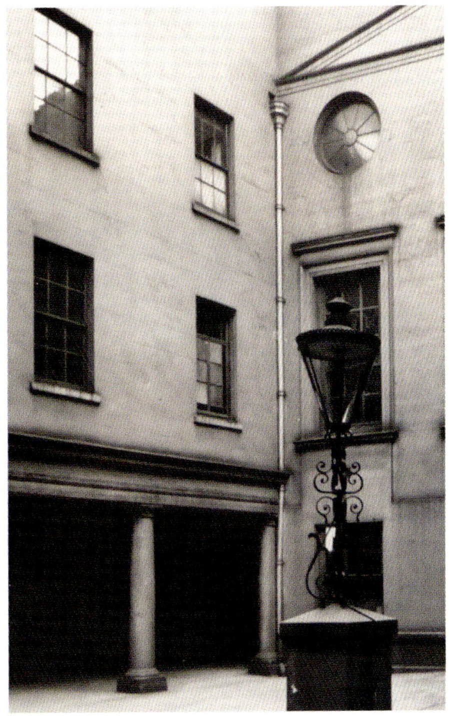

1911

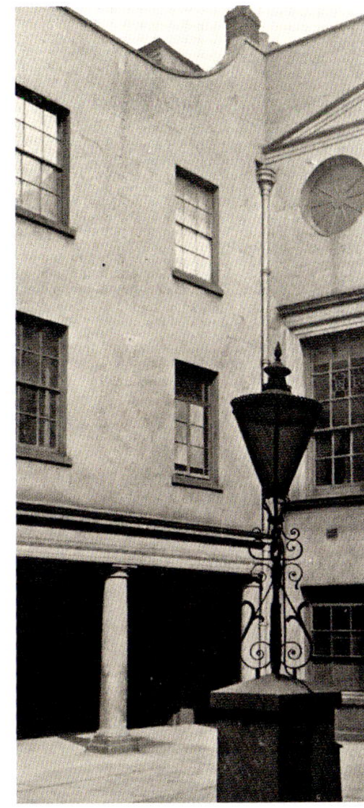

1917

10.7 The window at the end of the first floor 'corridor' on the right above the colonnade in 1910, 1911 and 1917

Firstly, the window is only two-panes wide (comparison with the window above confirms this); secondly, the top pane of the window seems to be a single pane extending across the whole width of the window; and thirdly, it appears to have a border of glass of a different 'colour'. In a pamphlet in the Society's Archive entitled 'The Apothecary Ancient and Modern of the City of London' by George Corfe MD (Master 1884–85), the contents of the Hall are listed, including the stained glass.[9] One item is a panel in the 'passage' (which must mean the first-floor landing 'main corridor' to which Barrett refers), which Corfe describes as showing the 'Arms of the Society' and mentions that it was presented to the Society by Richard Strong Eyles (Master 1852–53). If this is the panel described by Barrett, which seems very likely, then it must now be considered lost. Although there is no archival evidence to support this, it is likely that this window was widened at the time of the 1928–29 major refurbishment.

CHAPTER 11

Heraldic Strays

'Heraldic stray' is an informal term for finding Arms in an unexpected place. In this chapter strays will be considered in two parts: non-Society Arms found in the Hall, and Society's Arms found outside the Hall.

Heraldic Strays in the Hall

The Entrance Hall

As a result of a very close relationship with two livery companies, the Worshipful Company of Turners and the Worshipful Company of Spectacle Makers, permission to install stained glass panels of their Arms in the Hall was granted by the Court in 1961.[1] The panels were made at the Hall by Carl Edwards (see Chapter 7).

The Arms of the Company of Turners, which received its Royal Charter in 1604 and which ranks in the City as Company number 51, just ahead of the Society at number 58, are displayed in the Entrance Hall in a window to the east of the double Courtyard doors (Figure 11.1).

The Society has had a strong relationship with the Turners since 1945, when the Masterships of the Society, the Company of Barbers and the Company of Turners were held simultaneously by Sir Stanley Woodwark. The Turners had sold their second Hall on College Hill in 1766 and with the destruction of most of the Halls in the Second World War, Sir Stanley invited the Turners to use Apothecaries' Hall for Court meetings and social functions, an arrangement which continues to this day.

The Turners' Arms, which were granted in 1634, are:

Azure, a Catherine Wheel between two Columns, in chief an Imperial Crown Or and in base a Hatchet fesswise to the sinister, head downwards, Argent, handled Or. And for the Crest, upon a helm, mantled Azure doubled Or, on a wreath Or and Azure, the figure of St. Catherine crowned Or with a nimbus, wearing a Gown Gules with a Girdle Or about her Waist beneath a Mantle Azure furred Ermine, holding in the dexter hand a Catherine Wheel Or and in the sinister a Sword Argent, hilted Or, the point downwards. St Catherine is the patron Saint of Turners.

Supporters were not granted and the motto, which is not shown, is *'By faith I obteigne'*.

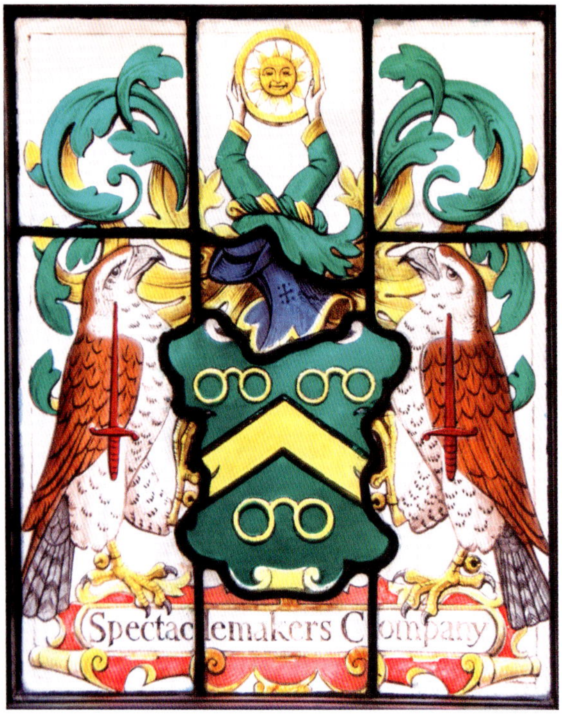

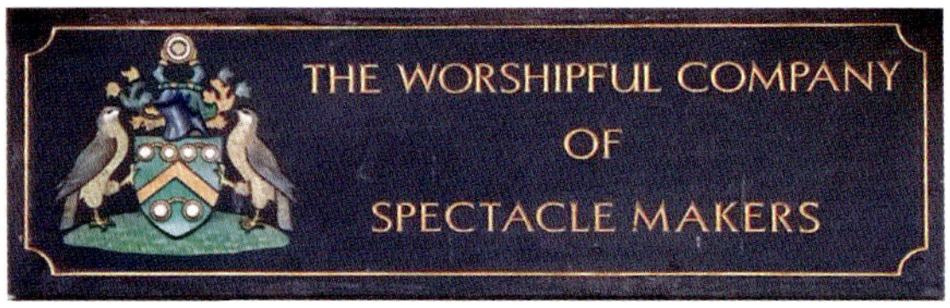

11.2 The Arms of the Worshipful Company of Spectacle Makers in the Entrance Hall

11.3 The plaque above the door of the offices of the Worshipful Company of Spectacle Makers in the Courtyard

The Turners still maintain a display cabinet in the Entrance Hall which contains some outstanding examples of the art and craft of turning.

The Arms of the Company of Spectacle Makers, which received its Royal Charter in 1629 and which ranks in the City as Company number 60, just behind the Society, are displayed in the Entrance Hall in a window to the west of the double Courtyard doors (Figure 11.2).

The Society has had a close relationship with the Spectacle Makers since 1946, when they became our tenants and have remained so ever since. The Company has never owned its own Hall. The Spectacle Makers' Arms, which were granted in 1950, are:

Vert, a Chevron Or between three pairs of Nose-Spectacles proper framed of the second. And for the Crest, upon a Helm, mantled vert doubled Or, on a Wreath Or and Vert, two Arms embowed vested Vert cuffed Or, the Hands proper holding a Sun in splendour within an Annulet gold. For Supporters on either side a Falcon proper belled Or charged with a Sword erect Gules.

Interestingly, the Company had two previous unofficial devices, the first coming into use in the period 1629–66 and the second in 1810. Both of these designs were similar to the later official Arms but did not include the chevron. No motto was granted in 1950 but traditionally the words 'A blessing to the Aged' are used.

The Arms of the Spectacle Makers are also displayed in slate over the door to their offices in the Courtyard (Figure 11.3). These are more accurate in that the nose-spectacles show a glass lens as they are blazoned '*Proper* [that is, in real-life colours], *framed Or*'.

Tucked away on the west side of the entrance Hall is a pair of late seventeenth-century oak hall chairs. The chairs were presented to the Society in 1921 by Court Assistant Dr H. J. W. Martin. Henry Joseph Walklate Martin was admitted to the Society in 1880, promoted to the Livery in 1890 and elected to the Court in 1917. He died in 1924 before

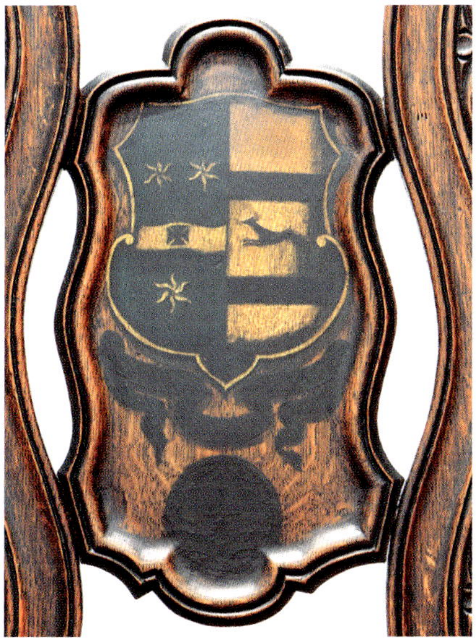

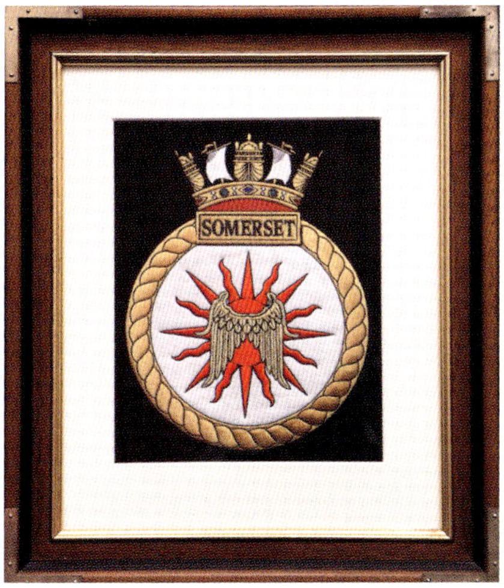

11.4 Unknown impaled Arms on Entrance Hall chairs

11.5 The badge of HMS *Somerset*

serving on the Private Court. He was a GP and Medical Officer at Mill Hill School and several other local organisations, although in his younger days he was Surgeon to the Blue Funnel Line's SS *Telamon*.

Dr Martin was a benefactor of the Society, also donating two silver salvers in his lifetime, and half of his residual estate of £13,814 was left to the Hall once his widow had enjoyed the liferent. She died in 1938.

The chairs have backs that are scroll shaped with a carved crest rail and a cartouche painted with a coat of Arms (Figure 11.4). The Arms are an impaled coat of husband and wife, viz.:

Dexter: *Vert, on a Fess between three Estoiles Or a Cross pattée Sable*

Sinister: *Or, a Greyhound courant between two Bars Sable*

There is also a motto which is illegible but it is not recorded where the chairs came from and it has not been possible to trace whose Arms they are.

The Landing

In 1996, HMS *Somerset*, a recently commissioned Type 23 (Duke class) frigate, became affiliated to the Society and at a subsequent social exchange presented a plaque of her Arms for display in the Hall (Figure 11.5).

Ships' badges are the direct descendants of figureheads and, since 1918, ships of the Royal Navy have been issued with Arms under the auspices of the Ships' Badges Committee to replace the unofficial and often frivolous designs previously chosen by ships. Nowadays, a member of the College of Arms serves on this Committee. All the Arms have as a crest the naval crown, which is said to be a representation of the Armada of 1588 – showing the smaller and more manoeuvrable English sails amongst the hulls of the Spanish galleons.

The shape of the badge was dependent on the type of ship which it represents, namely circular for battleships and battlecruisers, pentagonal for cruisers, shield-shaped for destroyers and diamond-shaped for aircraft carriers, submarines and auxiliaries. The available shapes represented the Fleet in 1918 and the original shape is kept by succeeding ships of the same name regardless of their current type.[2] Since there was no *Somerset* in commission in 1918, as the previous ship of the name had been wrecked in 1778, she was issued with a circular badge on commissioning in 1996.

The blazon of *Somerset*'s Arms is: *Argent, two Wings conjoined in lure, the tips downwards, Or, en soleil Gules*. The wings come from the coat of Arms of the Seymour family, the Dukes of Somerset.

The Parlour and the Cloakroom

On top of the bookcase in the Parlour are five large glass specie jars with gold tops and in the Cloakroom are six smaller glass specie jars also with gold tops. These were used for display purposes in pharmacists' shops.

Two of the Parlour jars (Figures 11.6a and b) display the Arms of the Royal College of Physicians of London, one with the label 'Magnesia' below and one with no label. The College was founded in 1518 and granted the following Arms, without supporters or crest, in 1546:

> *Sable, a Border with demi-fleur-de-lys Or, in Chief an arm Proper with a Cuff Ermine issuing out of a Cloud Argent and Azure, rayonne Or, the Hand feeling the pulse of an Arm in fesse Proper, in base a Pomegranate Gold.*

Difficult to make out and in classical Greek, the motto is Ο ΒΙΟC ΒΡΑΧΥC Η ΔΕ ΤΕΧΝΗ ΜΑΚΡΗ (Life is short, Art is long). In the examples on these jars the fleurs-de-lys are incorrectly depicted in the wrong colour metal and as four full flowers in the field rather than the demi-flowers on the border stated in the blazon.

The hand feeling the pulse is an obvious diagnostic medical act, its descent from the sky indicating divine authority for both the profession and the institution. The pomegranate is a symbol of fertility and regeneration in classical mythology and also has medicinal properties, particularly in the treatment of tapeworm (see Chapter 6). The Greek author Dioscorides mentions its use for a range of other conditions using various parts of the plant.[3]

11.6 Specie jars in the Parlour

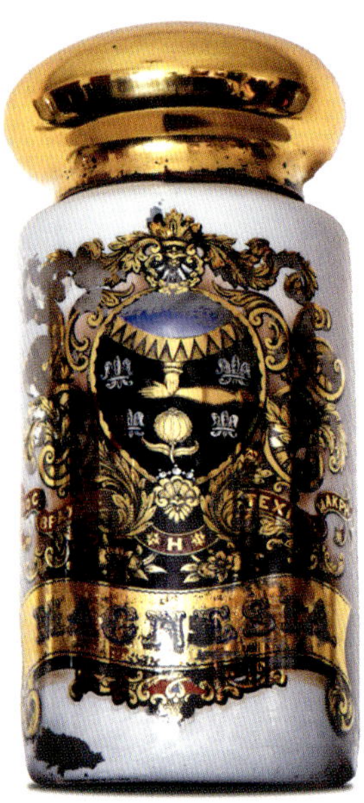

A. Royal College of Physicians of London

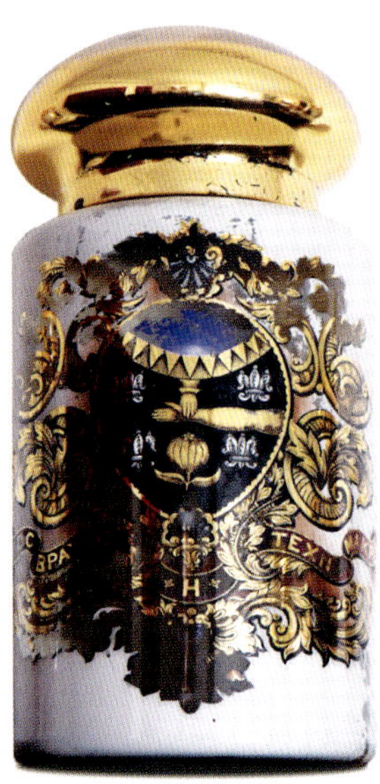

B. Royal College of Physicians of London

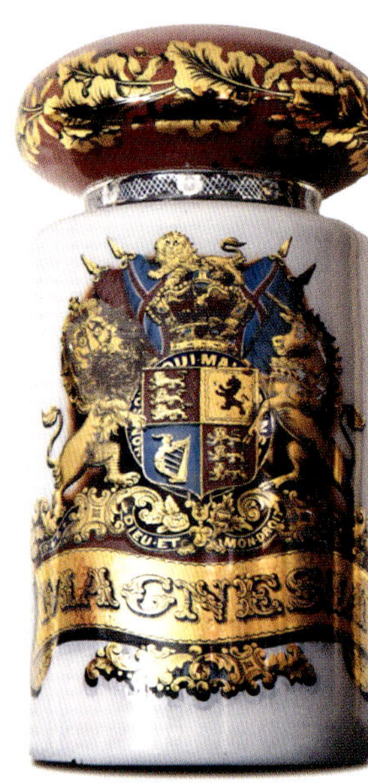

C. The Royal Arms

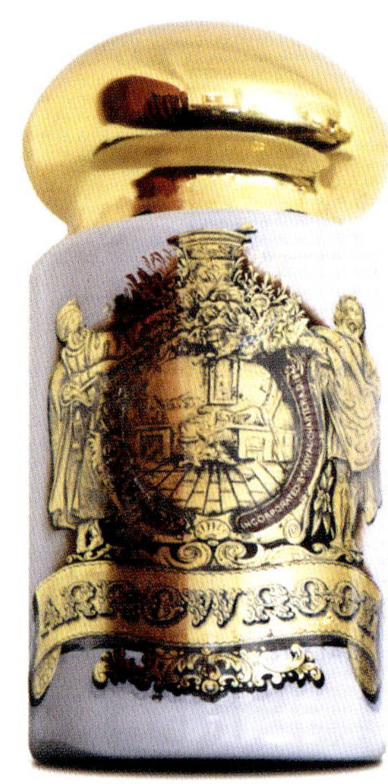

D. A non-heraldic design

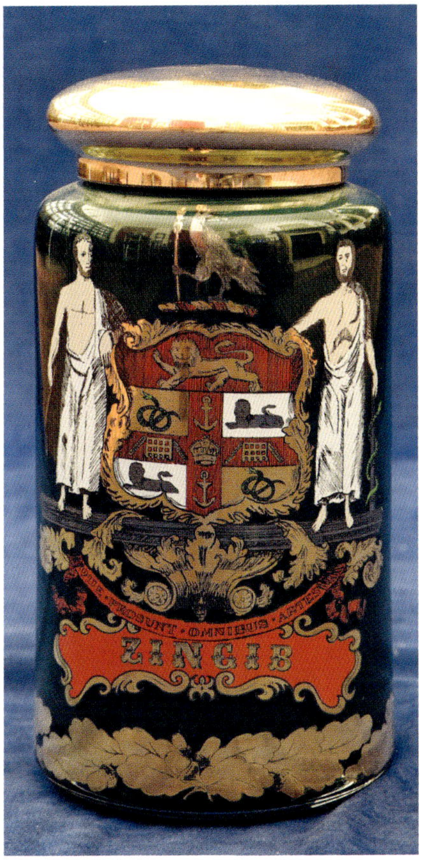

11.7 Arms of the Royal College of Surgeons of England

A third jar (Figure 11.6c) displays the current Royal Arms, also with the label 'Magnesia' below and the fourth jar (Figure 11.6d) displays a fanciful, and definitely non-heraldic, image of what is probably an apothecary's shop, with the label 'Arrowroot' below. A fifth jar displays the Society's Arms.

The six jars in the Cloakroom are all connected with medical or pharmaceutical bodies.

A dark green jar (Figure 11.7) displays the Arms of the Royal College of Surgeons of England with the label 'Zingib'. Zingib or 'Pulvis Zingiberis' is ginger in powder form and was used mainly to calm the stomach and prevent colic but it is also still used as a flavouring agent.

The College was formed from the split of the Company of Barbers and Surgeons in 1745 into the Company of Barbers and a company which never took livery but which in due course was to become the Royal College of Surgeons of England. A private artist was paid to design the College's coat of Arms, which were not made official by the College of Arms until the grant of a supplementary Royal Charter in 1822. The blazon of the Arms is:

> *Quarterly Or and Argent, a Cross Gules thereon the Imperial Crown Proper between two Anchors erect in pale and two Portcullises in fess of the first, in the first and fourth quarters a Serpent nowed and in the second and third a Lion couchant guardant Proper; on a Chief of the third a Lion passant guardant of the first being part of the Royal Arms of England. For the Crest, on a Wreath of the colours, an Eagle regardant imperially crowned proper, the dexter Claw supporting a Mace erect gold; for Supporters, dexter a figure representing Machaon habited in a robe, holding in the exterior hand a Dart broken, the point downwards; sinister a figure representing Podalirius, habited as the dexter, holding in his exterior hand a Staff entwined by a Serpent, all Proper.*

The motto is *Que Prosunt Omnibus Artes* (The Arts which are of service to all). The knotted serpents represent healing and the smaller lions professional vigilance. The portcullises may represent the City of Westminster and also the role of examining surgeons for the Army. The anchors may represent the parish of St Clement Danes and also the role of examining surgeons for the Navy. The eagle crest symbolises fortitude. Machaon's dart, extracted from the side of King Menelaus, represents healing and Podalirius, his brother, was a physician.

With the Royal Charter, additions to the Arms were made in the form of a St George's cross bearing the imperial crown and the lion of England and a mace and crown were given to the Eagle crest – all representing the Royal connection.

A white jar (Figure 11.8) displays the Arms of the Royal College of Surgeons of Edinburgh with the label 'Colocynth'. The ripe fruit of *Citrullus colocynthis* is a poison and was used as a drastic purgative for treating constipation, liver and gallbladder ailments.

The College, which was granted its Royal Charter in 1778, can trace its origins to the Incorporation of Surgeons and Barbers in 1505 and recorded its Arms with Lord

Lyon King of Arms in 1672 as:

> *Azure, a Human Body fesswise between a dexter Hand having an Eye in the Palm issuing out of a Cloud downwards and a Castle situate on a Rock proper, within a Bordure Or charged with several Instruments peculiar to the Art; on a Canton of the first a Saltire Argent surmounted of a Thistle Vert crowned of the 3rd. For the Crest, on a Peer's helm mantled Azure doubled Argent, on a Wreath of the colours, a Sun in splendour; for Supporters, dexter a figure representing Asclepius; sinister a figure of Hippocrates.*

The motto is *Hinc Sanitas* (From Here, Health). It is unusual that the colour of the several instruments is not stated – probably because it is not allowed heraldically to place metal on metal (for example, a *silver* knife on a *gold* background). Possibly this is why the border in this example is incorrectly painted as white, not gold as stated in the blazon.

The hand, cloud, body and instruments are similar references to surgery and divine assistance as shown on the Royal College of Physicians of London's Arms. The castle in base represents Edinburgh castle and the saltire is a very Scottish symbol. The supporters are Asclepius (dexter) the Greek God of Medicine and Hippocrates (sinister) the Greek Father of Medicine.

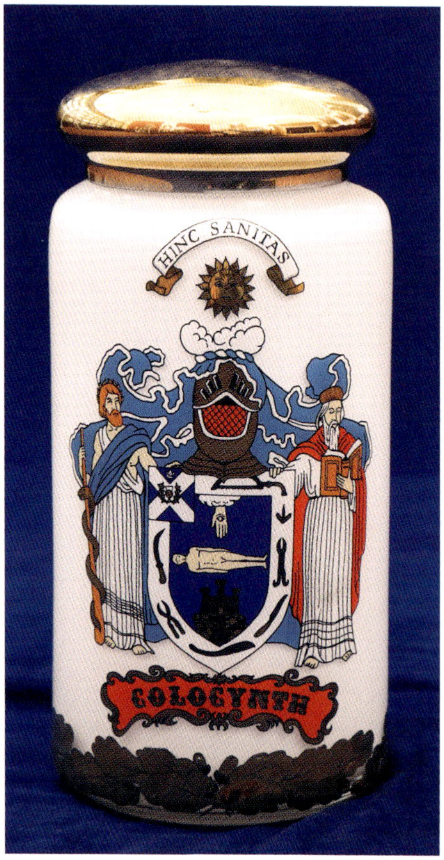

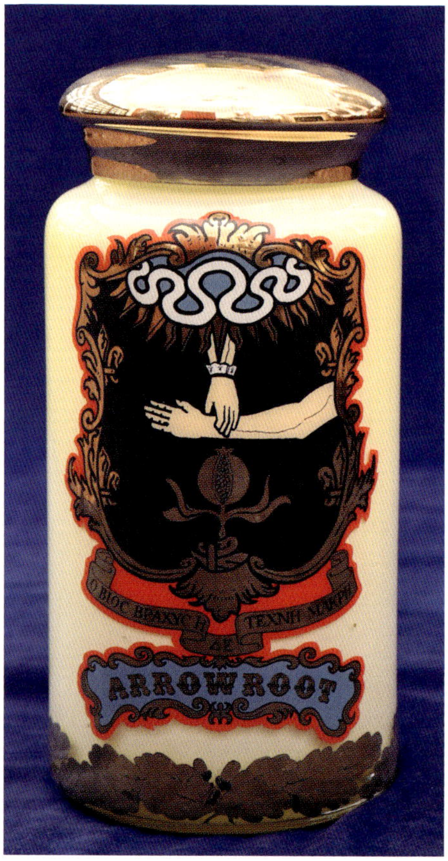

11.8 Arms of the Royal College of Surgeons of Edinburgh

11.9 Arms of the Royal College of Physicians of London

11.10 Arms of the Royal Society of Medicine

11.11 Arms of the Royal Pharmaceutical Society of Great Britain

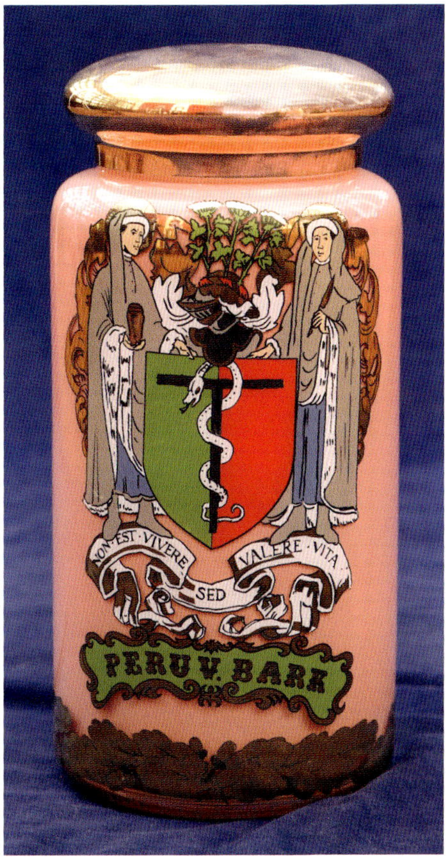

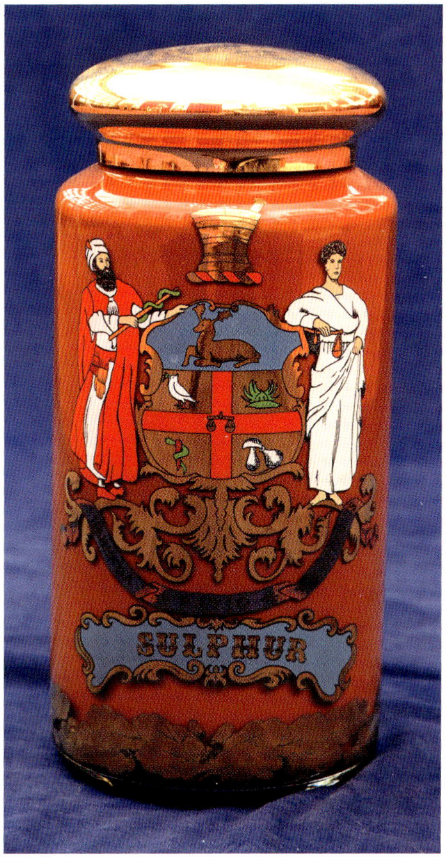

A cream-coloured jar (Figure 11.9) with the label 'Arrowroot' displays the Arms of the Royal College of Physicians of London. Arrowroot, or *Maranta arundinacea*, was used for its demulcent properties as an easily digested, nourishing diet for convalescents, especially in bowel complaints.

These Arms have already been encountered in the Parlour but this time the fleurs-de-lys are correctly painted.

A pink jar (Figure 11.10) with the label 'Peruv. Bark' shows the Arms of the Royal Society of Medicine. Peruvian Bark, or *Cinchona succirubra*, and related species were a source of quinine for treating malaria and was, at one time, used as an antipyretic, a tonic and an astringent for influenza, neuralgia and debility.

The Society was established in 1805, received its Royal Charter in 1834, and the Arms were granted in 1927. The blazon is:

> *Per pale Vert and Gules, the Serpent of Moses Or entwined around a Tau cross Argent. For the Crest, on a Peer's helm mantled Or doubled Argent, on a Wreath of the colours, three Sprigs of the herb "All Heal" Proper; for Supporters, dexter a representation of St. Cosmas; sinister a representation of St. Damian, both Proper.*

The motto is *Non est vivere sed valere vita* (It is not sufficient in life merely to exist, but rather to flourish).

The divided field of green and red indicates physicians and surgeons respectively. The Arms are based on a rod of Asclepius, the typical symbol for medicine, but here described as a Tau Cross for St Anthony and a Serpent of Moses. These charges are painted incorrectly on the jar, with the snake being shown as Argent and the cross a non-heraldic brown. The supporters are the well-known martyrs St Cosmas and St Damian, often considered patron saints of physicians. St Cosmas bears a drug jar and St Damian holds a surgeon's knife.

A brown jar (Figure 11.11) with the label 'Sulphur' shows the Arms of the Royal Pharmaceutical Society. Sulphur is used as an active ingredient in many medicated ointments, soaps and lotions due to its antifungal, antibacterial and keratolytic properties, thus speeding up the process of wound healing.

The Society was founded in 1841 as the Pharmaceutical Society of Great Britain and received its Royal Charter in 1843, although it did not use the prefix Royal until 1988. It was granted Arms in 1844 with the blazon:

> *Or, on a Cross Gules between a Dove holding in the mouth an Olive Branch in the first quarter, an Aloe in the second, a Staff erect entwined by a Serpent in the third, and an Alembic and Receiver in the fourth, all proper, a Pair of Scales of the first; on a Chief Azure a Stag lodged also of the first. For the Crest, on a Wreath of the colours, a Mortar, therein a Pestle Or; for Supporters, dexter a figure intended to represent Avicenna, habited in a dark red Robe with a white Under Vest, his Shoes red, around his waist a Shawl also red fringed gold, and upon his head a white Turban, in his right hand a Staff gold entwined with a Serpent Proper; sinister a figure intended to represent Galen, habited in a long white Vest and loose Robe, his Sandals red, and holding in his right hand a Steelyard Or.*

The motto is *Habenda ratio valetudinis* (Taking account of health). The charges on the Arms and the crest all represent aspects of pharmacy with the supporters being patriarchs of modern medicine, Avicenna (sinister), an eleventh-century Persian polymath of the Islamic Golden Age, and Galen (dexter), the third-century Greek physician and philosopher.

A sixth jar has the Society Arms on it. It is a light blue jar with the label 'Rhubarb' in addition to the Arms. Rhubarb is the rhizome of different species of the genus *Rheum* and was used as an astringent, tonic, stomachic and appetite stimulant, especially useful as a simple and safe purgative.

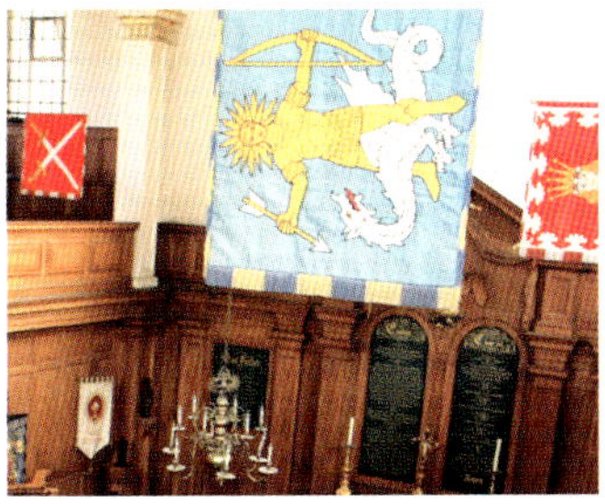

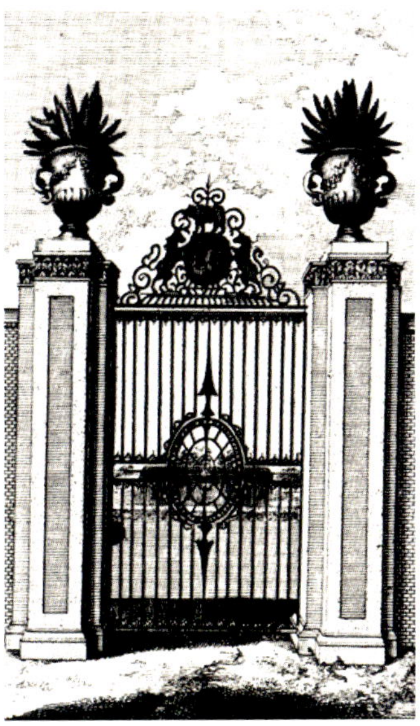

11.12 The Society Banner in the church of St Andrew-by-the-Wardrobe

11.13 The river gate of the Chelsea Physic Garden in 1730

Displays of the Society of Apothecaries Arms Outside the Hall

St Andrew-by-the-Wardrobe

In 1907 the Society presented a stained glass window to St Andrew-by-the-Wardrobe. However, it is possible that this was part of a programme of donation from all the church's regular users. It may also be relevant that the gift was made during the year in which James Henry Jeffcoat, the initiator of the Great Hall stained glass windows (see Chapter 4), was the Immediate Past Master (1906–07).

This window was destroyed in 1941 when the church was gutted in the Blitz and only the walls and tower remained standing.[4] There is no record of what form the window took, but it is presumed to have included the Society's Arms.

In 1988 the Court agreed that the shield of the Society's Arms could be displayed as a banner in the Church of St Andrew-by-the-Wardrobe, which the Society has used as its Livery Church for many years.[5] It is displayed alongside banners bearing the Arms of St Paul's Cathedral, the City of London, the Worshipful Company of Mercers (which has the Advowson or Patronage of the Living of the Church), the Worshipful Company of Blacksmiths and the Company of Parish Clerks.

The banner shows Apollo supplanting the serpent in the correct colours but improperly has a bordure company (alternate rectangles) in blue and gold added to three of the edges.

Chelsea Physic Garden

The Society's Arms appear on gates in the Chelsea Physic Garden. The Society established the Garden in 1673 initially on a lease from Lord Cheyne. In 1713 Sir Hans Sloane bought the land from Lord Cheyne and in 1722 conveyed the freehold to the Society. The Society administered the Garden until 1899, when it was transferred to the City Parochial Foundation. It is now run by a Trust which was established in 1981.

The first mention of gates in the records does not occur until 1723, when a new gate was required in the West wall but it is probable that the Society's Arms were always only displayed on the River Gate, in the south-west wall, which was the ceremonial entrance. Figure 11.13 shows the frontispiece to Philip Miller's 1730 *Catalogus Plantarum Officialium quae in Horto Botanico Chelseyano aluntur.* He was the Gardener and this was his catalogue of the plants in the Garden. It shows the Society's Arms on the gate but the iron scrollwork is entirely different to that seen today.

In 1771 the Society embanked the river outside the Garden, raising the wall by five feet and constructing new piers for the river gate, in order to protect the Garden from the wash of passing boats and the general scour of the tides.[6] Figure 11.14 shows the river gate in 1790 after this work was completed but before the next major engineering project; it is not possible to detect any Arms on the gates at this period.

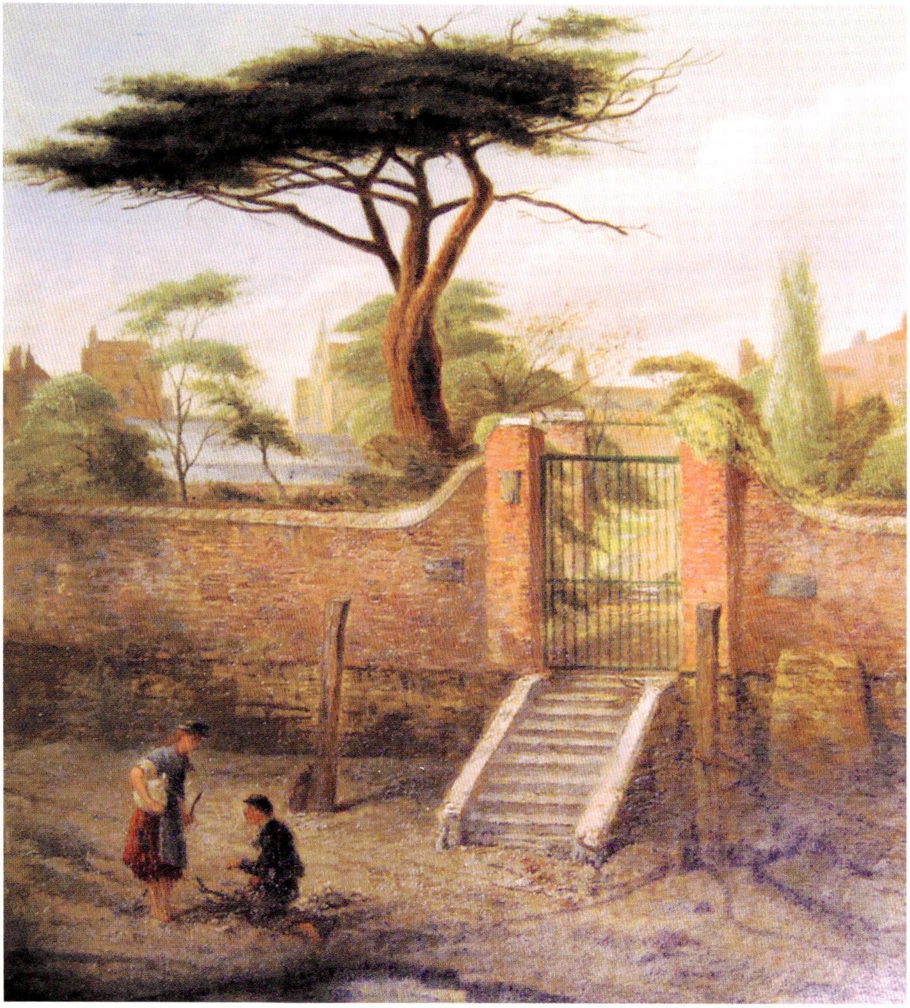

11.14 The river gate of the Chelsea Physic Garden in 1790, after the Society's embanking works

Barrett reports that in 1857 a gang of young Chelsea thieves stole the bell and mutilated the iron scrollwork over both gates.[7] The Arms are not mentioned, possibly because there were not any, and this is also implied by the fact that the Curator then had the gates spiked. This incident may be connected with the Curator's complaints in the 1860s that the derelict barge houses were being haunted by ragamuffins and ne'er-do-wells.

The Thames Embankment Act 1868 required the Society to give up riverside land for the construction of the Embankment. Work on this project adjacent to the Garden took place between 1871 and 1874. This involved the loss of access to the river both from the gate and from the barge houses. The boundary wall was realigned and in 1877 new gates and piers were installed to give access to the Embankment road: these are the ones seen today.

Two sets of Arms in metal are displayed on these riverside gates (Figure 11.15) and they are back-to-back so that they face both the Garden and the Embankment. These

Arms depict the charges of the shield and the crest but without any mantling, helm or supporters, and the shape of the shield is somewhat elaborate. Bizarrely, they have been constructed with the rhinoceros facing the wrong way on both sides.

In 2009 the Society paid for the Arms to be taken down, refurbished and re-gilded, but the error with the crest could not be corrected and remains a curiosity.

The Guildhall

In the Great Hall of the City of London Guildhall, the Arms of all 110 livery companies are displayed high above the windows. Each company's Arms displays the shield only, without supporters, helm or crest and the Azure shield of the Apothecaries bearing Apollo slaying the dragon of disease can be found in its due place at number 58.

St Mary's Church, Battersea

In the eighteenth-century St Mary's Church, Battersea, there is a stained glass panel commemorating William Curtis FLS (1746–1799), who was an apothecary before concentrating on botany and entomology. Curtis became the Praefectus Horti (Superintendent of the Garden) and Demonstrator of Botany at the Chelsea Physic Garden in 1771.

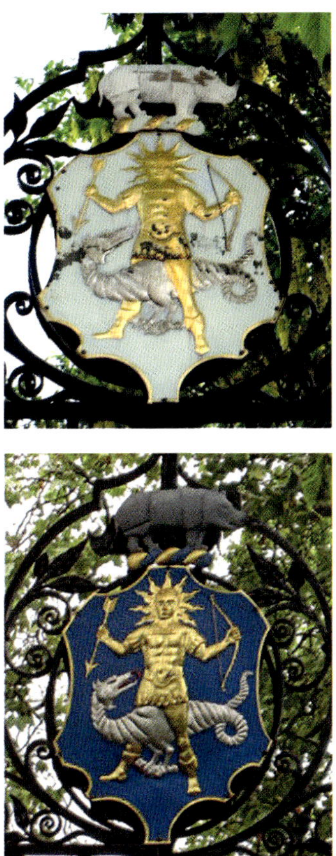

11.15 The Arms on the Gates at the Chelsea Physic Garden before (above) and after (below) restoration in 2009

His duties required him to supervise the Garden, to encourage the study of botany, to demonstrate plants to students at least once a month, to conduct five herbarising expeditions annually, to organise general herbarising for members of the Society, to attend to international correspondence, to improve the Garden and to prepare fifty plant specimens annually for the Royal Society and a further twenty for the late Mr Rand's collection (a previous Director of the Garden).[8] All of this proved too much for him and he resigned in 1777.

He went on to construct his own garden, to write the *Flora Londiniensis* and to found the *Botanical Magazine*. The genus *Curtisia* is named in his honour, the sole species in this genus being *Curtisia dentata* (the assegai tree) a flowering tree from South Africa.

As many of his samples were collected from the churchyard of St Mary, a modern memorial stained glass panel made by John Hayward (1929–2007) was installed in 1982 (Figure 11.16). The portrait of Curtis is framed with a chaplet of flowers from his *Flora Londiniensis*. Below the portrait is the epitaph of the original headstone over his grave in the churchyard and above is the fructed tree badge of the Royal Horticultural Society.

To the right are the Arms of the Linnaean Society, of which he was a founder member, and to the left are the Arms of the Society of Apothecaries commemorating his time at the Physic Garden. Neither sets of Arms show the supporters to which both bodies are entitled, probably for lack of space. The Society Arms are otherwise correct, except that the mantling is of the Society's colours rather than the red and silver specified by Camden.

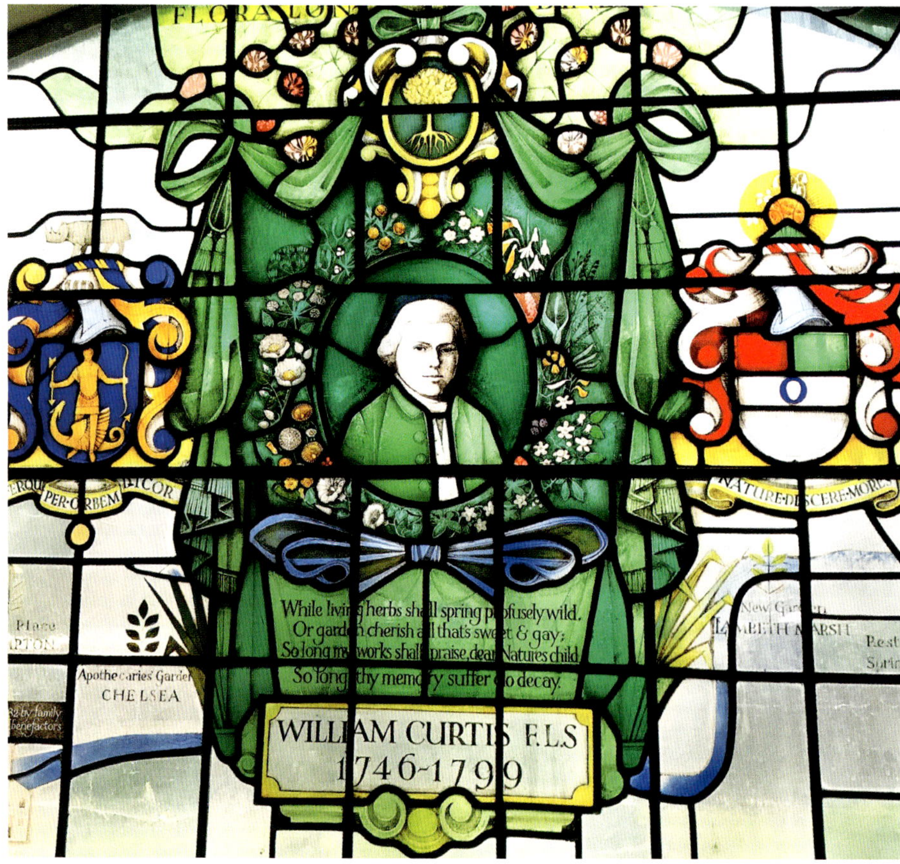

11.16 Memorial window to William Curtis in St Mary's Church, Battersea

Guildford Cathedral

Guildford was made a diocese in 1927. Its cathedral was designed by Sir Edward Maufe (1883–1974) and construction started in 1936. Building work was suspended during the Second World War and the cathedral was finally consecrated in 1961. In the north and south aisles, there are a number of windows commemorating the professions of teaching, nursing, dentistry, physiotherapy and the law, together with the armed forces.

Amongst these is the doctors' window which consists of four lights in one bay in the centre of the south aisle. The lower two lights were paid for by the dentists, the left-upper light by the British Medical Association and the right-upper light by the Society (Figure 11.17).

The Society's window shows St Luke below a shield of the Arms without crest, helm, mantling or supporters. Appropriately for a cathedral, Apollo's sunburst looks more like a halo!

The panel was executed by Moira Forsyth (1905–1991) in 1961 and paid for by the Society's Court, liverymen, yeomen and members of the Faculty of the History of Medicine and Pharmacy.[9] Forsyth, who made all the glass in these lights, also worked in the Glass-House studio in Fulham to which Carl Edwards moved in 1972. Other artists who worked on Guildford Cathedral windows included Francis Spear, Lawrence Lee and James Powell & Sons, all of whom have made panels for the Hall.

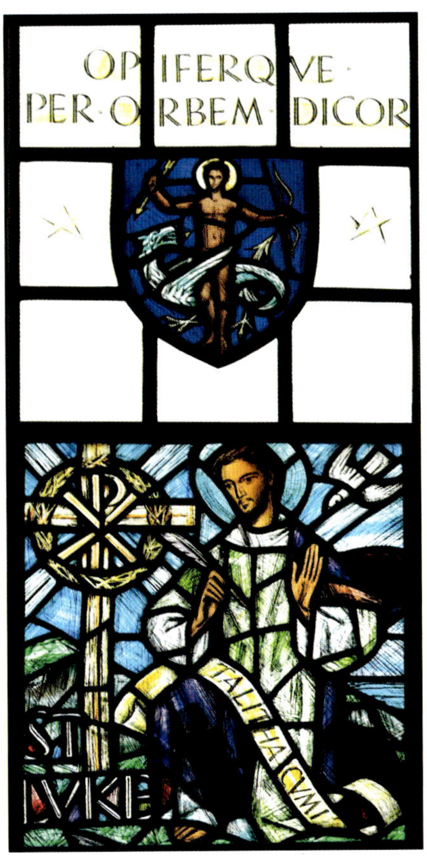

11.17 The doctor's window in Guildford Cathedral

Bolling Hall, Bradford

Bolling Hall dates from the fourteenth century, with additions from every succeeding century. The Bolling family owned the estate from the fourteenth to late fifteenth centuries and was briefly deprived of the estate 1461–72 as Lancastrian supporters. The Hall passed to the Tempests by marriage in *c.*1502 and they held it until 1649, when Richard Tempest had to sell it to pay his debts incurred as a Royalist during the Civil War. Between 1649 and 1912 the Hall was owned by the families of Saville, Lindley, Pigott, Wood, Mason and Paley. Bolling Hall was presented to Bradford Corporation in 1912 and is now a museum.

Part of the collection in the Hall consists of twenty-four stained glass panels depicting the coats of Arms of leading northern families dating from *c.*1500. In addition, there are four larger armorial panels, two with shields of Arms and two with crests and mottoes dated 1695, each within an ornate non-heraldic cartouche (Figure 11.18). One shield and one crest are the Society's and all four were made by Henry Gyles (1645–1709), who was based in York, one of the leading and much-admired stained glass artists of his time.[10]

The Society's shield is a dramatic display with a deep blue field and a bright gold Apollo and dragon, who is a large and dangerous opponent in this representation. Unfortunately, the figures of Apollo and the dragon are reversed. The second panel carries a bold image of Dürer's gomda, complete with dorsal horn, on a white background, with the date 1695 below and the motto in an elaborate label above. The supporters, helm and mantling have been omitted from both panels.

For reasons unknown, all the stained glass was removed from Bolling Hall in about 1825 and taken to Copt Hewick Hall near Ripon. The glass was returned to Bolling Hall in 1949 and underwent some restoration by John Alder Knowles (1881–1961).[11] Part of the collection, including three of the four panels in Figure 11.18, are now on display in Cliffe Castle Museum, Keighley. The fourth panel remains in store at the Bolling Hall Museum in Bradford.

Why the Society's Arms were ever in Bolling Hall and to whom the other Arms belong is unknown, but the two must be connected as they are dated in the same year and surrounded by almost identical cartouches. The second Arms are an impaled coat representing a husband and wife, viz.:

Dexter: *Sable, five fusils in fess Argent*

Sinister: *Argent, on a Chevron Sable, between three Shamrocks Vert, three Crescents Or.*

The family of Lindley owned Bolling Hall in 1695 but neither theirs nor any of the other families' Arms resemble the impaled window. One theory is that this was a Master Apothecary celebrating his year in glass, but neither Sir John Clarke (Master 1694–95) nor John Danson (Master 1695–96) seem to be associated with Yorkshire. It is not even clear that these four panels were ever actually installed at Bolling Hall and there is no hint of where else they may have been used; so, despite extensive research the mystery remains unsolved.

Christ's Hospital

Christ's Hospital School was established at the Grey Friars in Newgate Street in 1552. It burnt down in the Great Fire of 1666 and was rebuilt on the site in 1705. Between 1793 and 1836, there was a further major rebuilding programme which included a new Great Hall. The Society had supported Christ's Hospital since at least 1803 and in recognition of this the Society's Arms were placed in this Hall in 1831.[12]

In 1902 the school moved from the City to a new site in Horsham.[13] The Arms shown in Figure 11.19 are currently in a window in the dining room at Horsham, but it is not clear if these Arms were moved from the City site in 1902 or are a new installation for a new site. On balance, it is likely that they were made in 1831 but the artist is unknown.

Although near faithful to the Camden grant, it is an unusual display of the Arms within an octagonal boundary. The helm and mantling are missing but the proportions are otherwise good. The artist has become slightly carried away with the scroll for the motto, on which the unicorns usually stand, and has created a separate ground for the unicorns which looks a little like nowed snakes – perhaps a medical reference? The blank cartouche at the top of the piece is also crying out for a year of presentation or similar information to balance the lower one.

Westminster Hospital

Sir Stanley Woodwark (Master for the three years 1941–44) was appointed to the staff of the Westminster Hospital in 1919 as Physician to the Hospital and Dean of the Medical School, appointments he retained until his retirement in 1934.[14] After his death in 1945, the Court agreed to the Hospital's request to include the Society's Arms in a memorial window to Sir Stanley in the Hospital.[15]

At that time the Westminster Hospital was in Horseferry Road, a site which had opened in 1939. This was closed in 1994 when the Hospital became the Chelsea and Westminster Hospital on a new site on the Fulham Road. The Horseferry Road site has since been developed into luxury flats and it is not clear whether the memorial remained on site, as it cannot be traced. It was not transferred to the new Chelsea and Westminster Hospital.

Glossary of Stained Glass and Heraldic Terminology

Stained Glass

The following terms related to stained glass are expanded to give an overview of the techniques involved.

ABRASION: The selective removal of the coloured layer of flashed glass (see below) by scratching or grinding with a metal tool to reveal the underlying clear glass, a technique which preceded acid etching.

ACID ETCHING: The selective removal of the coloured layer of flashed glass (see below) with hydrofluoric acid to reveal the underlying clear glass, a technique not widely used until the nineteenth century.

CEMENTING: The technique of making a leaded panel waterproof by introducing black putty between the edge of each piece of glass and its surrounding lead.

ENAMELLED GLASS: Glass painted with a mixture of ground glass of a specific colour, metallic oxides and an organic medium, which is then fired in a kiln, during which process the medium burns off and the enamel fuses onto the surface of the underlying glass. Sometimes, after many years the enamel may peel off as it is only fused to the surface of the underlying glass – in contrast to silver stain (see below). This defect may be due to the differing coefficients of expansion and contraction of the base glass and the components of the enamel. This technique became popular in England from the seventeenth century onwards, having been introduced by Flemish glaziers who came from the continent to teach English glaziers the techniques of stained glass window-making which had been lost as a result of the Reformation.

FLASHED GLASS: A sheet or base of clear glass to which a thin layer of coloured glass has been fused when both the clear and the coloured glass are molten on the glass-blower's blow-pipe, before being blown into a cylinder which is then cooled, cut and allowed to fall flat by reheating in the kiln. The underlying base glass can also be coloured.

LEADING: The assembly of the pieces of a stained glass panel in a network of lead strips which are H-shaped in section and are soldered together on both sides of the panel at the meeting points. The 'arms' of the 'H' can be of different widths depending upon the design of the panel.

LIGHT: A column of glass in a window, often made up of several panels. If the window is made up of more than one vertical column it is described, for example, as a two-light or a three-light window. If the vertical column is broken by a horizontal stone mullion, the window is described as tiered.

PAINTED GLASS: Glass painted with a mixture of iron or copper oxide and a flux which is applied with a brush, the panel then being fired in a kiln. The result is almost invariably permanent but if the firing temperature is not high enough the paint can in due course flake off.

QUARRY: A small diamond-shaped piece of glass, often bearing a single motif and often used as background decoration in a larger panel.

SILVER STAINING: A technique developed in the early fourteenth century whereby a yellow or gold stain is produced on the base glass after painting with a compound of silver, for example silver nitrate, and firing in a kiln. During firing the silver ions migrate into the glass and thus produce colouring which is permanent. This is the origin of the term 'stained glass'.

TRACERY: A pattern of small panels within stonework above a multi-light window.

Heraldry

This is not a comprehensive explanation of heraldry and all its terms but merely a glossary to explain the expressions used in this book.

In England and Wales, heraldry is controlled by the College of Arms under the direction of the hereditary Earl Marshal, the Duke of Norfolk. All the officers of the College are styled Heralds in Ordinary and are organised at three levels. Annual salaries range from £13.95 for a Pursuivant to £49.07 for Garter – enhanced by professional fees from their private practices in heraldry and genealogy, principally by designing achievements of arms for personal and corporate use. In special circumstances, Heralds Extraordinary are appointed to supplement the College.

There are three Kings of Arms, who anciently conducted county visitations to check and record armorial bearings and pedigrees:

> GARTER KING OF ARMS – the principal King of Arms
> CLARENCEAUX KING OF ARMS – jurisdiction in England south of the River Trent
> NORROY AND ULSTER KING OF ARMS – jurisdiction in England north of the Trent and in Northern Ireland

They have authority to grant arms under approval from the Earl Marshal and serve as heralds for the orders of chivalry.

Below them there are six Heralds:

> LANCASTER HERALD, WINDSOR HERALD, SOMERSET HERALD, RICHMOND HERALD, YORK HERALD, CHESTER HERALD

They are employed to oversee state ceremonial and deal with matters of precedence; they regulate the use of armorial bearings and (historically) make proclamations and carry official messages.

The four Pursuivants at Arms are the junior officers of Arms with similar duties to the Heralds:

> PORTCULLIS PURSUIVANT, ROUGE CROIX PURSUIVANT, ROUGE DRAGON PURSUIVANT, BLUEMANTLE PURSUIVANT

In Scotland there is a similar hierarchy under Lord Lyon King of Arms:

> ROTHESAY HERALD, SNAWDOUN HERALD, MARCHMONT HERALD; ORMOND PURSUIVANT, DINGWALL PURSUIVANT, UNICORN PURSUIVANT.

ARMORIAL BEARINGS Armorial bearings, also described as an achievement of Arms, comprise: a shield with emblems which are known as charges; a helm with mantling; a crest on a wreath or torse; a motto in a compartment; and supporters which are animals or human figures that support the shield on each side. Supporters are granted to peers, the higher ranks of orders of chivalry, civic institutions and certain incorporated bodies. Anyone receiving a grant of arms is an armiger.

The Arms are described or blazoned in order as follows: the colour of the field of the shield; the principle charge; secondary charges; cadency marks (see below); the crest; the motto (if described); the supporters (if granted). Tinctures in the blazon refer to everything described before the tincture. Where the tincture needs to be repeated 'of the 1st/2nd/3rd [tincture]' is used. The term 'canting' indicates tinctures or charges alluding to the grantee's name or profession.

In English heraldry any legitimate male descendent of an armiger may bear those Arms undifferenced. In Scotland this is not the case and younger sons must difference their Arms with a cadency mark or a difference such as a bordure [border] or change of tinctures. Cadency marks distinguish sons in order of seniority. The marks are: 1st son – a label of three points in the lifetime of his father; 2nd son – a crescent; 3rd son – a mullet [star]; 4th son – a martlet [a heraldic bird]; 5th son – an annulet [ring], and so forth.

HERALDIC TINCTURES

Colours

Azure	Blue
Gules	Red
Purpure	Purple
Sable	Black
Vert	Green

Metals

Argent	Silver
Or	Gold

Stains (rare)

Murrey	Mulberry
Sanguine	Blood red
Tenne	Orange/Tawny

Furs (uncommon)

Ermine	Black spots on white
Ermines	White spots on black
Erminois	Black spots on gold
Pean	Gold spots on black

Proper the natural colours of a charge

Counter changed when the field is in two colours and the charges placed upon it are in the opposite colours

As it was difficult and expensive to illustrate arms in colour, a system of hatching which came to be known as the Petra Sancta method was developed in the mid-seventeenth century and this convention is still used today. Each tincture is represented by hatching as indicated below:

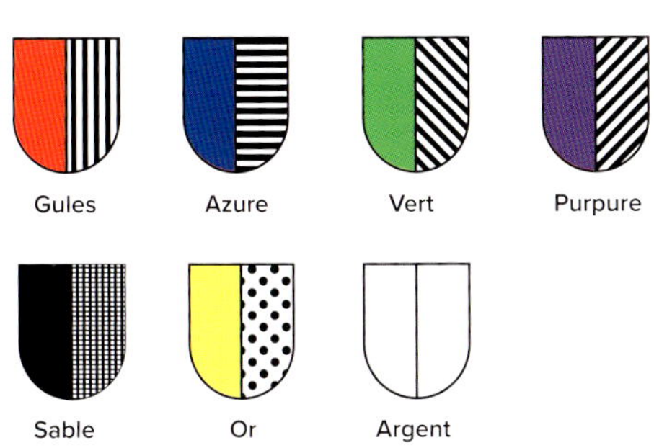

POINTS OF THE SHIELD

The shield is described from the bearer's point of view, so the dexter (although meaning right) side is on the left as the observer sees it and the sinister side is on the right. The upper part of the shield is the chief and the lower part the base.

FORMS

Fess	a horizontal form
Pale	a vertical form
Bend	a diagonal top left to bottom right viewed by the observer
Bend Sinister	the opposite diagonal to Bend
Chevron	an inverted V
Tierce	in three parts
Saltire	as a St Andrew's cross
Gyron	divided into eight
Quarter	divided into four and numbered 1 top left, 2 top right, 3 bottom left, 4 bottom right, viz:

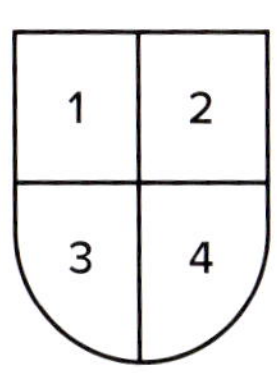

ATTITUDES

Unless otherwise stated, all beasts face/move to the observer's left. When an animal's head or an object faces the observer full on it is said to be affronté. Common forms of stance are:

Couchant	lying down
Courant	running
Dormant	asleep
Embowed	in a semi-circular shape
Forcene	a horse rearing
Guardant	head turned to look at the observer
Hauriant	swimming in pale (rising)
Naiant	swimming fesswise
Nowed	knotted (snakes)
Passant	walking with front right paw raised
Rampant	standing on its hind legs

Reguardant	head looking back over the shoulder
Salient	springing
Sejant	sitting
Sejant erect	sitting with forepaws raised
Soaring	upwards flight
Statant	standing still
Trippant	a walking stag
Urinant	swimming in pale (diving)
Volant	horizontal flight
Vulning	wounding its breast

OTHER TERMS

Addorsed	back to back
Appaumé	open hand showing the palm
Armed	concerning horns, tusks or claws
Attired	a stag's antlers
Barbed	concerning thorns of a plant
Caboshed	an animal's full face with no neck
Caparisoned	with bridle, saddle and horse trapper
Close	bird with wings folded
Couped	cut straight
Crined	concerning the hair or bristles
Debruised	one charge placed on another
Displayed	bird with wings extended
Embowed	bent at the elbow
Erased	cut with three ragged edges
Flexed	bent at the knee
Fructed	with fruit
Furnished	with bridle, saddle etc.
Gorged	encircled about the neck
Langued	concerning the tongue
Maned	concerning the mane
Radiant	encircled with rays
Seeded	concerning sepals of a flower
Slipped	concerning leaves
Unguled	concerning the hoof
Vambranced	in armour

HELMS The helm or helmet sits above the shield on a wreath of colours and is used to carry the crest and to distinguish the rank of the armiger. It is not used in ladies' Arms.

The shape of the helm is not significant but the metals, which way it faces and whether or not the visor is open are important. The crest must also be designed to suit the way the helm faces – i.e. a crest in profile on a helm affronté is quite wrong. The various grades of helm are:

The Sovereign & Princes	Barred helm of gold placed affronté
Peers	Barred helm of silver, decorated with gold and placed sideways
Baronets & Knights	Visored helm of steel with the visor open, usually placed affronté
Esquires & Gentlemen	Visored helms of steel with the visor closed, usually placed sideways
Corporate body	as for an Esquire

Abbreviations

ACIS — Associate of the Chartered Institute of Secretaries & Administrators
ADMS — Assistant Director of Medical Services
AE — Air Efficiency Medal (RAFVR)
AKC — Associate of King's College London
Bart/Bt — Baronet
BDS — Bachelor of Dental Surgery
BIR — British Institute of Radiology
BM BCh — Bachelor of Medicine and Surgery (University of Oxford)
BM BS — Bachelor of Medicine and Surgery (Universities of Brighton Sussex, Exeter, Nottingham, Plymouth, Southampton)
BMA — British Medical Association
BPharm — Bachelor of Pharmacy
BSMGP — British Society of Master Glass Painters
BUPA — British United Provident Association
CB — Companion of the Most Honourable Order of the Bath
CBE — Commander of the Most Excellent Order of the British Empire
CChem — Chartered Chemist
CH — Companion of Honour
CIE — Commander of the Most Eminent Order of the Indian Empire
CIMgt — Companion, Institute of Management
CMLJ — Commander of Merit, Order of St Lazarus of Jerusalem
CO — Commanding Officer
CStJ — Commander of the Most Venerable Order of the Hospital of St John of Jerusalem
CVO — Commander of the Royal Victorian Order
DBA — Doctor of Business Administration
DFFP — Diploma in Fertility and Family Planning
DHMSA — Diploma in the History of Medicine of the Society of Apothecaries
DIH — Diploma in Industrial Health
DL — Deputy Lieutenant
DMJ — Diploma in Medical Jurisprudence
DMRE — Diploma in Medical Radiology and Electrology
DO — Diploma in Ophthalmology
DObstRCOG — Diploma in Obstetrics of the Royal College of Obstetricians & Gynaecologists
DPMSA — Diploma in the Philosophy of Medicine of the Society of Apothecaries
DSc — Doctor of Science
ERD — Emergency Reserve Decoration
FACP — Fellow of the American College of Physicians
FACR — Fellow of the American College of Radiology
FCIS — Fellow of the Institute of Chartered Secretaries & Administrators
FCRA — Fellow of the College of Radiologists of Australia
FDS RCS — Fellow in Dental Surgery of the Royal College of Surgeons of England
FFCM — Fellow of the Faculty of Community Medicine
FFLM — Fellow of the Faculty of Legal Medicine
FFOM — Fellow of the Faculty of Occupational Medicine
FFPHM — Fellow of the Faculty of Public Health Medicine
FFPM — Fellow of the Faculty of Pharmaceutical Medicine
FFR — Fellow of the Faculty of Radiology
FIPharmM — Fellow of the Institute of Pharmaceutical Medicine
FKC — Fellow of King's College London
FMedSci — Fellow of the Academy of Medical Sciences
FRACO — Fellow of the Royal Australian College of Obstetricians
FRACP — Fellow of the Royal Australian College of Physicians
FRCGP — Fellow of the Royal College of General Practitioners
FRCOG — Fellow of the Royal College of Obstetricians & Gynaecologists
FRCOphth — Fellow of the Royal College of Ophthalmologists
FRCP — Fellow of the Royal College of Physicians
FRCPath — Fellow of the Royal College of Pathologists
FRCPCH — Fellow of the Royal College of Paediatrics and Child Health
FRCPI — Fellow of the Royal College of Physicians of Ireland
FRCPS — Fellow of the Royal College of Physicians Surgeons of Glasgow
FRCPsych — Fellow of the Royal College of Psychiatrists
FRCR — Fellow of the Royal College of Radiologists
FRCS — Fellow of the Royal College of Surgeons
FRGS — Fellow of the Royal Geographical Society
FRIC — Fellow of the Royal Institute of Chemistry
FRIPHH — Fellow of the Royal Institute of Public Health and Hygiene
FRPharmS — Fellow of the Royal Pharmaceutical Society
FRS — Fellow of the Royal Society
FRSA — Fellow of the Royal Society of Arts
FRSC — Fellow of the Royal Society of Chemistry
FRSH — Fellow of the Royal Society for the Promotion of Health

FRSM	Fellow of the Royal Schools of Music
FRSPH	Fellow of the Royal Society for Public Health
FSA	Fellow of the Society of Antiquaries
FSLCPaed	Fellow of the Sri Lanka College of Paediatrics
GBE	Knight Grand Cross of the Most Excellent Order of the British Empire
GCMG	Knight Grand Cross of the Most Distinguished Order of St Michael and St George
GCVO	Knight Grand Cross of the Royal Victorian Order
GSM	Guildhall School of Music and Drama
GStJ	Bailiff Grand Cross of the Most Venerable Order of the Hospital of St John of Jerusalem
Hon Caus	Honoris Causa
HQ	Headquarters
JP	Justice of the Peace
KBE	Knight Commander of the Most Excellent Order of the British Empire
KCB	Knight Commander of the Most Honourable Order of the Bath
KCMG	Knight Commander of the Most Distinguished Order of St Michael & St George
KCVO	Knight Commander of the Royal Victorian Order
KHP	Honorary Physician to the King
KLJ	Knight of the Order of St Lazarus of Jerusalem
KStJ	Knight of the Most Venerable Order of the Hospital of St John of Jerusalem
LAH	Licentiate of Apothecaries' Hall, Dublin
LCh	Licentiate in Surgery
LDS RCS	Licentiate in Dental Surgery of the Royal College of Surgeons of England
LLB	Bachelor of Laws
LLM	Master of Laws
LMSSA	Licentiate in Medicine and Surgery of the Society of Apothecaries
LRCP MRCS	Licentiate of the Royal College of Physicians of London and Member of the Royal College of Surgeons of England (the Conjoint qualification)
LSA	Licentiate of the Society of Apothecaries
LVO	Lieutenant of the Royal Victorian Order
MA	Master of Arts
MB BCh	Bachelor of Medicine and Surgery (Universities of Cardiff and Swansea)
MB BCh BAO	Bachelor of Medicine, Surgery and Obstetrics (Queen's University Belfast)
MB BChir	Bachelor of Medicine and Surgery (University of Cambridge)
MB BS	Bachelor of Medicine and Surgery (Universities of London, Hull York, Newcastle, East Anglia)
MB ChB	Bachelor of Medicine and Surgery (Universities of Aberdeen, Birmingham, Bristol, Dundee, Edinburgh, Glasgow, Keele, Lancaster, Leeds, Leicester, Liverpool, Manchester, Sheffield, St Andrews, Warwick)
MBA	Master of Business Administration
MC	Military Cross
MCh	Master in Surgery
MCPP	Member of the College of Pharmacy Practice
MD	Doctor of Medicine
MFCM	Member of the Faculty of Community Medicine
MFOM	Member of the Faculty of Occupational Medicine
MFPM	Member of the Faculty of Pharmaceutical Medicine
MIBiol	Member of the Institute of Biology
MMSA	Mastership in Midwifery of the Society of Apothecaries
MRCGP	Member of the Royal College of General Practitioners
MRCOG	Member of the Royal College of Obstetrics and Gynaecology
MRCP	Member of the Royal College of Physicians
MRCPath	Member of the Royal College of Pathologists
MRCS	Member of the Royal College of Surgeons of England
MRCS and LM	Member of the Royal College of Surgeons of England and Licentiate in Midwifery
MS	Master of Surgery
MVO	Member of the Royal Victorian Order
NUI	National University of Ireland
OBE	Officer of the Most Excellent Order of the British Empire
OStJ	Officer of the Venerable Order of the Hospital of St John of Jerusalem
PC	Privy Councillor
PhD	Doctor of Philosophy
PLAB	Professional & Linguistic Assessments Board (of the GMC)
QHP	Honorary Physician to the Queen
RAFVR	Royal Air Force Volunteer Reserve
RAMC	Royal Army Medical Corps
RAMC(V)	Royal Army Medical Corps (Territorial Army Volunteer Reserve)
RMO	Regimental Medical Officer
RN	Royal Navy
RNVR	Royal Naval Volunteer Reserve
ScD	Doctor of Science
TA	Territorial Army
TD	Territorial Decoration
VR	Volunteer Reserve Medal
WHO	World Health Organisation

APPENDICES I-IV

APPENDIX I

Description and Explanation of the Individual Stained Glass Panels in the Great Hall

Introduction

At the time of writing, seventy-seven of the ninety panels in the Great Hall contain Arms and two further panels contain the remaining blank Type A and Type B cartouches. All of the West windows are filled, the remaining spaces being on the East side.

The majority of the filled windows, fifty-six, display the armiger's full Arms and four of these have supporters; a further eleven have the Type A cartouche design and eight the Type B, each showing only the shield of the Arms. One panel shows the crest only; the Bristow panel is unique.

Interestingly, not all of the Arms are authentic – that is to say, they are not all correctly registered at the College of Arms and borne by a legitimate descendant. Some of the early installations are creative, although unsurprisingly, the first three to be installed are absolutely correct. Of the fourteen incorrect Arms, eight are legitimate but without any apparent connection to the original grantee and six are simply fictitious, some with heraldic errors.

A curious feature in several cases is the grant of retrospective Arms, in that the grantee asked the College to grant the Arms to the descendants of a deceased father or grandfather so that his brothers or uncles would also be entitled to bear them.

In fifty-three cases the Arms displayed are contemporary, having been granted to the individual commemorated rather than inherited from an ancestor. Many of these show 'borrowings' from the Society's Arms:

18	use the Society colours of Or and Azure
8	feature Dürer's Gomda (Indian rhinoceros) or part of it
8	include unicorns or their heads or horns
2	display a dragon or a wyvern
2	contain Apollo or a sun in splendour

Each window is examined in Appendix 1 and the formal blazon, along with the creation process, the personal meaning of the charges and a Society-based CV of the individual is given. However, for some of the older Arms and also for individuals whose connection with the Society died with them, it has not been possible to assemble a comprehensive entry.

Note on sources and interpretation

In interpreting the heraldry discussed in this book, the authors have had to start from the standpoint that the strict rules of heraldry have been followed. This must be tempered by human imperfections in that the rules may not have been so strictly applied in times gone by; individuals may have been ignorant of these rules, families could appropriate heraldic or genealogical status with less chance of discovery and litigation concerning inheritance could be generations long. As a result, there are large numbers of inconsistencies or oddities in the work that are not easily explained (e.g. Chapter 5 the Lorymer Arms, Chapter 9 the Bristow Royal Arms and several of the Arms discussed in Appendix 1).

With regard to sources, references have been made to the various directories of armory and genealogy edited by Sir Bernard Burke, A. C. Fox-Davies and others in researching the window panels in this Appendix and elsewhere in the book, and it is acknowledged that their sources were usually the family concerned. Ancient Arms and a long pedigree were an important component of social standing, and unsurprisingly, some of these accounts contained embellishments or outright fiction to enhance that standing. The ultimate authority in these matters rests with the College of Arms in London or the Lyon Office in Edinburgh, but in the distant past these bodies were not infallible, nor were Heralds' Visitations without recrimination. Proving a negative is always a difficult task and this accounts for the major scattering of 'likely', 'possible' and 'probable' in the work.

Cartouche Type A (floral vase design)

Made by W. B. Simpson & Sons between 1920 and 1922 and identical to the 1906 design by James Powell & Sons.

This panel was originally installed in a West window and removed to window East 1, panel 3 at some stage after 2000. It is the last remaining blank Type A cartouche on display.

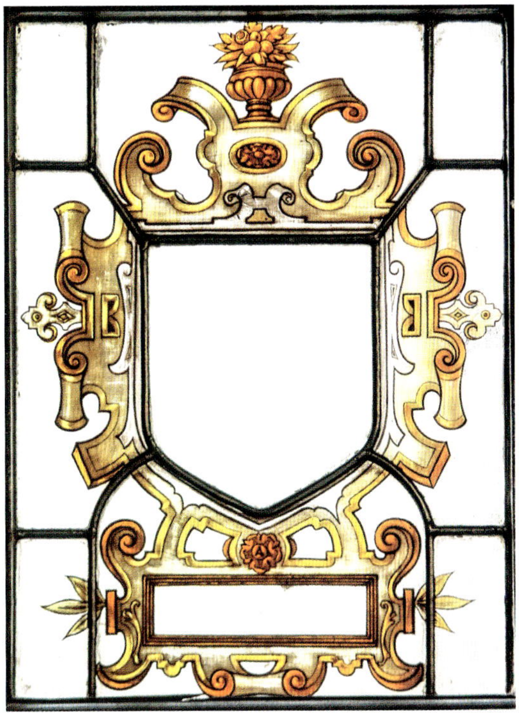

Cartouche Type B (covered cup design)

Made by W. B. Simpson & Sons between 1920 and 1922 and identical to the 1906 design by James Powell & Sons.

This panel was originally installed in a West window and removed to window East 1, panel 1 at some stage after 2000. It is the last remaining blank Type B cartouche on display.

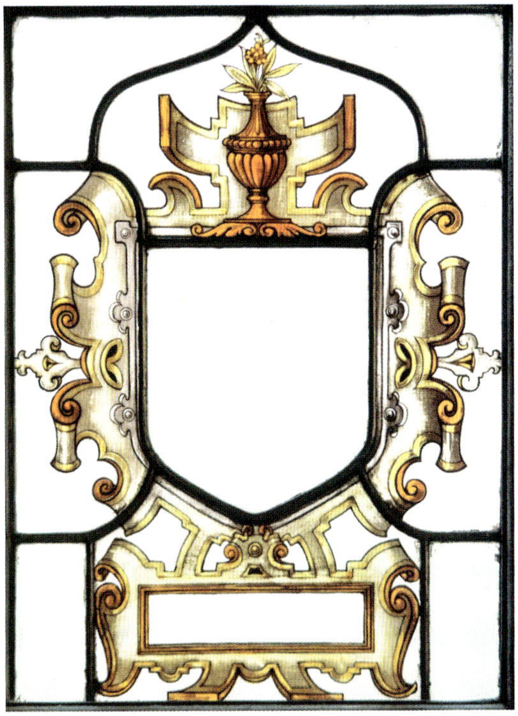

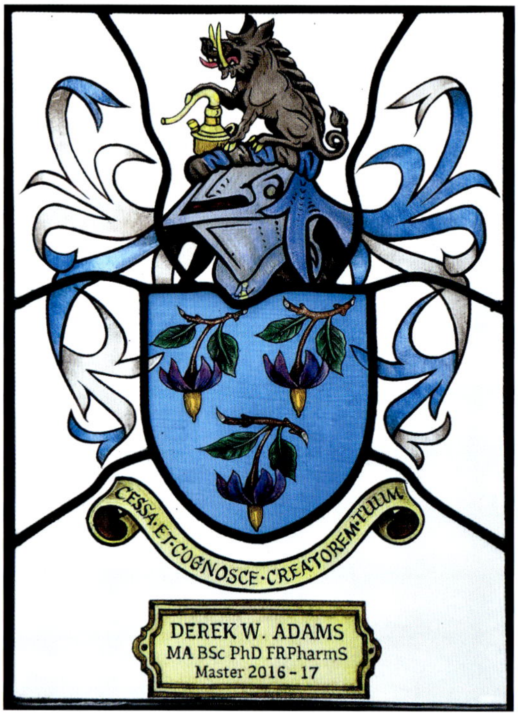

Bleu Celeste, three Deadly Nightshade Flowers each suspended from a Tendril slipped and leaved proper; And for the Crest upon a Helm, mantled Bleu Celeste doubled Argent, on a wreath of the colours, a Boar sejant Argent armed and unguled Or resting the dexter Foreleg on the brass condenser of a Copper Alembic Still proper

Motto: *Cessa et Cognosce Creatorem Tuum*

Dr Derek Westwood ADAMS, MA, BSc, PhD, FRPharmS

The Arms were designed by Thomas Woodcock, Garter Principal King of Arms, in 2010 and are recorded at the College of Arms in Volume Gr 179, Folio 73.

The stained glass panel was made by Richard Scowen and was installed in window E1-6 in 2017, showing the full Arms and motto without a cartouche.

The light blue field reflects the University of Cambridge and the deadly nightshade flowers allude to the skill of the pharmacist in taking a poisonous plant and preparing a useful medicine from it.

The white boar indicates Yorkshire origins. The copper alembic is a link to pharmacy and to the alembic in the Society's Court Room. Philosophically, the alembic illustrates the separation of materials into fraction and dross, or the division of good and evil.

The motto *Be still and know your creator* is an adaptation of Psalm 46:10, 'Be still, and know that I am God.'

BORN Leeds 13 Apr 1941; *s* of Ernest Wilfred Adams and Hilda Wightman; *m* 1972 Kathryn Robinson.

EDUC U Manchester (BSc Pharmacy); U Cambridge (MA); U Hertfordshire (PhD).

QUALIFICATIONS BSc 1966; MRPharmS 1967; FRPharmS 1989; MA 2007; PhD 2010.

CAREER Merck, Sharp & Dohme Ltd: Pharmaceutical Research & Development 1966–78; Manufacturing Manager 1978–79; Production Manager 1979–84; Distribution services Manager 1984–87; Group Quality Control Manager 1987–92; Director Quality Operations (Gt Britain & Ireland) 1992–94; Director External Quality Operations 1994–96; Director of Compliance for Europe 1996–99.

HON APPTS EEC Authorised Person to release medicines for sale or supply 1980–d; Assessor for EEC Authorised Persons 1980–99; Antibiotics Sub-Cttee British Pharmacopeia Commission 1988–89; Court U Hertfordshire 2012–17.

SOCIETY Proposed for the Society by Prof Peter Roylance and Dr Brian Wills. Yeoman 1994; Liveryman 1999; Chairman Livery Cttee 2004–07, *ex officio* Court Assistant 2005–07 *vice* Prof Barrie Jay. Chairman Charity Cttee 2005–15; Elected to the Court 2014 *vice* Mr John Missen. Junior Warden 2014–15, Senior Warden 2015–16, Master 2016–17. Hon Treasurer 2019–d.

CITY AND CIVIC Barbers' Company: Freeman 2018.

Presented his miniature portrait and his stained glass Arms panel.

Professor Trevor BEEDHAM, BDS, LDS RCS, MB BS, LRCP MRCS, DObstRCOG, MIBiol, FRCOG

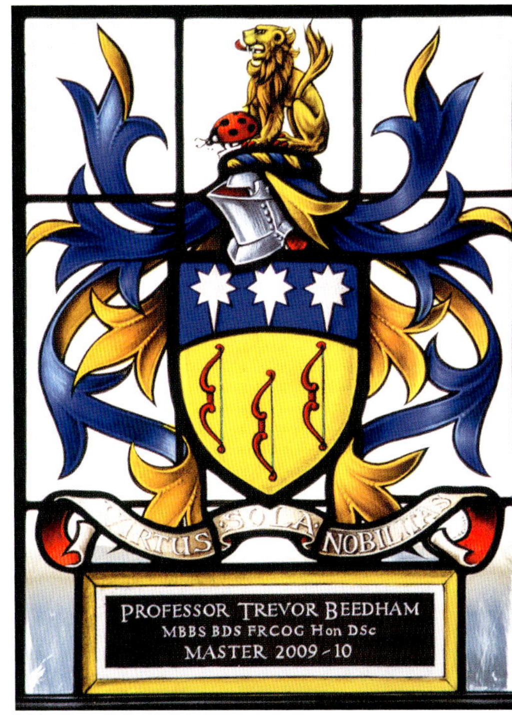

Or, three Bowes Gules stringed Azure on a Chief enarched also Azure three Mullets of eight points the lowest points extended Argent; And for the Crest upon a Helm, mantled Azure doubled Or, on a wreath of the colours, a Lion sejant between the Forepaws a seven spot Ladybird proper

Motto: *Virtus Sola Nobilitas*

The Arms were designed by Timothy Duke, Chester Herald, in 2010 and are recorded at the College of Arms in Volume 177, Folio 86.

The stained glass panel was made by Leonie Seliger of Canterbury and was installed in window W3-3 in 2014, showing the full Arms and motto without a cartouche.

The three bows with their strings are a two-fold allusion to his home town of Nottingham and to Apollo. In chief are three mullets with an extended limb (the natal star) taken from the Arms of the Royal College of Gynaecologists. The three stars also represent his three children. The curved line of the chief imitates the sky line at dawn which, as an obstetrician, he has witnessed many times.

A lion sejant is for his birth sign, with a ladybird between its feet as a symbol of his wife's love of gardening.

The motto translates as *Virtue alone is noble* and was used by his school, High Pavement Grammar School Nottingham.

BORN 30 Jul 1942; *s* of Herbert Beedham and Olive Spikings; *m* 1966 Anne Darnbrough-Cameron, two sons, one dau.

EDUC Royal Dental Hosp (BDS); the London Hosp Medical Coll (MB BS).

QUALIFICATIONS BDS 1965; LDS RCS Eng 1965; MB BS 1972; LRCP MRCS 1973; DObstRCOG 1975; MIBiol 1977; MRCOG 1977; FRCOG 1989.

CAREER Cons Gynaecologist & Obstetrician Barts & the Royal London Hosps 1981–2009: Clin Director 2003–08, Divisional Dir 2006–09, Dep Medical Dir 2007–09; Hon Sen Lecturer 2005–08, Assoc Dean 2006–09, Hon Professor 2008–d; Q Mary Sch of Medicine & Dentistry: Examiner for the MB BS, LMSSA, DObstRCOG, MRCOG, PLAB.

HON APPTS Chairman NE Thames Obs & Gynae Higher Trg Cttee 1991–94; Chairman Continuing Medical Education Cttee RCOG 1998–2002; General Medical Council Medical Schools Visitor 2001–13; Assessor Postgraduate Medical Education & Trg Board & GMC Appeals 2002–13; UK Forensic Regulators Cttee 2010–17.

SOCIETY Proposed for the Society by Dr David Hughes. Yeoman 1984; Liveryman 1988; United Examining Board 1993–2007, Chairman UEB Examinations Committee 1997–2007; elected to the Court 1996 *vice* Prof Paul Turner: Chairman Examinations Committee 2004–18. Junior Warden 2007–08, Senior Warden 2008–09, Master 2009–10. Inaugural Dean of the Society 2012–16; Past Master Emeritus 2018.

CITY AND CIVIC City Livery Club Council 2014–17; President, Friends of the Royal London Hospital 2015–d.

HONOURS AND AWARDS Hon DSc U Buckingham 2010.

Presented several books to the Library, a silver butter dish, his miniature portrait and his stained glass Arms panel.

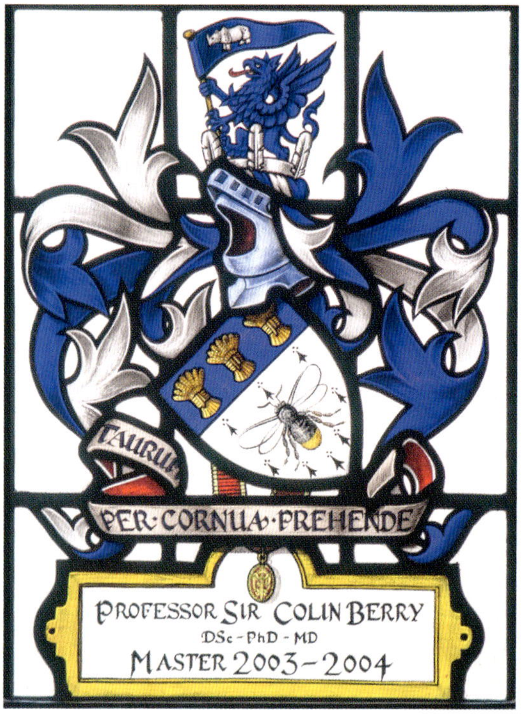

Ermine, a Bombus Lucorum proper, on a chief Azure three Garbs of Wheat Or; And for the Crest, upon a Knight's Helm mantled Azure doubled Argent, on a wreath of the colours, rising from the Circlet set on the side three of four Quills Argent (three manifest) a Griffin segrant Azure langued Gules supporting with the Foreclaws a Staff proper flying therefrom a Pennon also Azure, charged with a Rhinoceros statent Argent

Motto: *Taurum Per Cornua Prehende*

Professor Sir Colin Leonard BERRY, MB BS, MD, PhD, FRCPath, FFPM, DSc, FRCP, FRCP Ed, FFOM

The Arms were designed by Peter Gwynne-Jones, Garter King of Arms, in 2005 and are recorded at the College of Arms in Volume 161, Folio 56.

The stained glass panel was made by Leonie Seliger of Canterbury and was installed in window W2-6 in 2005 showing the full Arms and motto without a cartouche.

The bumble-bee (*Bombus lucorum*) and the sheaves of wheat recall that he both kept bees and was much involved with the safety of crops, the ermine tails are a reference to Charing Cross medical school and are seen in Redvers Ironside's window, from the same source.

The griffin is the emblem of the old London Hospital Medical College of which he was the last Dean. The three feathers in the chaplet are a reference to the Three Feathers, the pub where the London Hospital was founded in 1740. The rhinoceros on the flag refers to the Society.

The motto translates as *Take the bull by the horns.*

BORN 28 Sep Oct 1937; *s* of Ronald Berry and Peggy Caroline Benson; *m* 1960 Yvonne Waters, two sons.

EDUC Charing Cross Hosp Medical Sch (MB BS).

QUALIFICATIONS MB BS 1962; MD 1968; PhD 1970; MRCPath; FRCPath 1979; FFPM 1991; DSc Lond 1993; FRCP Lond 1993; FFOM 1995; FRCP Edin 1997.

CAREER Senior Lect Inst of Child Health 1964–70; Reader in Pathology Guy's Hosp Med Sch 1970–76; Prof Morbid Anatomy London Hosp Med Coll 1976–2002; WHO Toxicology Review Panel 1976–84; Chairman Cttee on Dental & Surgical Materials 1982–92; Adv Cttee on Pesticides MAFF/DHSS 1988–99; Cttee on Safety of Medicines DoH 1990–92; Dean London Hosp Med Coll 1994–95; Warden Barts & London Sch Med and Dent 1995–96.

HON APPTS Royal College Pathology, Treasurer 1988–93; General Medical Council 1993–96 & 1998–2003; Review of Coroner Service Home Office 2001–03; Pres British Acad Forensic Med 2002–03.

SOCIETY Gillson Scholar in Pathology 1967–68 & 1970–72. Proposed by Dr B. Kiernander and Dr Christopher Scott. Yeoman 1967; Liveryman 1971; elected to the Court 1990 *vice* Prof J. A. Dudgeon. Junior Warden 2001–02, Senior Warden 2002–03, Master 2003–04. Hon Treasurer 2004–14; Past Master Emeritus 2014.

CITY AND CIVIC Imperial Society of Knights Bachelor: Council 1997; Treasurer 2006–12; Knight Principal 2012–19. Knight President 2019–d.

HONOURS AND AWARDS Kt Bachelor 1993; Hon MD U Ioannina 2003.

Presented various books for the Library, a twentieth-century Wedgewood pestle and mortar, a bowl commemorating the London Hospital anniversary, a silver butter dish, the ironstone rhinoceros, an oriental rug, the Treasurer's badge, his miniature portrait and his stained glass Arms panel.

Dr Robert George Hankin BETHEL, MA, MB BChir, MRCGP, FRSH

The Arms were designed by David White, Somerset Herald, in 2010 and are recorded at the College of Arms in Volume 176, Folio 45.

The stained glass panel was made by Leonie Seliger of Canterbury and was installed in window W2-3 in 2015, showing the full Arms with motto without a cartouche.

The field is from the Arms of the University of Cambridge; the sword is for the City of London and the snake for medicine. The stag beetles are a canting reference to Bethel. The wreath and mantling are in the Society colours.

The seahorse is from Eastbourne and Eastbourne Grammar School. The shamrock garland is for an Irish maternal grandfather and the gavel is for the auctioneer paternal grandfather and for masonry.

The motto translates as *Caring for throughout life* (I shall take care of while life remains) and is a reference to his work as a GP.

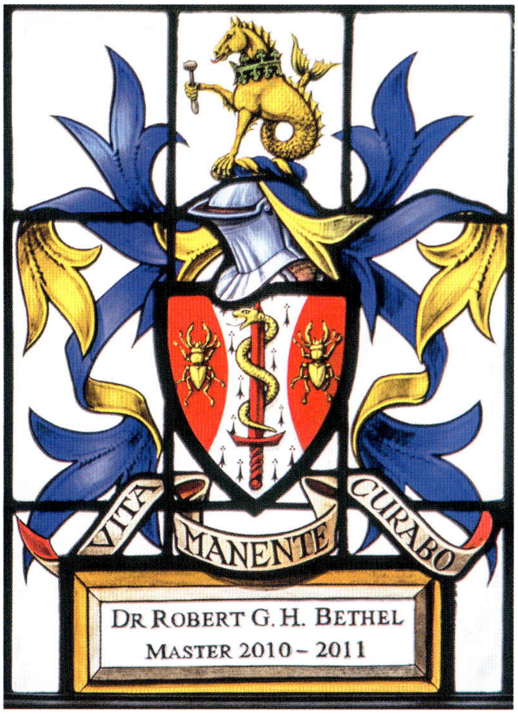

Ermine, between two Flaunches Gules each charged with a Stag Beetle palewise Or, a Sword in pale Gules the Blade entwined by a Serpent Or. And for the Crest, upon a helm mantled Azure doubled Or, on a wreath Or and Azure, a Seahorse sejant Or gorged with a Collar trefoiled on both edges Vert holding in the dexter foot a Gavel Sable

Motto: *Vita Manente Curabo*

BORN London, 7 Jun 1948; *s* of Horace Hankin Bethel and Mollie Motyer.
EDUC Pembroke Coll Cambridge (BA, MA, MB BChir); St Mary's Hosp Medical Sch.
QUALIFICATIONS BA 1969; MB BChir 1972; MA 1973; MRCGP 1979; FRSH 1990.
CAREER GP Englefield Green & Old Windsor 1976–2005; Rheumatologist Heatherwood Hosp Ascot 1976–92; Course Tutor Open U 1979–80; GP Trainer (Oxford) 1984–2005; Assoc Teacher ICSTM 1989–2004; Med Officer Brunel U 1993–98; GMC Performance Assessor & Examiner 2002–d; GP Appraiser 2004–d.
SOCIETY Proposed for the Society by Dr Phillip Willcox, Junior Warden. Yeoman 1977; Liveryman 1981; elected to the Court 2000 *vice* Dr James Fisher. Chairman of the Charity Cttee 2007–10. Junior Warden 2008–09, Senior Warden 2009–10, Master 2010–11. Hon Treasurer 2014–19.
CITY AND CIVIC Member Guild of Freemen 1979; Trustee Curriers' Company Millenium Bursary 2002–d; Liveryman Company of Curriers 2011; Wandsman St Paul's Cathedral 1987–d; Governor Corporation of the Sons of the Clergy 2011–d; Life Governor Royal Humane Soc 2011–d.
Presented his miniature portrait and his stained glass Arms panel.

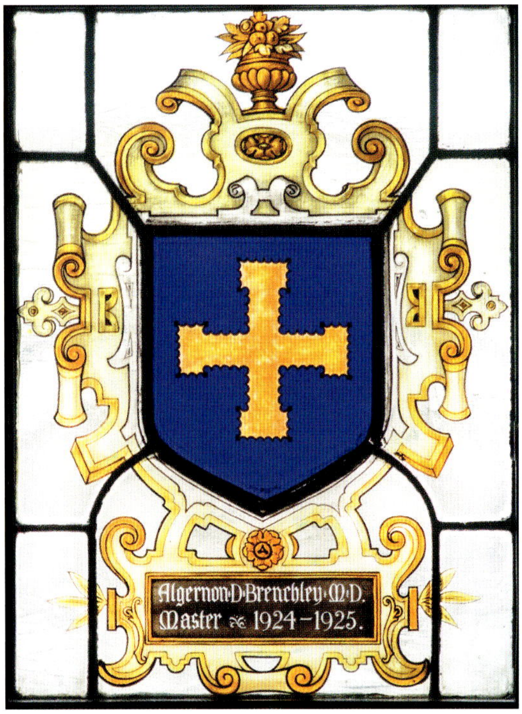

Azure, a Cross Potent engrailed Or

Dr Algernon Dutton BRENCHLEY, LSA, MRCS, MB ChB, MD

The Brenchleys of Brenchley County Kent were granted a simple cross *temp* Edward III and over the years differences for cadet branches were made with the colours and style of cross.

Brenchley of Maidstone, to whom he is related, was granted *Azure, a Cross Patonce engrailed Or,*[1] and these Arms change the cross to one potent but on what authority is not known and they are not recorded at the College of Arms.

It is possible that the stained glass panel was made by Francis Spear as it was installed by him in window W3-15 in 1931, showing the shield in Cartouche A. From Sep 1941 to Jan 1946, all stained glass was removed from the Hall during hostilities and on return in 1946 these Arms were replaced in window W3-15.

BORN Brighton 4 Apr 1854; *s* of Horatio Coare Brenchley LSA and Sarah Dutton; *m* 1887 Marion Spurling, *no children*; *ob.* 6 Dec 1940.

EDUC Guy's Hosp Medical Sch; U Aberdeen Medical Sch (MB ChB, MD).

QUALIFICATIONS LSA 1875; MRCS 1875; MB ChB 1877; MD 1880.

CAREER GP Denmark Hill; Medical Officer Camberwell Provident Dispensary in succession to his father 1886.

SOCIETY Yeoman 1876; Liveryman 1889; elected to the Court 1916 *vice* Albert Bryan Day. Examinations Cttee 1921–27. Junior Warden 1922–23, Senior Warden 1923–24, Master 1924–25. Society Representative on the Management Cttee of the Chelsea Physic Garden 1928–34.

In 1925 he donated 5 guineas to the Widows' Fund and he presented a modern Japanese silver pint mug and his stained glass Arms panel. He left a bequest of £1,200 which was used to buy candelabra for dinners.

Dr John Hubert Daly BRISCOE, LVO, MA, MB BChir, DObstRCOG, FRCGP, Hon LAH Dublin

The Arms were designed by Thomas Woodcock, Norroy and Ulster King of Arms, in 2001 and are recorded at the College of Arms in Volume 162, Folio 293.

The stained glass panel was made by Leonie Seliger of Canterbury and was installed in window W2-7 in 2001, showing the full Arms and motto without a cartouche. Suspended from the shield is the LVO medal.

Red is for blood with silver for contrast. The battlements represent Windsor Castle. The lily is from the Arms of Eton College. The cornflower is associated with his school, Winchester College. A Saracen's head is the crest of the Irish Briscoes but the change to a moor indicates his time in Basutoland. The torch symbolises learning and is also the emblem of the Medical Officers of Schools Association with a serpent entwined for medicine. The rhinoceros and the serpent also feature in the Society's Arms.

The motto *Faithful to one* is feminine to signify his wife, his Queen and his profession.

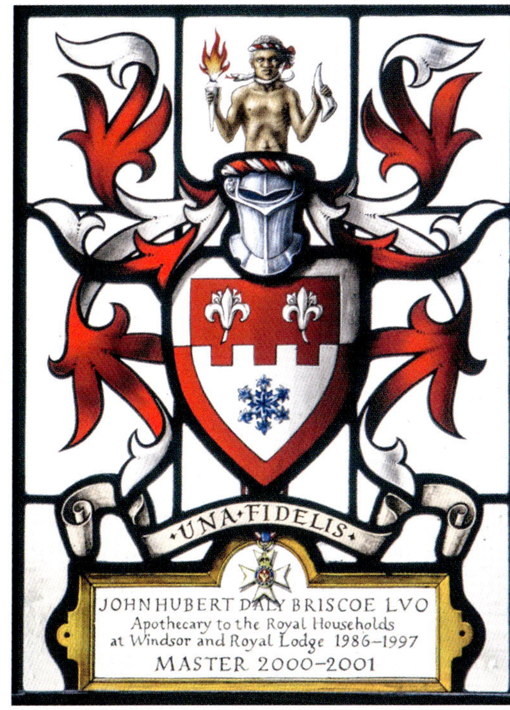

BORN 19 Mar 1933; *s* of Dr Daly Briscoe and Doris Nicholson; *m* 1958 Anne Earlham, one son, four daus.

EDUC St John's Coll Cambridge (BA, MA, MB BChir); St Thomas's Hosp Medical Sch.

QUALIFICATIONS MA 1957; MB BChir 1957; DObstRCOG 1959; MRCGP 1968; FRCGP 2006.

CAREER Med Offr Overseas Civil Service Basutoland 1959–62; Asst GP Aldeburgh 1963–65; GP Eton 1965–97; Med Offr Eton Coll 1965–97; Med Offr St George's Sch 1976–97; Apothecary to HM Household Windsor & to HM The Queen Mother's Household at Royal Lodge 1987–97.

HON APPTS Pres MOs of Sch Assoc 1989–91.

SOCIETY Proposed for the Society by Dr Daly Briscoe. Yeoman 1956; Liveryman 1960; elected to the Court 1984 *vice* Dr E. G. Grey-Turner. Junior Warden 1998–99, Senior Warden 1999–2000, Master 2000–01. Past Master Emeritus 2008.

FAMILY LIVERYMEN (father) Dr Daly Briscoe, (son) Dr James Briscoe.

HONOURS AND AWARDS LVO 1997; Hon LAH Dublin.

Presented a photograph of three generations of Briscoe Liverymen and Yeomen, a foetal stethoscope, a mahogany table, his miniature portrait and his stained glass Arms panel.

Per fess embattled Gules and Argent, a Bordure counter-changed, in chief two Lilies Argent and in base a Cornflower Azure; And for the Crest, upon a Helm mantled Gules doubled Argent, on a wreath of the colours a Demi-Moor affrontée proper, wreathed about the temples Argent and Gules, grasping in the dexter hand a Torch enflamed and in the sinister hand a Rhinoceros Horn proper, coiled around the neck a Serpent Argent langued Gules

Motto: *Una Fidelis*

Dr Uriah BRISTOW

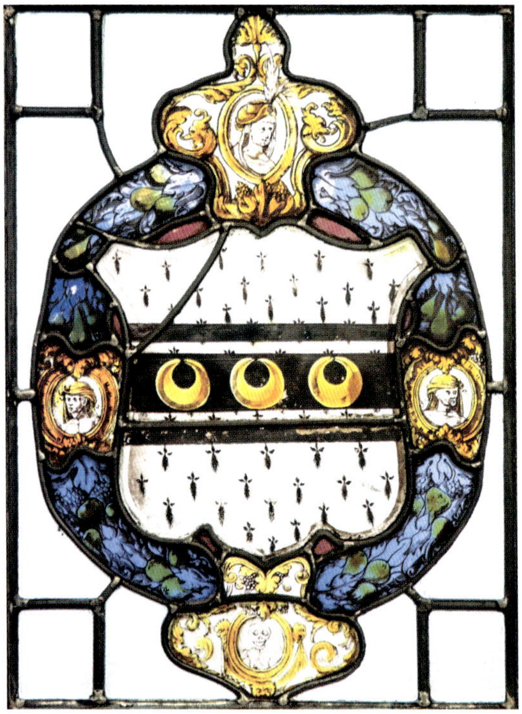

Ermine, on a Fess cotised Sable, three Crescents Or

Crest (not shown): *upon a Helm on a wreath Argent and Sable, out of a Crescent Or a demi-Eagle displayed Azure*

The Arms are recorded at the College of Arms in Vincent 162.100 (Dethick's Grants) and the grant was to Nicholas Bristowe of Ayot, Hertfordshire in 1544.

The manor of Ayot St Lawrence was held by the Bristowes from 1572 to 1714. This stained glass panel originally came from the disused church at Ayot St Lawrence and was presented to the Society in May 1980 by Bristow's great-great-grandson Lt Col P. F. White & great-great-granddaughter Mrs D. Bousted.

The stained glass panel was restored by Carl Edwards and was installed in window E2-14 in 1980. It shows the shield within a floral surround with four small cartouches.

See Chapter 9 for a full discussion of this panel.

BORN Clerkenwell 1734; *s* of Edward Bristow and Elizabeth Slindall; 1766 married his second cousin Elizabeth Bristow, two daus; *ob.* 23 Dec 1812.

EDUC Apprenticed to his father 1749.

CAREER Apothecary in St John's Wood.

SOCIETY Yeoman 1757; Liveryman 1779; Treasurer Chemical Dept 1798–1800; Treasurer Navy Stock 1800–; elected to the Court 1795. Renter Warden 1801–02, Upper Warden 1802–03, Master 1803–04.

FAMILY LIVERYMEN (father) Dr Edward Bristow.

The Society also holds his mourning ring and seal (given by Mr T. B. Hughes in 2006) and a book entitled *The Doctrine of Morality* which belonged to his stepmother Lydia (given by Col P. F. White in 1982).

Dr Frederick Gordon BROWN
LSA, MRCS

The Arms are of the colours and charges of Brown families (cf. Buckston Browne W2-8) but with the tinctures reversed compared to those of his elder brother T. E. B. Brown. This is reasonable when differencing cadet branches except that he now has a silver chief on a silver field which is horribly wrong. Oddly, despite the reversal of tinctures, he still uses the annulet as a cadency mark (for a fifth son). These are unofficial Arms probably designed by himself.

The stained glass maker is unknown but may have been W. B. Simpson & Sons. The panel was installed in window W3-11 between 1917 and 1922, showing the shield in Cartouche A. From Sep 1941 to Jan 1946, all stained glass was removed from the Hall during hostilities and on return in 1946 these Arms were placed in window W2-15.

The patterns showing on the corners of the field and in the chief and the black edgings to compartments of the charges are the glassmaker's stylised work and should not appear heraldically.

The motto translates as *Let us be judged by our actions.*

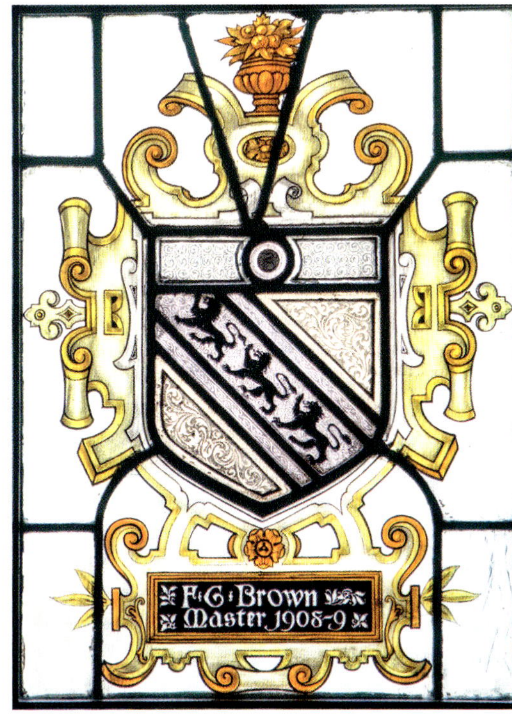

Argent, three lions passant in bend between two pairs of bendlets Sable; on a chief a pellet charged with an annulet of the field

Crest (not shown): *on a helm on a wreath of the colours an eagle displayed*

Motto (not shown): *Spectemur Agendo*

BORN London 10 Mar 1843; *s* of Dr Thomas Brown and Mary Denny; *ob.* 15 Jan 1928.

EDUC St Thomas's Hosp Medical Sch.

QUALIFICATIONS MRCS and LM 1863; LSA 1863.

SERVICES Medical Officer to 7th Bn Royal Fusiliers 1882.

CAREER Finsbury Circus partnership with Dr AP Gibbons; Medical Officer City of London Union (workhouse) 1865–1916; Surgeon City of London Police 1885–1914, in which capacity he examined some of the Ripper victims in 1888; Surgeon of the Guildhall School of Music 1880; Medical Officer of the Central Markets 1890.

HON APPTS President Hunterian Society 1892–94.

SOCIETY Apprenticed to his father; Yeoman 1863; Liveryman 1880; elected to the Court 1897 *vice* Thomas Dickinson. Junior Warden 1906–07, Senior Warden 1907–08, Master 1908–09. Examinations Cttee 1910–17; Society Representative on the Management Cttee of the Chelsea Physic Garden 1910–18.

FAMILY LIVERYMEN (father) Thomas Brown; (bro) Dr Thomas Edwin Burton Brown, Master 1901–02; (nep) Dr Frederick Hewlett Burton Brown; (nephew) Arthur Thomas Brown FRCS; (nephew) Surg Capt Gerald Burton Brown RN.

(Cashell states that the Brown brothers were relatives of Sir Hugh Lett. If so, they must have been distant relatives of Lady Lett who was the dau of Sir Buckston Browne but in what way has not been established.)

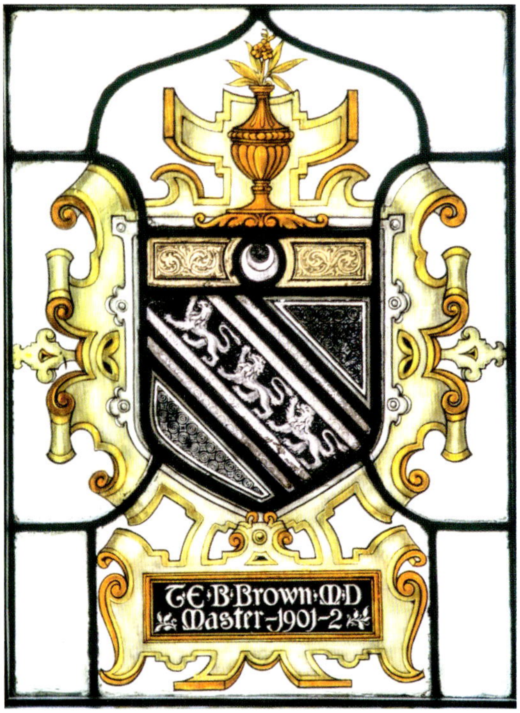

Dr Thomas Edwin Burton BROWN, CIE, LSA, MRCS, MD

The Arms are of the colours and charges of Brown families (cf. Buckston Browne W2-8) but it is very strange to use a Chief simply to display a cadency mark (The crescent is the mark of a second son). Fox-Davies in 1895 describes the Arms and goes on to remark 'for which no authority has been established'.[2] These are unofficial Arms likely to have been designed by his brother F. G. Brown.

The stained glass panel-maker is unknown but may have been W. M. Simpson & Son. The panel was installed in window W3–10 between 1917–22, showing the shield in Cartouche B. From Sep 1941 to Jan 1946 all stained glass was removed from the Hall during hostilities and on return in 1946 these Arms were placed in window W2-13.

The patterns showing on the corners of the field and in the chief and the edgings to compartments of the charges are the glassmakers stylised work and should not appear heraldically.

The motto translates as *Let us be judged by our actions.*

Sable, three lions passant in bend between two pairs of bendlets Argent; on a chief of the second a pellet charged with a crescent of the second

Crest (not shown): *upon a helm on a wreath of the colours an eagle displayed*

Motto (not shown): *Spectemur Agendo*

BORN 8 Feb 1833; *s* of Dr. Thomas Brown and Mary Denny; *m* 1862 Mary Caroline Hewlett, four sons, one dau; *ob.* 28 Jun 1911.

EDUC Guy's Hosp Medical Sch (MB).

QUALIFICATIONS LSA 1854; MRCS 1854; MB 1856; MD 1857.

SERVICES Bengal Army: Asst Surg 1858, Surg 1870, Surg Major 1873, Brigade Surg 1885.

CAREER Demonstrator in Anatomy at Guy's until 1858; Professor of Medicine and Principal Lahore Medical College.

SOCIETY Apprenticed to his father 1848; Yeoman 1855; Liveryman 1878; Court of Examiners 1892–93; elected to the Court 1893 *vice* Edwin Chalbot. Junior Warden 1899–1900, Senior Warden 1900–01, Master 1901–02. Examinations Cttee 1905–09; Society Representative on the Management Cttee of the Chelsea Physic Garden 1906–10.

FAMILY LIVERYMEN (father) Dr Thomas Brown; (bro) Dr Frederick Gordon Brown, Master 1908–09; (son) Dr Frederick Hewlett Burton Brown; (son) Arthur Thomas Brown FRCS; (son) Surg Capt Gerald Burton Brown RN.

(*Cashell states that the Brown brothers were relatives of Sir Hugh Lett. If so, they must have been distant relatives of Lady Lett who was the dau of Sir Buckston Browne but in what way has not been established.*)

HONOURS AND AWARDS CIE 1891.

In 1902 donated 10 guineas to the Distressed Members' Fund.

Sir George Buckston BROWNE, FRCS, Hon LMSSA, Hon LLD Aberd

The Arms were designed by Richard Graham-Vivian, Bluemantle Pursuivant, in 1939 and are recorded at the College of Arms in Volume Gr 105, Folio 296.

The stained glass panel was made by James Powell & Sons and was probably installed in window W4-7 in 1939, showing the full Arms and motto without a cartouche. From Sep 1941 to Jan 1946 all stained glass was removed from the Hall during hostilities and on return in 1946 these Arms were placed in window W2-8.

The same colours, lions and bendlets were used by the Brownes, Marquesses of Sligo. It is likely that when the Arms illustrated were created for Sir Buckston he chose a variation of Arms that had been used by Brownes in the past.

The motto translates as *The lively impetus of genius conquers all.*

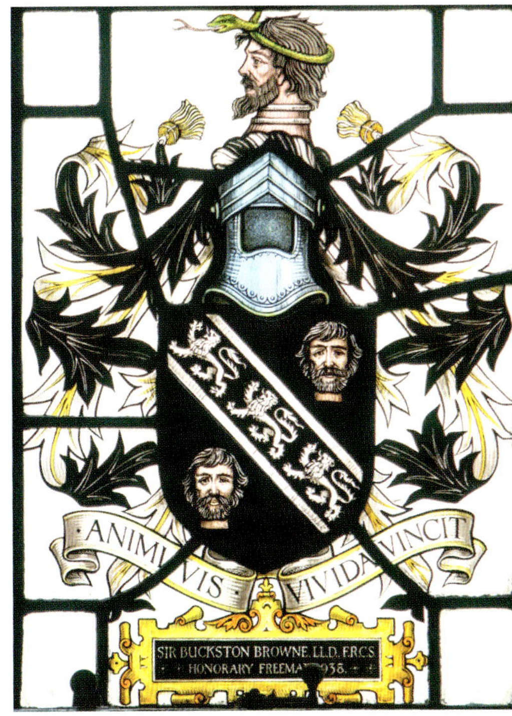

Sable, within two Bendlets three Lions passant Argent, between two Saracen's Heads affrontée couped at the neck proper; And for the Crest upon a Knight's Helm, mantled Sable doubled Argent, on a wreath of the colours a Saracen's Head in profile wreathed about the temples by a Serpent proper and gorged with a Collar gemel Argent

Motto: *Animi Vis Vivida Vincit*

BORN Manchester 13 Apr 1850; *s* of Dr Henry Browne and Ann Hadfield; *m* 1874 Helen Vaine, one son, one dau: *ob.* 19 Jan 1945. His son was killed in the Great War and his only grandson died of enteric fever in 1924. His dau Helen married Sir Hugh Lett (Master 1937–38, PRCS 1938–40).

EDUC University Coll London Medical Sch.

QUALIFICATIONS MRCS 1874; FRCS Eng 1926.

CAREER Private Asst to surgeon Sir Henry Thompson 1870–1884; own private urological surgical practice 1884–1909.

RETIREMENT in retirement he devoted himself to public benefactions especially the promotion of surgical science. In 1928 he bought Charles Darwin's house for preservation by the British Association and in 1931 gave £100,000 for the Buckston Browne surgical-research farm on the estate. He was a benefactor to University College Hosp, Wesley House Methodist Theological Coll Cambridge, the Royal College of Surgeons of England, and the Society of Apothecaries.

In 1927 he endowed the annual Buckston Browne dinner for fifty Fellows and fifty Members at the RCS which brought members back into contact with College affairs and in 1928 an annual dinner for the Harveian Society.

SOCIETY Honorary Freeman 1938 in the Mastership of Sir Hugh Lett; Honorary LMSSA 1944 in the Mastership of Sir Stanley Woodwark.

HONOURS AND AWARDS Kt Bachelor 1932, Hon LLD U Aberdeen 1932.

Presented a silver octofoil salver dating from 1860, a silver wine jug from 1895, two silver goblets from 1897 and a silver biscuit box of 1901.

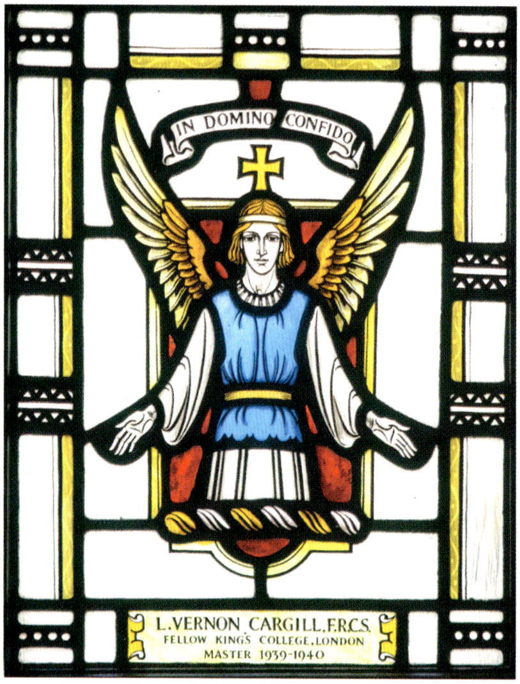

Mr Lionel Vernon CARGILL, LSA, LRCP MRCS, FRCS, FKC

The stained glass panel was made by James Hogan of James Powell & Sons in 1948 and was installed in window W4-2 in 1948 showing the Crest and motto only, without a cartouche.

The Cargills were a Scottish family whose cadets used a variant of *Gules, three Martlets Or* and one branch certainly used this crest.[3]

Mr Cargill's branch of the family moved to Nottinghamshire from Perthshire in the seventeenth century.

It is not clear why the full achievement of Arms was not used and it may be that he was not directly related to the armigerous branches of the family.

The motto translates as *In the Lord I trust.*

Main blazon unknown; on a Wreath Or and Argent, a demi-Maiden affrontée Arms outspread vested Azure and Argent, winged proper, bearing on her Head a Cross Patté Or

Motto: *In Domino Confido*

BORN London 27 Jun 1866; *s* of William and Annie Cargill; *m* 1897 Emma Shearwood, three daus; *ob.* 13 Dec 1955.

EDUC Salter's University Scholarship to King's College Hosp Medical Sch.

QUALIFICATIONS LSA 1890; LRCP MRCS 1890; FRCS Eng 1892.

SERVICES Ophthalmic Surg Imperial Yeomanry Hosp 1899–1900; Hon Ophthmalic Cons 4th Gen Hosp 1914–18.

CAREER Ophthalmic Surgeon to King's College Hosp 1894–1931, the Royal Eye Hosp 1896–1931 and the Seamen's Hosp Greenwich 1889; Lecturer in Ophthalmology King's Coll Medical Sch; Examiner U Oxford.

HON APPTS Council Ophthalmological Soc of UK.

SOCIETY Yeoman 1897; Liveryman 1908; elected to the Court 1931 *vice* Francis de Haviland Hall. Junior Warden 1937–38, Senior Warden 1938–39, Master 1939–40.

CITY AND CIVIC Cttee of Management Chelsea Physic Garden 1941–55.

HONOURS AND AWARDS Fellow of King's College London 1939.

He paid for the decoration of the Parlour after the fireplace was installed and presented the gilt-framed mirror; he also presented a pair of George III silver fruit spoons, a silver sugar bowl and sifter of 1888, a 1937 silver cream jug, his miniature portrait, his stained glass Arms panel and a bequest of £80,000.

Mr Geoffrey Thomas Willoughby CASHELL, KStJ, LMSSA, LRCP, MB BS, FRCS Ed, FRCS, FRCOphth, AKC

The Arms were designed by John Brooke-Little, Richmond Herald, in 1971 and are recorded at the College of Arms in Volume Gr 134, Folio 191.

The stained glass maker is unknown but the panel was installed in window E1-5 in 1972 showing the shield in Cartouche A.

The minutes of the Future Activities Committee suggest that the panel was originally installed in one of the West window cartouches and moved to the East side in 1980 but this cannot be confirmed.[4]

It is not known what the charges and colours signify.

The motto translates as *Time is a great healer of the eyes* – adapted from Ovid's *Remedia Armoris.*

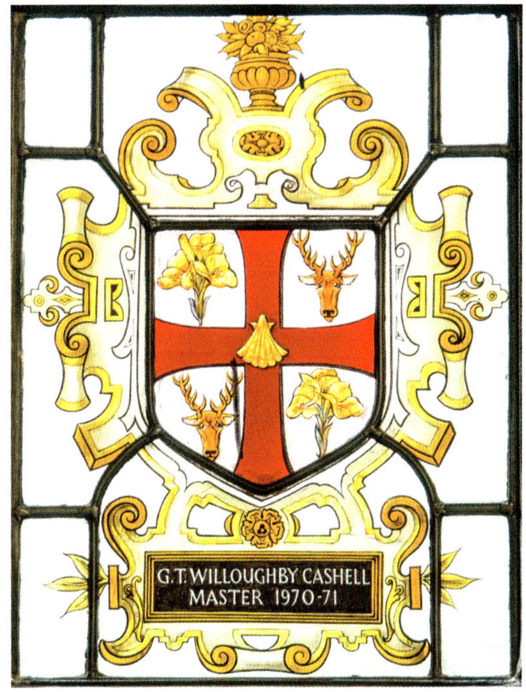

Argent, on a Cross formy throughout Gules, between in the 1st and 4th quarters the head of a Yellow Iris and in the 2nd and 3rd quarters a Stag's Head cabossed all proper, an Escallop Or

Crest (not shown): *upon a Helm, on a Wreath Argent and Sable, a demi-Horse Argent issuant from Rays of the Sun and supporting between the Forelegs a Unicorn's Horn erect Or*

Motto (not shown): *Temporis Ars Medicina Oculorum Fere Est*

BORN Beckenham 2 Sep 1905; *s* of Alfred Ernest Cashell and Minnie Barbara Lyle; *m* 1933 Hilda Kinmont, two sons; *ob.* 21 Jan 1994.

EDUC King's Coll Hosp Medical Sch (MB BS).

QUALIFICATIONS LMSSA 1930; LRCP MRCS 1930; MB BS 1933; FRCS Edin 1933; FRCS Eng 1952; FRCOphth 1988.

SERVICES Sqn Ldr RAF; Wing Cdr RAFVR 1954; Cons in Ophthalmology to RAF.

CAREER Cons Ophthalmic Surgeon Royal Berkshire Hosp 1933–70; Director Orthoptic Training Sch Reading 1935–70; Chairman British Orthoptic Board, examiner 1952–59; Area Clinical Tutor Reading U Oxford 1970.

HON APPTS Chairman Medical Advisory Cttee 1959–69; Treasurer Faculty Ophthalmology.

SOCIETY Yeoman 1931; Liveryman 1934; elected to the Court 1959 *vice* Cornelius Ver Heyden de Lancy, who had resigned on not being elected Junior Warden. Junior Warden 1968–69, Senior Warden 1969–70, Master 1970–71. Hon Treasurer 1975–85; Assistant Emeritus 1990.

HONOURS AND AWARDS Hon DSc U Reading 1976; Hon FRACO 1976; CStJ 1976; KStJ 1981.

He produced in 1984 a loose-leaf catalogue of the stained glass windows. Presented various books for the Library, two silver medals commemorating Keats' death, a silver beaker commemorating the City's 800th anniversary, his miniature portrait and his stained glass Arms panel. He also left a bequest of £1,000.

Sir Leonard John CHALSTREY, MA, LRCP MRCS, MB BChir, MD, FRCS, FRSA

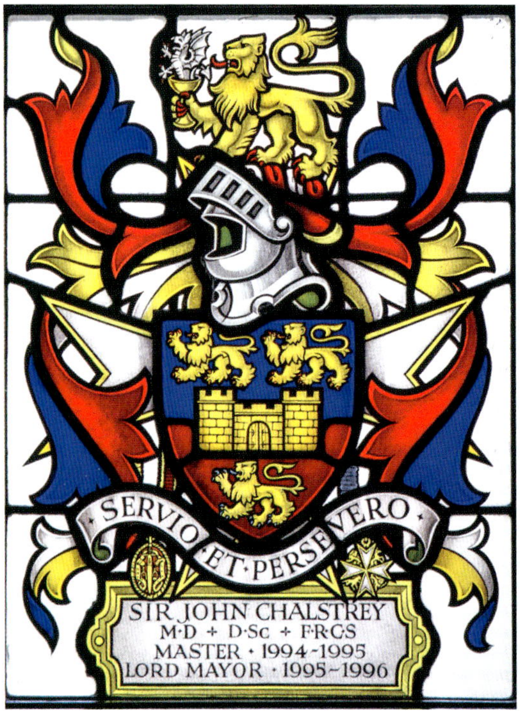

Per fess Azure and Gules, a Roman fort, the Entrance Way closed and on each side a Tower, all Or masoned between three Lions passant of the last. And for the Crest, upon a Knight's Helm mantled Gules and Azure doubled Or and Argent, on a wreath Argent and Gules, a Lion statant holding in the dexter Paw a Chalice Or issuant therefrom a Dragonet Argent

Motto: *Servio et Persevero*

The Arms were designed by Peter Gwynne-Jones, Garter King of Arms, in 1998 and are recorded at the College of Arms in Volume 149, Folio 159.

The stained glass panel was made by Goddard & Gibbs of Bow and was installed in window W2-12 in 1998, showing the full Arms and motto without a cartouche. Suspended from the shield is the badge of a Knight Bachelor and the star of a Knight of St John. The panel was deliberately placed next to Sir Thomas Crosby the only other former Lord Mayor in the Hall.

The fort represents the family's origins in the Roman hamlet of Cholstrey and the lions to its connection with Leominster. They are also a pun on the family name of Leonard.

In the crest, the goblet refers to his Aldermanic seat in Vintry and the dragon refers both to St John the Apostle and the Society Arms.

The motto translates as *I serve and I persevere.*

BORN Tipton 17 Mar 1931; *s* of Leonard Chalstrey and Frances Mary Lakin; *m* 1958 Aileen Bayes, one son, one dau; *ob.* 12 Mar 2020.

EDUC Queen's Coll Cambridge (BA, MA, MB BChir, MD) and St Bartholomew's Hosp Medical Coll.

QUALIFICATIONS MA 1954; LRCP MRCS 1957; MB BChir 1957; MD 1967; FRCS Eng 1962; FRSA 1996.

SERVICES National Service Welch Regiment and Royal Army Education Corps 1949–54; Major 357 Field Surg Team RAMC TA 1991–96; Hon Col 256 (City of London) Field Hosp RAM C (V) 1996–2000.

CAREER Cons Surgeon Barts, Hackney & Homerton Hosps 1969–96; Hon Cons Surgeon St Luke's Hospital for the Clergy 1975–93.

SOCIETY Proposed for the Society by Prof EW Walls and Mr Ivo Smith. Yeoman 1972; Liveryman 1976; elected to the Court 1984 *vice* Sir Ronald Gibson. Junior Warden 1991–92, Senior Warden 1992–94, Master 1994–95. Monckton Copeman Lecturer 1998; Past Master Emeritus 2006. He served for two years as Senior Warden in order not to be Master whilst also Sheriff.

CITY AND CIVIC Parish Clerks Company 1993–2007; HAC 1995–d; Company of Barbers: Freeman 1982, Liveryman 1984, Court 1987, Master 1998–99; Common Councillor for Langbourn 1981–1984; Alderman for Vintry 1984–2001; JP 1984; Aldermanic Sheriff 1993–94; Lord Mayor 1995–96. He was the first Apothecary Lord Mayor as Sir Thomas Crosby's mother company was the Turners.

FAMILY LIVERYMEN (wife) Aileen Chalstrey, (dau) Ms Susan Chalstrey FRCS (Mrs Sullivan).

HONOURS AND AWARDS DSc Hon Caus (City U) 1995, KStJ 1995; Kt Bachelor 1996; Hon GSM 1996; Hon FRSPH 1996. Presented several books for the Library, nine lead planters, his shrieval chain for the Master's use, his miniature portrait and his stained glass Arms panel. The portrait which hangs on the Landing of Sir John in his mayoral robes was painted by June Mendoza in 1996.

Dr Timothy Lachlan CHAMBERS, OBE, JP, DL, VR, MB BS, FRCP, FRCP Ed, FRCPI, FRCPCH, KLJ

The Arms were designed by Patric Dickinson, Clarenceaux King of Arms, in 2010 and are recorded at the College of Arms in Volume 175, Folio 130.

The stained glass panel was made by Richard Scowen of Cornwall and was installed in window W2-1 *c.*2013, showing the full Arms and motto without a cartouche.

The red field, the unicorns, castle and hand with a serpent are all part of the City of Bristol's Arms.

A castle on a rock is the McLachlan crest.

Unicorn horns and the serpent represent medicine and the former also feature in the Society's Arms.

The shamrocks represent an Irish heritage.

The motto translates as *May Thy will be done.*

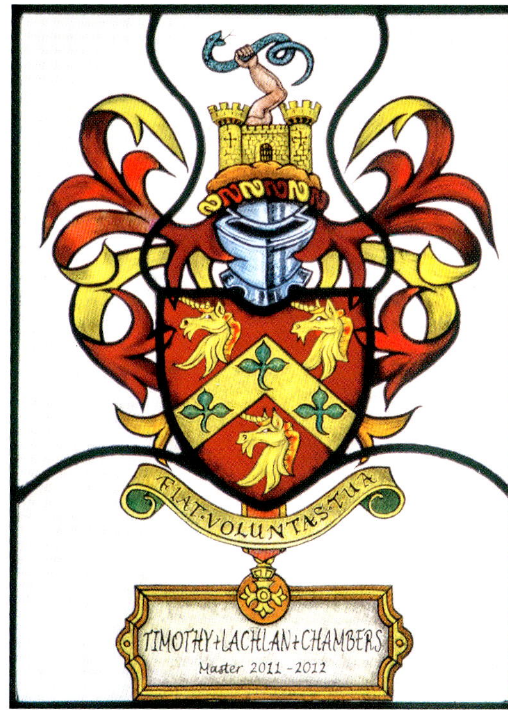

Gules, on a Chevron between three Unicorn's heads erased Or, armed Argent, three Shamrocks Vert: And for the Crest, upon a Helm mantled Gules doubled Or, on a wreath of the colours, upon a Rock a Castle issuant therefrom a sinister Arm embowed proper holding in the hand a Serpent Vert

Motto: *Fiat Voluntas Tua*

BORN 11 Feb 1946; adopted *s* of Victor Lachlan Chambers and Elsie Reynolds; *m* 1971 Joanna Ward, one son, two daus.

EDUC King's Coll Hosp Medical Sch (MB BS).

QUALIFICATIONS MB BS 1969; MRCP UK 1972; FRCP Lond 1983; FRCP Edin 1985; FRCPI 1995; FRCPCH 1997.

SERVICES Lt Col RAMC(V); OC Clin Sqn 243 Wessex Field Hosp (V) 2006–08; MO Somerset Cadet Bn ACF 1999–2012.

CAREER Phys & Nephrologist Derbyshire Children's Hosp 1976–79; Phys (General & Renal Med) Bristol Royal Hosp for Children & Paediatric Depts Southmead Hosp and Weston-super-Mare Gen Hosp 1979–2010; Sen Clin Lect in Child Health U Bristol 1979–2010; Clinical Dean Southmead Hosp 1983–90; Cons Paediatrician MoD 1985–2010.

SOCIETY Proposed for the Society by Sir Peter Tizard, Junior Warden. Yeoman 1982; Liveryman 1986; elected to the Court 2000 *vice* Mr Douglas Eadie: Examinations Cttee 2002–12; Chairman Academic & Resources Cttee 2003–08. Junior Warden 2009–10, Senior Warden 2010–11, Master 2011–12.

FAMILY LIVERYMEN (wife) Dr Joanna Chambers, (dau) Dr Catherine Chambers (Mrs Chapman) ob. 2007, (son-in-law) Dr Peter Chapman.

CITY AND CIVIC JP Bristol 1993; High Sheriff of the County & City of Bristol 2009–10; Vice Lord-Lieutenant of the County and City of Bristol 2012–d; Company of Barbers: Liveryman 2012.

HONOURS AND AWARDS Hon FSLC Paed 2002, OBE 2009, CMLJ 2013, KLJ 2017.

Presented various books for the Library, a bronze rhinoceros, a commemorative Barber's bowl, a silver quaiche in memory of Liveryman Dr Joy Edelman, a claret jug in memory of his daughter Catherine, the portrait of St James the Less, the miniature portrait of Sir Peter Tizard, his own miniature portrait and his stained glass Arms panel.

the Rt Hon Henry Cohen, Baron COHEN of Birkenhead, CH, KStJ, MB ChB, MD, FRCP, FRSH

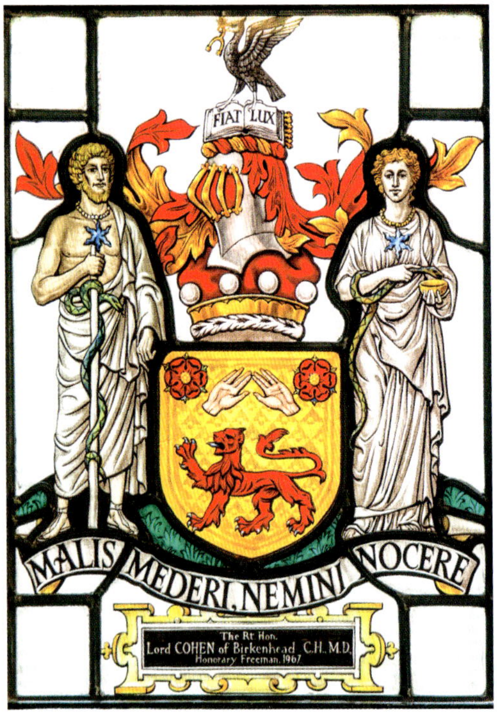

The Arms were designed by John Walker, Lancaster Herald, in 1957 and are recorded at the College of Arms in Volume Gr 120, Folio 87.

The stained glass panel was made by Carl Edwards in 1975 and was installed in widow E1-11 in 1975 showing the full Arms, supporters and motto without a cartouche.

Apart from the medical Supporters, the reason for the choice of charges and colours is unknown.

The motto translates as *To cure illness and harm no one.*

Or, a Lion passant Gules, in chief two Hands couped at the Wrist proper positioned as in the Priestly Blessing between as many Roses of the 2nd barbed and seeded also proper; And for the Crest upon a Peer's Helm, mantled Gules doubled Or, on a Wreath of the colours, perched on an open Book Argent with seven Clasps to the sinister Or, the Pages inscribed with the words Fiat Lux in letters Sable, a Cormorant wings elevated proper holding in the beak a Spur Or; for supporters: dexter a representation of Asclepius supporting in the exterior Hand his Rod proper; sinister a representation of Hygeia holding in the interior Hand a Serpent likewise proper and in the exterior hand a Bowl Or; both vested in white Robes also proper and gorged with a Chain gold pendant therefrom an Estoile Azure

Motto: *Malis Mederi, Nemini Nocere*

BORN Birkenhead 21 Feb 1900; *s* of Isaac Cohen and Dora Mendelson; *unmarried*; *ob.* 7 Aug 1977.

EDUC U Liverpool Medical Sch (MB ChB); U London (MD).

QUALIFICATIONS MB ChB 1922; MD 1924; MRCP 1926; FRCP Lond 1934; FRSH 1957.

CAREER Professor of Medicine U Liverpool 1934–65; Central Health Services Council – Vice Chairman 1949–57, Chairman 1957–63; Chancellor U Hull 1970–77.

HON APPTS Council Royal College of Physicians 1943–46; General Medical Council 1945, President 1961–73; President Royal Society of Medicine 1964–66; President BMA 1950–51; President Royal Society of Health 1958–77; President British Society for the History of Medicine.

SOCIETY Yeoman 1948; Gideon de Laune Lecturer 1962. Hon Freeman 1967 in the Mastership of Dr H. M. Sinclair as part of the 350th Anniversary celebrations.

CITY AND CIVIC JP for Lancashire; DL for Lancaster 1969.

HONOURS AND AWARDS Kt Bach 1949; Hon LLD U Liverpool 1950; Hon FRCGP 1952; Hon DSc NUI 1952; Baronage 1956; Hon FACP 1957; Hon FRIC 1959; Hon FRCPI 1959; KStJ 1961; Hon FPS 1962; Hon LLD U London 1963; Hon FFARCS 1963; Hon FRCPS Glas 1963; Hon FRCOG 1964; Hon LLD U Manchester 1966; Hon LLD U Hull 1966; Hon DSc U Sussex 1966; BMA Gold Medal 1967; Hon DCL U Oxford 1968; Hon FRCS Eng 1969; CH 1974.

Colonel Benjamin Bloomfield CONNOLLY, CB, MA, LSA, MRCS, MD BC, FRCSI

These Con(n)olly Arms were granted to William Conolly of Castletown, Speaker of the House of Commons in Ireland, *temp* Queen Anne; they were re-granted in 1821 to Edward Michael Pakenham of Castletown on assuming the name of Conolly by Royal licence and are recorded at the Ulster Office in Volume A25.[5]

The maker of the stained glass panel is unclear but may have been W. B. Simpson & Sons. The panel was installed in window W3-13 between 1919 and 1922, showing the shield in Cartouche A. From Sep 1941 to Jan 1946 all stained glass was removed from the Hall during hostilities and on return in 1946 these Arms were returned to window W3-13.

It is not known what the relationship to the original grantee was and it is likely that these Arms have simply been assumed. Also the artist has not engrailed the saltire.

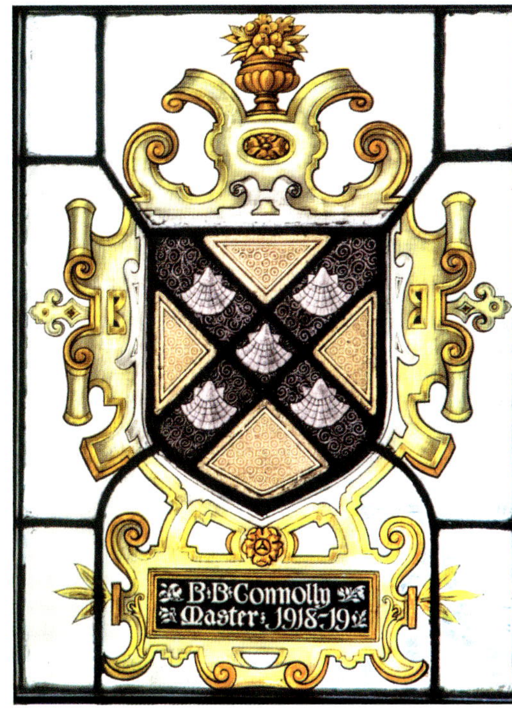

Argent, on a Saltire engrailed Sable, five Escallops of the field

---

BORN Woolwich 10 Sep 1845; *s* of Rev James Campbell Connolly RN and Dorothea Anne Handy; *m* 1881 Olivia Frances Potts, two sons, two daus; *ob.* 20 Jun 1924.

EDUC Gonville & Caius Coll Cambridge (BA, MA, MD & BC) and Guy's Hosp.

QUALIFICATIONS BA 1867; LSA 1869; MRCS Eng 1870; MA 1871; FRCSI 1889; MD & BC 1891.

SERVICES served in Franco-Prussian War 1870–71; Asst Surgeon AMS 40th Foot 1871; Zulu war 1879; Surgeon Major 1882; Egypt & Sudan 1882–89; Surg Lt Col and retired 1891; re-employed as principal MO at the Royal Arsenal & promoted Col 1902 for services in South African war; ADMS for Sussex 1914–18.

HON APPTS Society Representative on the General Medical Council 1918–24.

SOCIETY Yeoman 1869; Liveryman 1885; Court of Examiners 1914–21; elected to the Court 1907 *vice* F. R. Gibbes. Junior Warden 1916–17, Senior Warden 1917–18, Master 1918–19.

FAMILY LIVERYMEN (son) Dr Bloomfield George Connolly; (son) George Augustus Victor Connolly; (grandson) Rainier Campbell Connolly FRCS.

HONOURS AND AWARDS Order of Osmania 4th class, Turkey 1885; Khedive's Star 1882; CB 1900.

Presented a circular silver powder compact engraved with a rhinoceros and his stained glass Arms panel.

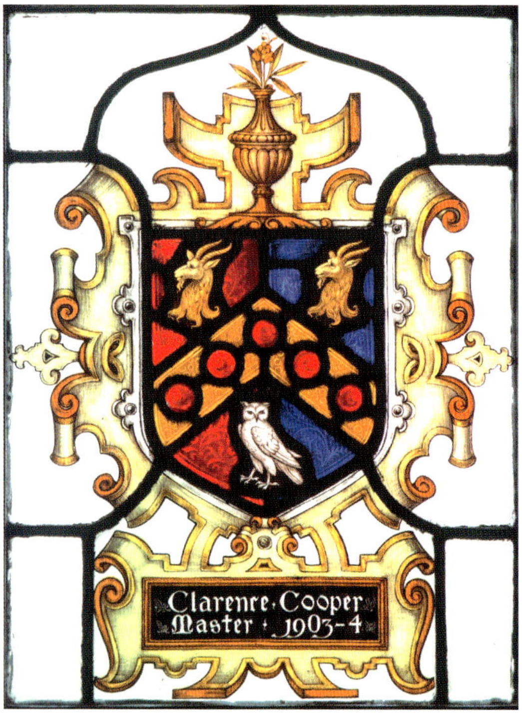

Per pale Gules and Azure, on a Chevron, between in chief two Goat's Heads erased Or and in base an Owl Argent, five Torteaux

Crest (not shown): *in front of a Cubit Arm holding a Scimitar, a Lotus Flower slipped all proper*

Mr Clarence COOPER, LSA, MD, MRCP, FRCS

The Arms were designed by Thomas King, York Herald, and Henry Molyneux-Seel, Bluemantle Pursuivant, in 1868 and granted to his father George Cooper FRCS of Egglesfield House, Hanwell. They are recorded at the College of Arms in Volume 57, Folio 39.

The stained glass panel was made by James Powell & Sons in 1906 and was installed in window W3-4 in 1906, showing the shield in Cartouche B, as one of the first three panels and paid for by Dr Jeffcoat. From Sep 1941 to Jan 1946 all stained glass was removed from the Hall during hostilities and on return in 1946 these Arms were placed in window W2-5.

BORN Brentford 28 Jun 1830; *s* of George Cooper FRCS and Charlotte Nicholas; *unmarried*; *ob.* 18 Dec 1924.

EDUC Guy's Hosp Medical Sch; U St Andrews (MD).

QUALIFICATIONS LSA 1852; MRCS 1852; MD 1853; MRCP Lond 1860; FRCS Eng 1867.

SERVICES Indian Medical Service 1853–81; Asst Surgeon 5th Native Infantry 1853; served in Labuan, Borneo as Colonial Surgeon, Coroner, Police Magistrate, Superintendent of Convicts, Colonial Secretary and Judge 1855–64; Surgeon 1865; Principal Medical Storekeeper Madras 1874–81, Brigade Surgeon 1879, Deputy Surgeon General IMS 1881–1924.

SOCIETY apprenticed to (f) George Cooper 1845; Yeoman 1853; Liveryman 1877; elected to the Court 1894 *vice* James Saner. Junior Warden 1901–02, Senior Warden 1902–03, Master 1903–04. Retired from the Court 1913.

FAMILY LIVERYMEN (father) George Cooper, Master 1866–67 and 1867–68; (bro) Dr George Francis Cooper.

Between 1901–05 donated 50 guineas to the Distressed Members' Fund and his stained glass Arms panel.

Dr William Sydney Charles COPEMAN, CBE,TD, JP, MA, LRCP MRCS, MB BChir, MD, FRCP, FSA Scot

The Arms were designed by Keith Murray, Portcullis Pursuivant, and granted in 1918 to his father Sydney Arthur Monckton Copeman and are recorded at the College of Arms in Volume Gr 86, Folio 41. The grant was extended to Sydney Arthur's deceased father, Arthur Charles Copeman, and his descendants.

The stained glass panel was made by Carl Edwards *c*.1960 and was installed in window W4-3 *c*.1960, showing full impaled Arms and motto without a cartouche.

The Copeman Arms are impaled with those of his wife's family which were granted to his mother-in-law Clara Louise Bourne for the descendants of her deceased husband Walter William Bourne. They were designed by Arthur Cochrane, Clarenceaux King of Arms in 1933 and are recorded in Volume Gr 100, Folio 112.

The motto translates as *I scarce call these deeds of our ancestors ours.*

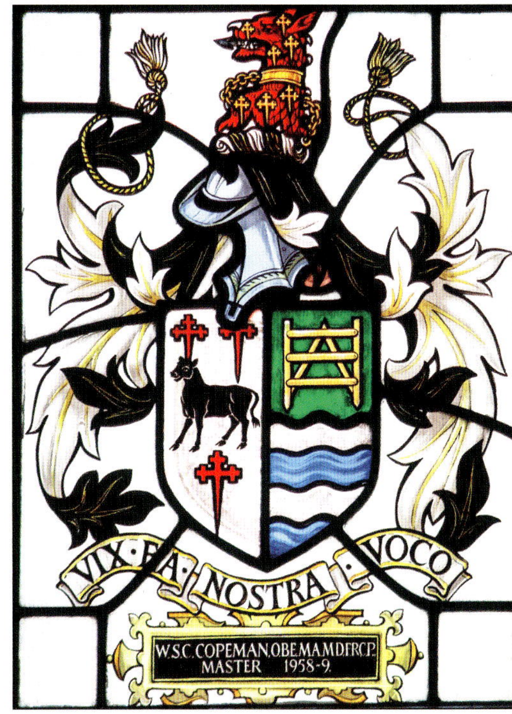

Argent, a Calf passant Sable between three Cross Crosslets fitchée Gules (Copeman) impaling per fess wavy Vert and barry wavy of four Argent and Azure, in chief a Hurdle Or (Bourne); And for the Crest upon a Helm, mantled Sable doubled Argent, on a wreath of the colours, a Dragon's Head erased Gules semee of cross crosslets fitchée collared and chained Or

Motto: *Vix Ea Nostro Voco*

BORN Ardingly 29 Jul 1900; s of Sydney Monckton Copeman FRCP and Ethel Boord; *m* 1931 Helen Bourne, one son, two daus; *ob.* 24 Nov 1970.

EDUC Gonville & Caius Coll Cambridge (BA, MA, MB BChir); St Thomas's Hosp Medical Sch.

QUALIFICATIONS LRCP MRCS 1924; BA; MA; MB BChir 1925; MRCP Lond 1926; MD 1936; FRCP Lond 1937; FSA Scot.

SERVICES Coldstream Guards 1914–18; Lt Col RAMC 1939–45.

CAREER Physician at the Middlesex and West London Hosps and the Hosp of St John and St Elizabeth; Chairman Kennedy Institute of Rheumatology 1967–70.

HON APPTS Heberden Soc – President 1949–50, Hon Librarian 1950–70; Royal College of Physicians – Council 1955–58, Library Cttee 1958–60, Vice President 1969; President British Society for the History of Medicine 1967–69; Arthritis and Rheumatism Council, Secretary then President.

SOCIETY Yeoman 1929; Liveryman 1930; elected to the Court 1951 *vice* Ronald Ogier Ward. Main instigator of the Faculty of the History of Medicine. Junior Warden 1956–57, Senior Warden 1957–58, Master 1958–59. Inaugural Chairman of the Faculty of the History of Medicine and Pharmacy 1959–64 and 1969–70; Sydenham Lecturer 1962; Gideon de Laune Lecturer 1967.

FAMILY LIVERYMEN (father) Dr Sydney Arthur Monckton Copeman; (son) Dr Peter William Monckton Copeman.

CITY AND CIVIC JP London 1950–62.

HONOURS AND AWARDS Heberden Gold Medal 1939; OBE 1945; TD 1948; CBE 1965. Presented the plaster bust of Charles I, the badge for the President of the Faculty of the History and Philosophy of Medicine and Pharmacy in 1950, the Worcester tea set, a gilt Hunt Cup, a carpet, his miniature portrait and his stained glass Arms panel. He wrote the History of the Society in 1967 and left a bequest of £250.

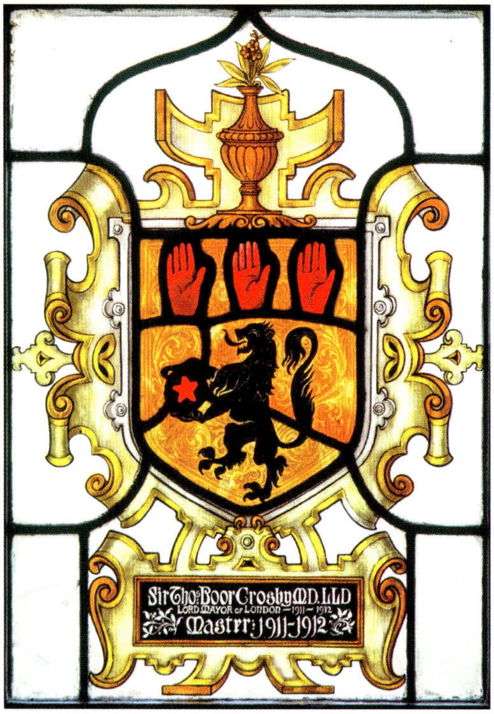
Sir Tho: Boor Crosby M.D. LLD
LORD MAYOR of LONDON —1911— 1912
Master: 1911-1912

Or, a Lion rampant Sable holding between the Forepaws a Mullet, in chief three dexter Hands couped apaumé Gules

Crest (not shown): *Three Swords, two in saltire hilts downwards and one in pale hilt upwards, proper pommels and hilts Or interlaced by a Serpent proper between two mullets Gules*

Sir Thomas Boor CROSBY LSA, MRCS, MD, FRCS, LLD

The Arms were designed by Charles Athill, Richmond Herald, in 1906 and are recorded at the College of Arms in Volume 76, Folio 300.

It is not known who commissioned the panel and the glassmaker is not known but may be W. B. Simpson & Sons. The panel was installed in window W3-12 between 1917 and 1922, showing the shield in Cartouche B. From Sep 1941 to Jan 1946 all stained glass was removed from the Hall during hostilities and on return in 1946 these Arms were placed in window W2-11.

Seventeenth-century Crosby Arms feature a lion rampant and two or three dexter hands.

BORN Gosberton 26 Oct 1830; *s* of William Crosby and Mary Boor; *m* 1859 Anne Ryan, two sons, one dau; *ob.* 7 Apr 1916.

EDUC St Thomas's Hosp Medical Sch; U St Andrews (MD, LLD); U Dublin (LLD).

QUALIFICATIONS LSA 1852; MRCS 1852; FRCS Eng 1860; MD 1862; LLD.

CAREER Fenchurch St General Practice with Charles Brodie Sewell 1852–?.

SOCIETY Yeoman 1906; He refused promotion to the Livery in 1909 but was then promoted to the Livery, elected to the Court *vice* Joseph Burton, and elected Master all in 1911 to coincide with his Mayoralty. Master 1911–12. Dr Arthur Long, the Master presumptive, stepped aside and acted as Deputy Master for the year, being awarded the status of Past Master on completion.

CITY AND CIVIC Liveryman, Company of Turners, Master 1900–01; Common Councillor for Langbourn 1877–1898; Alderman for Langbourn 1898–1916; JP; Aldermanic Sheriff 1906–07; DL 1907–; Lord Mayor 1911–12. First medical man to be Lord Mayor and, at 82, the oldest incumbent.

HONOURS AND AWARDS Kt Bachelor 1906, Officier de la Legion d'Honneur.

the Rt Hon Bertrand Edward Dawson, Viscount DAWSON of Penn, PC, GCVO, KCB, KCMG, BSc, LRCP MRCS, MD, FRCP

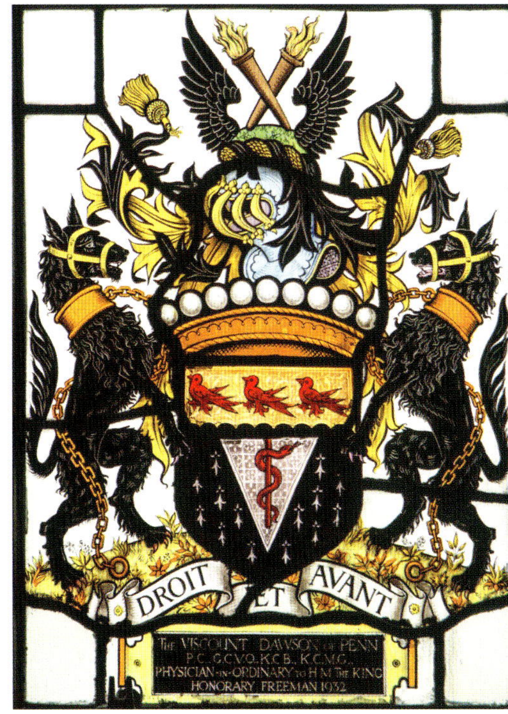
DROIT
ET
AVANT
THE VISCOUNT DAWSON OF PENN
P.C. G.C.V.O. K.C.B. K.C.M.G.
PHYSICIAN-IN-ORDINARY TO H.M. THE KING
HONORARY FREEMAN 1932

The Arms were designed by Arthur Cochrane, Clarenceaux King of Arms, in 1933 and are recorded at the College of Arms in Volume Gr 100, Folio 304.

The stained glass panel was made by James Powell & Sons in 1938 and was installed in window W4-8 in 1938, showing the full Arms with supporters and motto without a cartouche. From Sep 1941 to Jan 1946 all stained glass was removed from the Hall during hostilities and on return in 1946 these Arms were replaced in window W4-8.

The stained glass maker has used the wrong colours for the wreath (and possibly the mantling).

The motto translates as *Right and forward*.

BORN Croydon 9 Mar 1864; s of Henry Dawson and Frances Wheeler; *m* 1900 Minnie Ethel Yarrow, three dau; *ob*. 7 Mar 1945.

EDUC University Coll Hosp Medical Sch (BSc); London Hosp Medical Coll (MD).

QUALIFICATIONS BSc 1888; LRCP MRCS 1890; MRCP Lond 1893; MD 1893; FRCP Lond 1903.

SERVICES RAMC 1914–19; Col 1914, Hon Maj Gen 1919.

CAREER the London Hosp; Asst Physician 1896–1906, Physician 1906–30; Physician Extraordinary to Edward VII 1907–10; Physician in Ordinary to King George V 1914–36 (Extraordinary 1910–14); Council on Future Provision of Medical & Allied Services 1919–20; Physician in Ordinary to Edward VIII 1936; Physician in Ordinary to George VI 1936–45; Medical Research Council 1931–35; 1939 helped to organise the Emergency Medical Service.

HON APPTS President Royal Society of Medicine 1928–30; Royal College of Physicians – Senior Censor, President 1931–38; President British Medical Association 1932 and 1943.

SOCIETY Hon Freeman 1932 in the Mastership of Col Ernest Freeman.

HONOURS AND AWARDS KCVO 1911; KStJ 1916; CB 1916; GCVO 1918; KCMG 1919; Baron Dawson of Penn 1920; Hon LLD U McGill 1925; KCB 1926; Hon DCL U Oxford 1926; Hon LLD U Athens; Hon DCL U Durham; Hon LLD U Edinburgh 1927; PC 1929; Hon LLD U Leeds 1931; Hon FRCS Eng 1932; Hon LLD U Bristol 1933; Viscount 1936.

Ermines, on a Pile Argent a Rod of Asclepius Gules, on a Chief engrailed Or three Martlets of the 3rd; And for the Crest upon a Peer's Helm mantled Sable doubled Or, on a Wreath Argent and Sable upon a Mount Vert two Torches in saltire inflamed proper between as many Wings Sable; for supporters on either side a Wolf Sable, muzzled collared and chained, the chain reflexed over the back Or

Motto: *Droit et Avant*

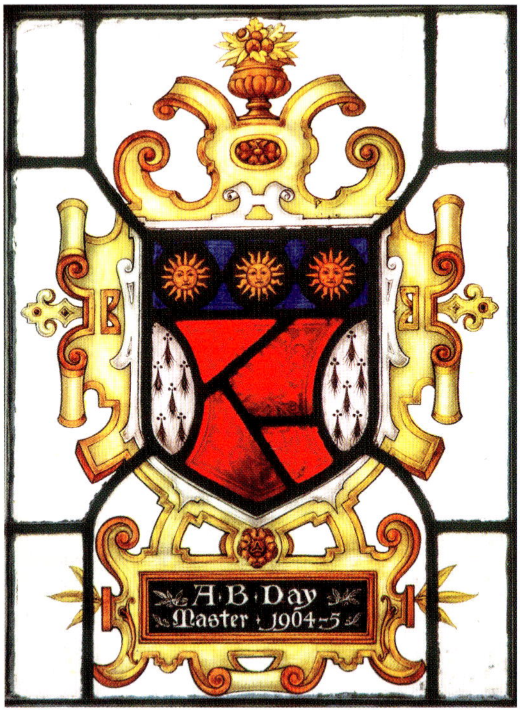

Gules, two Flaunches Ermine, on a Chief Azure three Suns Or

Crest (not shown): *a Greyhound's Head erased Argent, collared, ringed and lined Gules, the end nowed* [6]

Dr Albert Bryan DAY, LSA, MRCS

The Arms were confirmed to Edmond Day of London, gentleman, the son of Edmond, son of William Day of Derbyshire in 1582 and are recorded at the College of Arms in Volume 31, Folio 4.

The connection of Albert Day with the sixteenth-century family is unknown and these Arms are likely just to have been assumed.

The stained glass panel was made by James Powell & Sons and was installed in window W3-5 in 1906, showing the shield in Cartouche A, as one of the first three (the Private Court of 1903–04) and paid for by Dr Jeffcoat. From Sep 1941 to Jan 1946 all stained glass was removed from the Hall during hostilities and on return in 1946 these Arms were returned to window W3-5.

BORN Isleworth 1832; *s* of William Day and his 2nd wife, the dau of Bryan Donkin FRS; *ob.* 22 Jul 1912.

EDUC King's College Hosp Medical Sch.

QUALIFICATIONS MRCS 1854; LSA 1855.

CAREER Partnership practice with (½ bro) HG Day in Isleworth to 1867 then solo; Medical Officer to the Brentford Union Workhouse and District Schools; Cons Surgeon St John Hosp Twickenham; Medical Referee Norwich Union Assurance Co.

HON APPTS Friendly Medical Soc 1880–93.

SOCIETY Apprenticed to (½ bro) HG Day 1849; Yeoman 1856; Liveryman 1879; elected to the Court 1895 *vice* Montagu Champneys. Junior Warden 1902–03, Senior Warden 1903–04, Master 1904–05.

FAMILY LIVERYMEN (father) William Day; (½ bro) Horatio Grosvenor Day.

In 1904 he donated 10 guineas to the Widows' Fund and his stained glass Arms panel.

Sir Edward Charles DODDS, Bt. of West Chillington, MVO, MB BS, PhD, MD, DSc, FRCP, FRS Ed, FRS, FRIC

The Arms were designed by John Brooke-Little, Bluemantle Pursuivant, in 1965 and are recorded at the College of Arms in Volume 128, Folio 72.

The stained glass panel was made by Carl Edwards and was installed in window W2-14 *c.* 1965, showing the full Arms with motto without a cartouche.

The hand and the sunburst come from the Arms of the Royal College of Physicians and the swords and crabs are symbolic of the fight against cancer.

The formula on the crest commemorates his discovery and synthesis of diethylstilboestrol with Sir Robert Robinson and Wilfred Lawson which was used to treat prostate cancer.

The panel was damaged in 2019 with several pieces of glass broken but was restored.

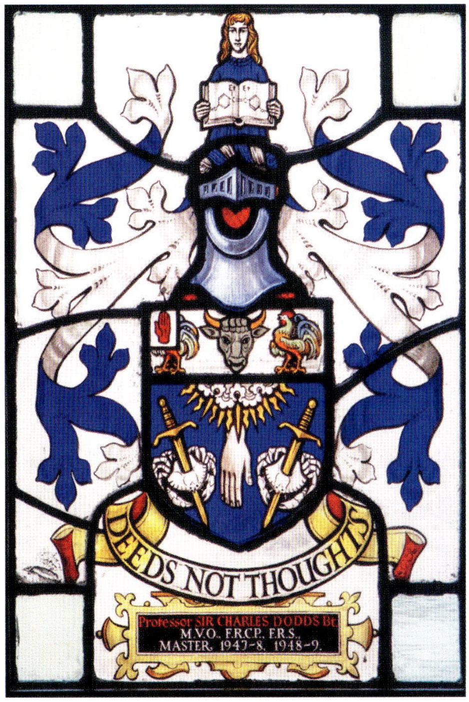
DEEDS NOT THOUGHTS
Professor SIR CHARLES DODDS Bt.
M.V.O. F.R.C.P. F.R.S.
MASTER. 1947-8. 1948-9.

Azure, issuant from a Chief Argent and out of a Sunburst a dexter Hand proper between two Crab's Heads downward Argent, each transfixed by a Sword Or; on the Chief a Steer's Head caboshed Sable, armed Or, between two Capons proper. The augmentation of a Baronet of the UK in the dexter Chief. And for the Crest, upon a Knight's Helm mantled Argent doubled Azure, on a Wreath of the colours, a demi-Woman affrontée proper, vested Azure, holding an open Book proper inscribed with the Chemical Formula for Stilboestrol Sable

Motto: *Deeds Not Thoughts*

BORN Liverpool 13 Oct 1899; *s* of Ralph Edward Dodds and Jane Pack; *m* 1923 Constance Elizabeth Jordan, one son; *ob.* 16 Dec 1973.
EDUC Middlesex Hosp Medical School (MB BS); U London (PhD, MD, DSc).
QUALIFICATIONS MB BS 1922; PhD 1924; MD 1926; DSc 1932; MRCP Lond 1927; FRCP Lond 1933; FRIC 1968.
CAREER Prof Biochemistry U London 1925–65; Director of the Courtauld Institute of Biochemistry 1927–65.
HON APPTS Royal College of Physicians of London: Harveian Librarian 1949–62; President 1962–66.
SOCIETY Yeoman 1934; Liveryman 1937; elected to the Court 1941 *vice* William Henry Kelson. Custodian of the Cellar for 23 years; Examination Cttee 1943–46. Junior Warden 1946–47. In 1945–46 Dr Ogier Ward had been Junior Warden but he was unable to proceed and Past Master John Hedley served as Senior Warden for 1946–47 but was not able to repeat the Mastership. For 1947–48 Sir Charles proceeded straight to Master, with Past Master Arthur Gibbons serving as his Senior Warden: Sir Charles then served his due term in 1948–49. Gideon de Laune Lecturer 1965.
FAMILY LIVERYMEN (son) Sir Ralph Dodds Bt.
HONOURS AND AWARDS MVO 4th class 1929 for services to King George V; FRS Edin 1941; FRS 1942; MD (Hon Caus) U Melbourne 1952; MD (Hon Caus) U Birmingham; Hon DSc U Cambridge 1954; Kt Bachelor 1954; Hon DSc U Bologna 1958; Hon DSc Chicago 1959; Hon FRCOG 1962; Baronet 1964; Hon LLD U Glasgow; Hon FRCPS Glas; Hon FRCS Eng 1970; Hon FRACP; Hon FACP; Hon FRCPath.
Presented a Lambeth delft blue and white octagonal pill slab of *c.*1750, a seventeenth-century oriental tray formerly the property of the last Sultan of Egypt, the Parlour candelabrum, his miniature portrait, his stained glass Arms panel and left a bequest of £500.

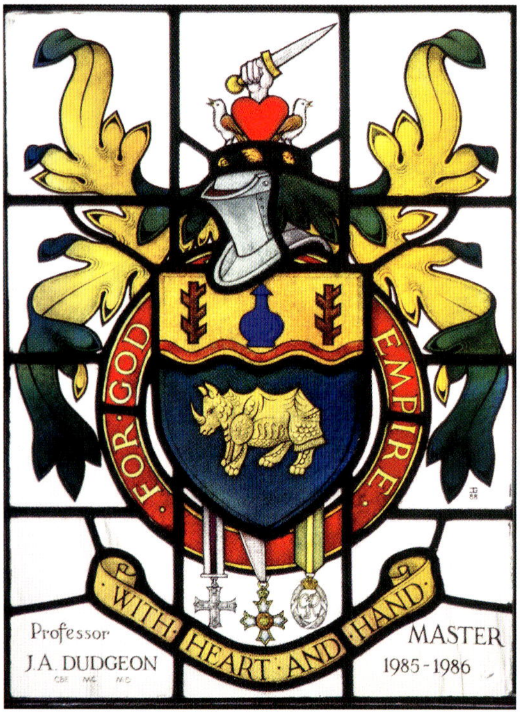

Per fess wavy Or and Vert, a Rhinoceros statant Or in base and in chief an Apothecary Jar Azure between two Staffs raguly proper and beneath them a Barrulet wavy Gules; And for the Crest upon a Helm mantled Vert doubled Or on a wreath of the colours, between two Nightingales each facing outwards proper a human Heart Gules from the top thereof a Hand grasping a short Sword both proper

Motto: *With Heart and Hand*

Professor John Alastair DUDGEON, CBE, OStJ, MC*, TD, DL, MA, MB BChir, MD, FRCPath, FRCP

The Arms were designed by Conrad Swan, York Herald, in 1987 and are recorded at the College of Arms in Volume 151, Folio 191.

The stained glass panel was made by Jane Gray in 1988 and was installed in window W4-9 in 1988 showing the full Arms surrounded by the insignia of the Most Excellent Order of the British Empire and motto without a cartouche. Also suspended from the shield are his Military Cross (without the Bar) and Territorial Decoration.

The rhino and field refer to the 1st Armoured Division, and the rhino also to the Society, the barrulet to blood, the jar to his collection of apothecary jars and the ragged staffs to his interest in woodworking.

The crest refers to the motto and the nightingales to his mother's and wife's nursing career at St Thomas', fledgling birds referring to child health. The sword alludes to his connection with the City of London and the heart is also an allusion to his work with the British Heart Foundation.

The colours in the stained glass are confusing as the green field and mantling look blue whilst the jar is a surprisingly bright blue.

BORN London 9 Nov 1916; *s* of Prof Leonard Stanley Dudgeon and Nora Edith Orpen; *m* 1st 1945 Patricia Joan Ashton (*ob.* 1969), two sons; *m* 2nd 1974 Joyce Kathleen Tibbetts; *ob.* 9 Oct 1989.

EDUC Trinity Coll Cambridge (MA, MB, BChir, MD); St Thomas's Hosp Medical Sch.

QUALIFICATIONS BA 1937; MA 1944; LRCP MRCS 1944; BChir MB 1944; MD 1947; FRCPath 1967; MRCP Lond 1970; FRCP Lond 1974.

SERVICES 7Bn Rifle Brigade TA 1935–43, RAMC 1944–47; RAMC(V) 1947–62, latterly ADMS 56 London Armoured Div; Hon Col 1977; Civilian Advisor in Pathology to the Army 1977–81.

CAREER Cons Virologist and Cons Microbiologist Hosp for Sick Children 1960–81; Professor of Microbiology U London 1972–81; Inst Child Health; Cttee 1966–81, Dean 1974–81; Dep Chairman Joint Cttee Vaccination and Immunisation; Chairman Cttee Rubella & Varicella Vaccines; Chairman Cttee on Complications of Vaccination.

HON APPTS British Heart Foundation, Council 1982–89; Foundation Fellow Royal College Pathologists.

SOCIETY Proposed for the Society by Dr Alan Reese and Dr CP Scott. Yeoman 1965; Liveryman 1969; elected to the Court 1974 *vice* Sir Edward Muir. Junior Warden 1983–84, Senior Warden 1984–85, Master 1985–86.

FAMILY LIVERYMEN (son) Dr Timothy Alastair Dudgeon.

CITY AND CIVIC Deputy Lieutenant for Greater London 1978.

HONOURS AND AWARDS MC 1942, and bar 1943; TD 1947; OStJ 1958; CBE 1977.

Presented the framed chart of London, the Thames and the East Coast, his miniature portrait and his stained glass Arms panel. He also created, with Past Master Col Neild, a bound record of the refurbishment of the Hall 1980–87.

Mr Douglas George Arnott EADIE, MB BS, MS, FRCS

The Arms were designed by Conrad Swan, York Herald, in 1991 and are recorded at the College of Arms in Volume 156, Folio 267.

The stained glass panel was made by Michael Bell of Clayton & Bell and is signed by him. The panel was installed in window W3-4 in 1992, showing the full Arms and motto without a cartouche.

The shield is in the Society colours with the wavy pale representing a blood vessel. The stags refer to his Scottish ancestry and interest in stalking.

The wyvern in the crest is from his step-father's Arms and is holding a fleam for surgery. The chaplet of white roses represents his Yorkshire youth and the pellets for his interest in shooting.

The motto translates as *Where there is blood let it flow* and was suggested to him by Enoch Powell.

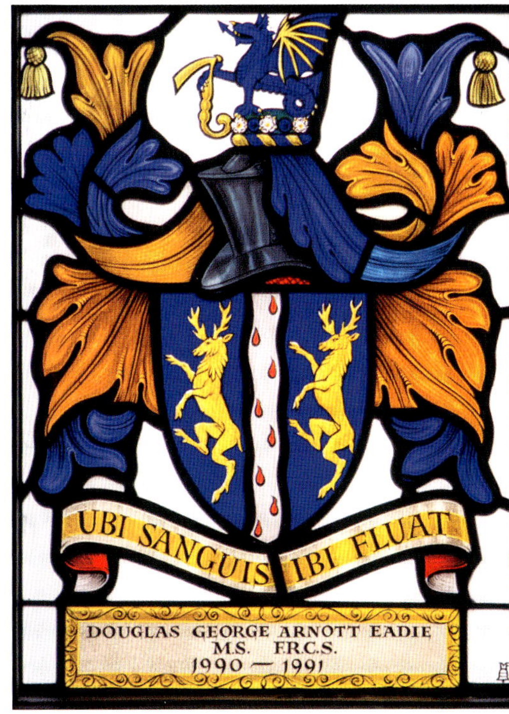

BORN 16 Jun 1931; *s* of Dr Herbert Arnot Eadie and Hannah Sophia Wingate; *m* 1957 Gillian Carlyon Coates, two sons, two daus; *ob.* 5 Dec 2000.
EDUC the London Hosp Medical Coll (MB BS); U London (MS).
QUALIFICATIONS MB BS 1955; FRCS 1962; MS 1969.
SERVICES Captain RAMC 1957–60.
CAREER Cons General & Vascular Surgeon, the London Hosp 1969–87; MB BS Exr U London 1976–84; Hon Surgeon King Edward VII Hosp for Officers 1978–87; Hon Cons Osborne House 1980; Cons to Royal Masonic Hosp 1980–82.
HON APPTS General Medical Council 1983–88.
SOCIETY Proposed for the Society by Mr AMA Moore. Yeoman 1962; Liveryman 1966; LMSSA Exr 1976–84; elected to the Court 1979 *vice* Sir John Butterfield. Junior Warden 1988–89, Senior Warden 1989–90, Master 1990–91.
FAMILY LIVERYMEN (dau) Lucy Jane Arnott Eadie.
Presented various books for the Library, a carved verdite rhinoceros, a pair of 1971 silver pepper mills marked JW and SW, his miniature portrait and his stained glass Arms panel.

Azure, a Pale wavy Argent, goutée de sang, between two Stags rampant Or; And for the Crest upon a Helm mantled Azure doubled Or, on a Wreath of the colours, a grassy Mound proper with a circle of Roses Argent, barbed and seeded proper and Pellets alternately, a Wyvern sejant Azure, armed Or the Wings spined and clawed also Or holding in the dexter Talon a Fleam Blade outwards also Or

Motto: *Ubi Sanguis Ibi Fluat*

Dr Ian Trevor FIELD, CBE, LRCP MRCS, MB BS, FFPHM, FFOM, CIMgt

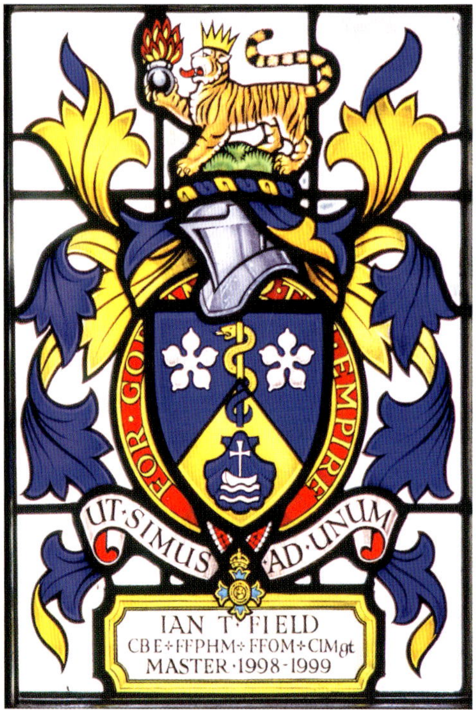

The Arms were designed by John Bedells, Howard Pursuivant Extraordinary, in 2000 and are recorded at the College of Arms in Volume Gr 163, Folio 147.

The stained glass panel was made at the Goddard & Gibbs Studio in Bow in 2000 and was installed in window W1-6 in 2000, showing the full Arms surrounded by the insignia of the Most Excellent Order of the British Empire and motto, without a cartouche.

The field per chevron is from the Arms of Guy's Hosp and the colours are from his school, Guy's, the BMA and the Apothecaries. The rod of Asclepius represents medicine and the cinquefoils are a pun on his wife's maiden name of Fraser. The shell and boat represent the family's commitment to ecumenism.

The green mound of the crest is a pun on Field, the tiger and eastern crown represent the family's long service in India. The bomb represents service in the Royal Engineers.

The motto translates as *That we may be one* – another reference to ecumenism.

Per chevron Azure and Or, a Rod of Asclepius counter-changed between, in chief two Cinquefoils Argent and in base an Escallop Azure charged with a Boat set upon the upper of two bars wavy couped, the Mast and Yard in cross formy Argent; And for the Crest upon a Helm, mantled Azure doubled Or, on a Wreath of the colours, upon a mount Vert a Bengal Tiger proper crowned with an eastern Crown Or and holding in the dexter Paw a Bomb Sable enflamed with nine Flames proper

Motto: *Ut Simus Ad Unum*

BORN 31 Oct 1933; *s* of George Edward Field and Bertha Davies; *m* 1960 Christine Osman; three sons, one dau; *ob.* 23 Dec 2012.

EDUC Guy's Hosp Medical Sch (MB BS).

QUALIFICATIONS LRCP MRCS 1960; MB BS 1960; FFPHM 1979; FFOM 1991; CIMgt 1993.

SERVICES Lieut Royal Engineers 1952–54.

CAREER GP Beckenham 1962–64; BMA – Asst Sec 1964–72, Under Sec 1972–74; Chief Medical & Health Services Adviser (Overseas Development) FCO 1978–83; WHO Global Adv Cttee on Malaria Control 1979–82; BMA – Dep Sec 1985–89, Sec 1989–93; Sec Gen World Med Assoc 1993–98.

HON APPTS Council Royal Vet Coll 1982–89.

SOCIETY Proposed for the Society by the Master, Sir John Richardson. Yeoman 1971; Liveryman 1976; elected to the Court 1986 *vice* Henry Thompson. Junior Warden 1996–97, Senior Warden 1997–98, Master 1998–99. Past Master Emeritus 2009.

FAMILY LIVERYMEN (son) Dr Giles Field.

HONOURS AND AWARDS CBE 1994.

Presented various books for the library, the framed LSA certificate of Henry Powell dated 1828, his miniature portrait and his stained glass Arms panel.

Dr James Frederick FISHER, JP, MA, MB BChir, FRCGP, DPMSA

The Arms were designed by Conrad Swan, York Herald, in 1984 and are recorded at the College of Arms in Volume 148, Folio 7.

The stained glass panel was made by Alfred Fisher of Chapel Studio, King's Langley, in 1990 and was installed in window W4-6 in 1990, showing the full Arms and motto without a cartouche.

The blue and gold represent the seaside, Mortimer ancestors and the Society's colours. The rose is for Yorkshire Haythornthwaite forebears. The serpent is for medicine, the maze for his son's professional work and the toad for his family nickname.

The panel also commemorates his father Dr Reginald Fisher (1884–1966), Master 1957–58.

The motto is translated as *Get it right first time.*

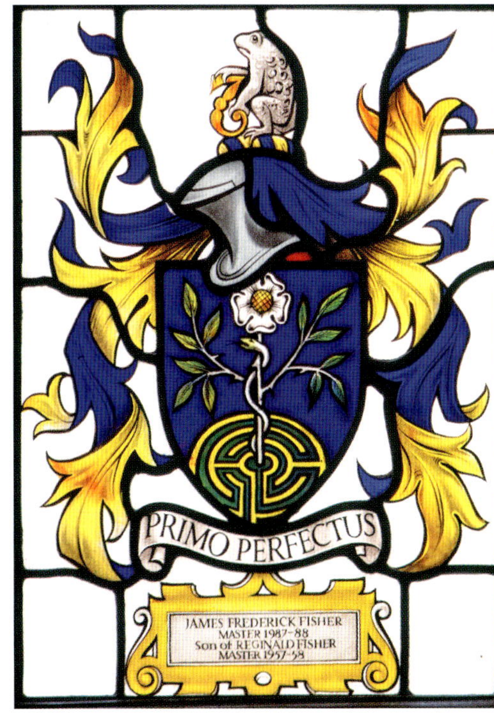

Azure, issuant from the midst of a Base enarched Or and from thereon a three-ring Maze throughout Vert a Rose Argent barbed, seeded and slipped its Leaves branching upwards and outwards and its Stalk erect proper environed by a Serpent Or; And for the Crest upon a Helm mantled Azure doubled Or, on a wreath of the colours, a Toad proper supporting a Fleam Gold

Motto: *Primo Perfectus*

BORN 9 Feb 1922; *s* of Dr Reginald Fisher and Grace Haythornthwaite; *m* 1950 Rosemary Hill, three sons, two daus; *ob.* 19 Dec 2012.

EDUC Sidney Sussex Coll Cambridge (MA, MB BChir); University Coll Hosp Medical Sch.

QUALIFICATIONS MB BChir 1945; MA 1947; FRCGP 1971; DPMSA 1984.

SERVICES Rifle Brigade TA 1936–44, RAMC 1944–47; RAMC(V) 1947–62, latterly ADMS 56 London Armoured Div; Hon Col 1977; Civilian Advisor in Pathology to the Army.

CAREER GP Bournemouth 1948–87; Provost Wessex Faculty RCGP 1976–79.

SOCIETY Proposed for the Society by his father. Yeoman 1948; Liveryman 1952; elected to the Court 1976 *vice* Dr Gordon Mitchell-Heggs. Junior Warden 1985–86, Senior Warden 1986–87, Master 1987–88. Sydenham Lecturer 1988; Assistant Emeritus 1996.

FAMILY LIVERYMEN (grandfather) Frederick Charles Fisher FRCS; (father) Reginald Fisher, Master 1957–58; (son) Adrian Roger Fisher; (dau) Sarah Rosemary Fisher.

CITY AND CIVIC JP for 33 years.

Presented various books for the Library, the Society's Arms embossing stamp, the cost of repair of several old record books, the library step chair, notes on John Hunter's lectures, his father's midwifery bag, his miniature portrait and his stained glass Arms panel.

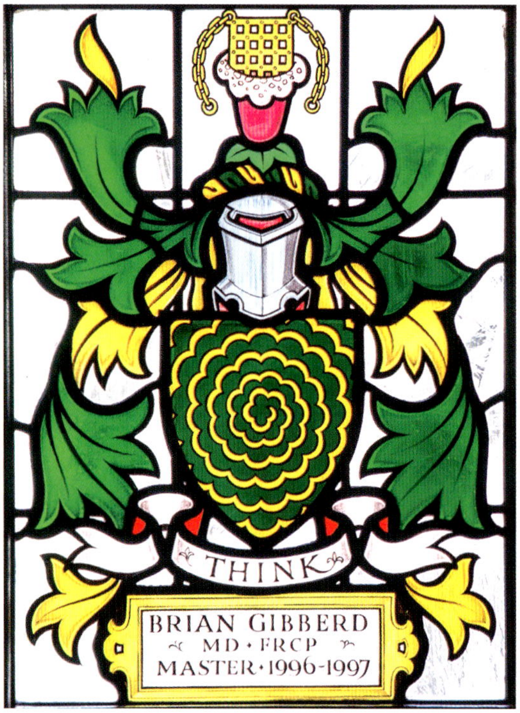

Dr Frederick Brian GIBBERD, LRCP MRCS, MB BChir, MD, FRCP, FRCP Ed

The Arms were designed by Timothy Duke, Chester Herald, in 1998 and are recorded at the College of Arms in Volume Gr 163, Folio 29.

The stained glass panel was made by John Lawson of Goddard & Gibbs Studios, London, in 1998 and was installed in window W1-12 in 1998 showing the full Arms and motto, without a cartouche.

The shield is a representation of the plant *Aeonium tabuliforme*, referring to his and his mother's interest in botany. It is also an allusion to the brain and his work as a neurologist.

The portcullis is from Palace of Westminster and his medical school. The foxglove signifies a physician who treats patients.

Vert, a spiral Gorge invected on the outer edge and engrailed on the inner edge Or; And for the Crest, upon a Helm mantled Vert doubled Or, on a Wreath of the colours, issuing from a Foxglove Flower erect with Calyx proper, a Portcullis chained Or

Motto: *Think*

BORN 7 Jul 1931; *s* of George Frederick Gibberd FRCOG and Margaret Erica Taffs; *m* 1960 Margaret Sidey; four daus; *ob.* 20 Feb 2006.

EDUC Gonville & Caius Coll Cambridge (MB BChir, MD) and Westminster Hosp Medical Sch.

SERVICES Trooper 14/20 Hussars & Lieut Royal Arty 1949–52.

QUALIFICATIONS LRCP MRCS 1957; MB BChir 1957; MD 1974; MRCP Lond 1960; FRCP Lond 1972; FRCP Edin 1993.

CAREER Physician in Neurology Queen Mary's Hospital Roehampton and Westminster & Chelsea Hosp 1965–1996; Examiner U London, LMSSA, RCP and PLAB.

HON APPTS Royal College of Physicians: Council 1970–72 & 1990–96, Censor 1991–92; Hon Librarian Royal Soc Medicine 1975–79; General Medical Council 1992–96; President Harveian Soc 1995; President Hunterian Soc 2003–04.

SOCIETY Proposed for the Society by Past Master Keith Lyle. Yeoman 1964; Liveryman 1968; elected to the Court 1986 *vice* Dr Macdonald Critchley. Junior Warden 1994–95, Senior Warden 1995–96, Master 1996–97. United Examining Board 1993–2006; Sydenham Lecturer 2005.

FAMILY LIVERYMEN (dau) Dr Lucy Gibberd.

HONOURS AND AWARDS Hon FFOM 1995.

Conserved and restored the Society's Ordinances, presented various books to the Library, his miniature portrait and his stained glass Arms panel.

Professor Tony William Alphonse GLENISTER, CBE, TD, OStJ, LRCP MRCS, MB BS, PhD, DSc

The Arms were designed by Sir Colin Cole, Garter King of Arms, in 1991 and are recorded at the College of Arms in Volume Gr 156, Folio 90.

It is unclear who made the stained glass panel but it may have been Messrs Goddard & Gibbs. The panel was installed in window E1-10 in 1993 showing the full Arms and motto without a cartouche.

No previous Arms are recorded for Glenister but it appears that Glenisters had been using similar Arms in these colours attributed to a fifteenth-century family called Gloucester (*Gules, on a fess indented Or a Lion passant Sable*).[7] Garter made variations to this blazon and Prof Glenister chose the boar as a crest from family silverware.

The motto is translated as *Openly and fairly*. Aperte is a pun on Aper (a goat), the main charge.

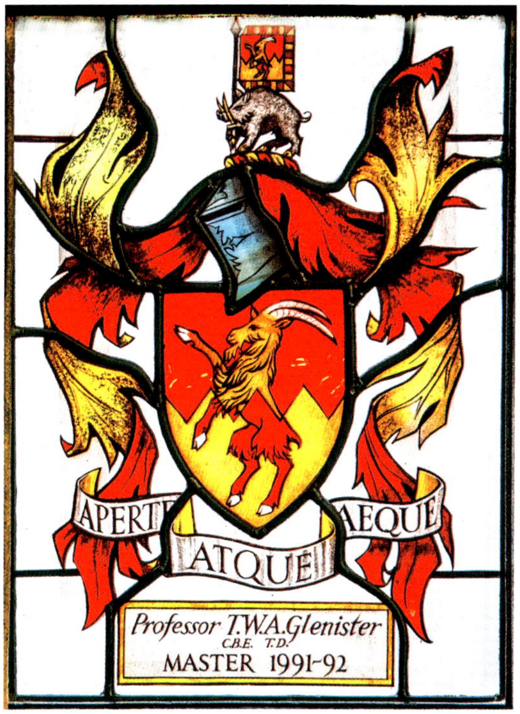

Per fess dancetty Gules and Or, a Goat salient horned and hooved Argent all Counterchanged; And for the Crest upon a Helm, mantled Gules doubled Or, on a Wreath of the colours, a Boar Sable tusked and hooved Or snout Gules supporting with dexter Foreleg a Banner of the Arms fringed Or and Gules, the shaft Or and lancehead Sable

Motto: *Aperte Atque Aeque*

BORN 19 Dec 1923; *s* of Dudley Stuart Glenister and Maria Leytens; *m* 1948 Monique de Wilde, four sons; *ob.* 1 May 1998.

EDUC St Bartholomew's Hosp Medical Coll (MB BS).

QUALIFICATIONS LRCP MRCS 1947; MB BS 1948; PhD 1955; DSc 1963.

SERVICES RAMC 1948–50; RAMC(V) 1963–(1978); ADMS 44 Div TA 1964–67; CO 217 (London) Gen Hosp 1968–72; Hon Col 220 Field Amb 1973–78; Hon Col 217 Gen Hosp 1981–86; Hon Brigadier.

CAREER Charing Cross Hosp Medical Sch: Lecturer & Reader in Anatomy 1950–57; Professor of Anatomy 1970–84 U London; Professor of Embryology 1967–70; Hon Cons in Clinical Anatomy & Genetics Charing Cross Gp of Hosps 1972–89; Dean Charing Cross & Westminster Medical Sch 1984–89; Examiner Us Cambridge, Liverpool, London, St Andrews, Singapore, NUI, RCS Eng, RCS Edin, RCPS Glas.

COMMITTEES General Medical Council 1979; General Dental Council 1983; Anatomical Soc GB & Ireland – Programme Secy 1961–65, Secy 1974–76, President 1979–81.

SOCIETY Proposed for the Society by KM Backhouse and WJ Hamilton. Yeoman 1969; Liveryman 1973; elected to the Court 1979 *vice* Mr AMA Moore. Junior Warden 1989–90, Senior Warden 1990–91, Master 1991–92.

HONOURS AND AWARDS TD 1963; OStJ 1967; QHP 1971–73; CBE 1979.

Presented several books for the Library, two silver pepper grinders for the Warden's use, a brass unicorn, two silver sweetmeat dishes each engraved with a rhinoceros, an 1858 watercolour of an Encorche by W. B. Richmond, his miniature portrait and his stained glass Arms panel.

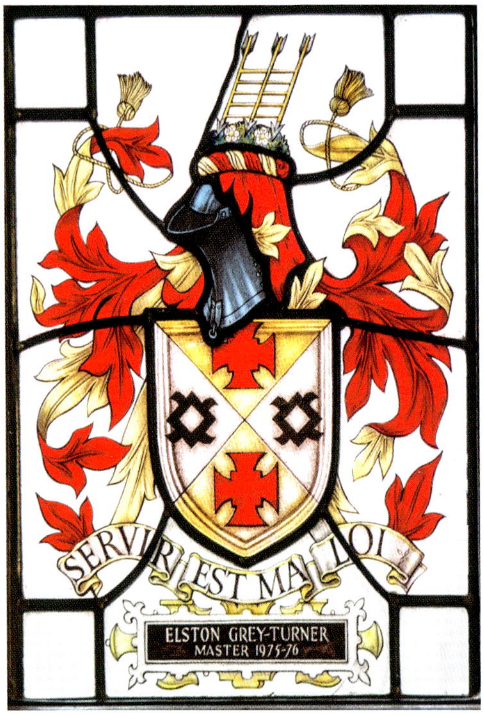

Dr Elston Grey GREY-TURNER, CBE, OStJ, MC, TD, LRCP MRCS, MB BChir, MA

The Arms were designed by the Hon Philip Cary, York Herald, for his father George Grey-Turner in 1931 and are recorded at the College of Arms in Volume Gr 99, Folio 119.

The stained glass panel was made by Carl Edwards in 1978 and was installed in window E2-14 in 1978, showing the full Arms and motto without a cartouche. It was moved to window E1-2 in 1980 to accommodate the Bristow stained glass.

The motto translates as *To serve is my rule*.

Per saltire Or and Argent, two Crosses patée quatrat in the centre in pale Gules and as many Millrinds in fess Sable; And for the Crest upon a Helm, mantled Gules doubled Or, on a Wreath of the colours, a Mount Vert charged with two Roses Argent, barbed and seeded proper, a Ladder Or the uprights consisting of three Arrows of the last, barbed and flighted Sable

Motto: *Servir Est Ma Loi*

BORN 16 Aug 1916; *s* of George Grey Turner FRCS and Alice Grey Schofield; *m* 1952 Lilias Tomlinson, two sons, one dau; *ob.* 20 Jan 1984. Between 1953–55 surname changed from Turner to Grey-Turner.

EDUC Trinity Coll Cambridge (BA, MA, MB BChir); St Bartholomew's Hosp Medical Coll.

QUALIFICATIONS BA 1938; MRCS LRCP 1942; MB BChir 1942; MA 1942.

SERVICES RMO 2nd Coldstream Gds 1942–46, RAMC(V) Lt Col 1956, Col 1958; Hon Col 257 Gen Hosp RAMC(V) 1973–78.

CAREER GP 1946; British Medical Association: Asst Secy 1948–60, Under Secy 1960–64, Deputy Secy 1964–76, Secretary 1976–79, Vice President 1982.

HON APPTS General Standing Cttee Doctors EEC 1979.

SOCIETY Yeoman 1945; Liveryman 1950; elected to the Court 1965 *vice* Edward Cullinan. Junior Warden 1973–74, Senior Warden 1974–75, Master 1975–76.

HONOURS AND AWARDS MC 1944; TD 1955; QHP 1960–62; OStJ 1961; Hon MD U Newcastle 1981; CBE 1981.

Presented various books for the Library, two lead crystal ship's decanters engraved with the Society Arms, his miniature portrait and his stained glass Arms panel.

Dr Samuel Clewin GRIFFITH, LSA, MRCS, MD

The College of Arms states firmly 'no entitlement to Arms' and so it must be assumed that these Arms were made up by Samuel Clewin Griffith. The style chosen but with gold passant guardant lions would be the Royal Arms of England. Similar Arms with silver lions are recorded for the twelfth-century Welsh Prince Griffith ap Cynan and in the time of Henry V and Henry VII there are records of these Arms being used by John Gifford of Whaddon and John Gyfford of Twyford as Sheriffs of Buckinghamshire.

The stained glass panel was made by James Powell & Sons in 1906 and was installed in window W2-6 in 1906, showing the shield in Cartouche A. It was moved to window W3-7 between 1917 and 1922. In May 1941 this panel was damaged in an air raid, prompting the removal of all stained glass from the Hall during hostilities and on return in 1946 these Arms were placed in window W1-14.

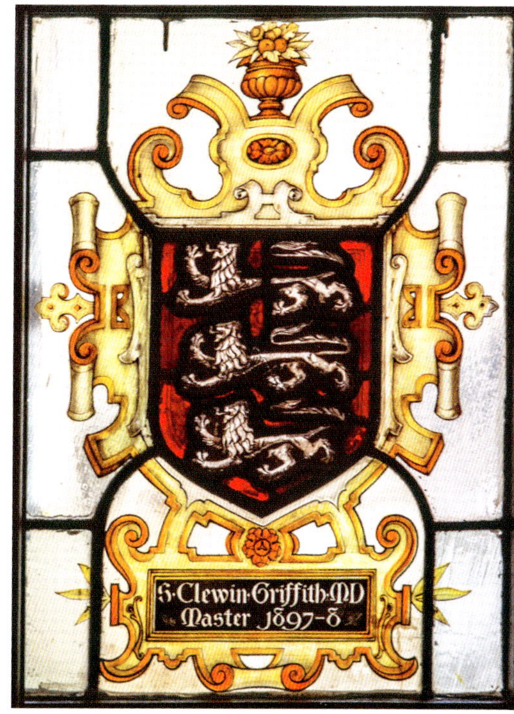

Gules, three Lions passant in pale Argent

BORN 1825; *s* of Richard Clewin Griffith and Eliza Cookson; *m* 1st Sarah Crookes, *ob. 1865*; *m* 2nd Caroline Hunter, one son: *ob.* 15 Mar 1909.

EDUC University College Hosp Paris; St Bartholomew's Hosp Medical Coll; St Andrew's U (MD).

QUALIFICATIONS MRCS 1846; LSA 1847; MD 1847.

CAREER Partner in Griffith & O'Flaherty at Portman Sq until partnership dissolved 1852.

HON APPTS Chairman Sanitary Board St Giles District 1897–99.

SOCIETY Apprenticed to his father in 1839. Yeoman 1847; Liveryman 1874; elected to the Court 1890 *vice* Thomas Skeel. Secy of Friendly Medical Soc 1893–1907. Junior Warden 1895–96, Senior Warden 1896–97, Master 1897–98. Examinations Cttee 1905–08; retired from the Court 1908.

FAMILY LIVERYMEN (grandfather) Samuel Griffith; (father) Richard Clewin Griffith, Master 1855–56; (uncle) Samuel Clewin Griffith; (bro) Richard Clewin Griffith; (bro) John Clewin Griffith; (bro) Daniel Clewin Griffith; (son) Revd Vere Yates Clewin Griffith. Nine of the Griffith family were members of the Society between the early eighteenth century and the early twentieth century.

In 1857 he gave £25 to the Widows' Fund and between 1863–98 he donated £31 to the Distressed Members' Fund. He presented the first Master's badge in 1898 and his stained glass Arms panel. A portrait of his father painted by Arthur Fisher, presented by his brother Richard, hangs in the Parlour.

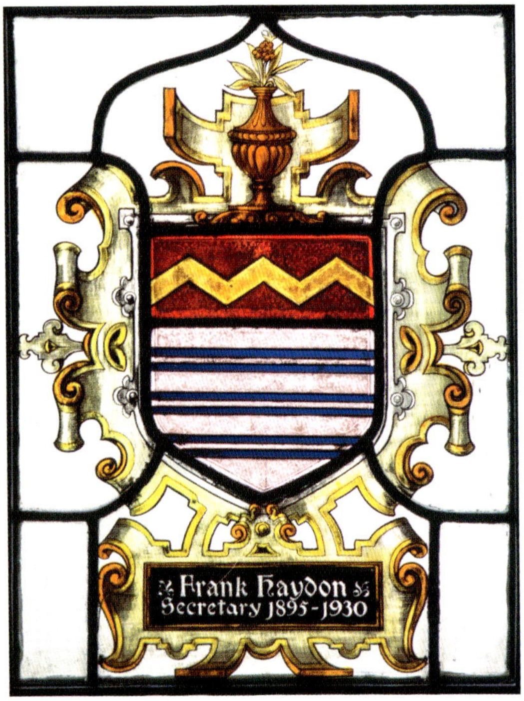

Argent, three bars gemels Azure, on a chief Gules a bar dancetty Or

Crest (not shown): *A Lion Argent seizing on a Bull courant Sable*

Dr Frank HAYDON, LRCP

These Arms are recorded in a visitation of Devon 1620 for Haydon of Bowood, Epford and Cadhay, County Devon.[8]

The maker of the stained glass panel is unknown, but might be James Powell & Sons. The panel was installed in window W4-11 in 1938 showing the shield in Cartouche B. From Sep 1941 to Jan 1946 all stained glass was removed from the Hall during hostilities and on return in 1946 these Arms were placed in window W4-15.

The connection of Frank Haydon with the seventeenth-century family is unknown.

BORN London 10 Sep 1861; *s* of George Henry Haydon and Clarissa Risdon; *m* 1904 Alice Waterfield, one son; *ob.* 1 Aug 1941.

EDUC Westminster Hosp.

QUALIFICATIONS LRCP 1891.

CAREER. Assistant Surgeon to the Royal London and Western Ophthalmic Hosps; Oculist to the London and South Western and Southern Railways for 45 years specialising in colour blindness.

SOCIETY Secretary to the Court of Examiners 1895–1930; title changed to Registrar after his retirement: Liveryman 1898 by gift.

FAMILY LIVERYMEN (son) Frank Risdon Haydon; (grandson) Hilary Risdon Haydon.

Presented a pair of oxidised fire-dogs and his stained glass Arms panel.

Dr Reginald Hewlett HAYES, LSA, LRCP MRCS

The Arms were granted by the Ulster Office under the auspices of Sir Bernard Burke, Ulster King of Arms in 1868 to his great uncle Henry Hayes for the descendants of his great-grandfather Andrew Hayes and are recorded at the College of Arms in the Irish records Volume G. 165.

The stained glass panel was made by James Powell & Sons in 1941 for installation after the War. The panel was installed in window W3-11 in 1946 showing the shield in Cartouche A.

The motto translates as *Renew your courage*.

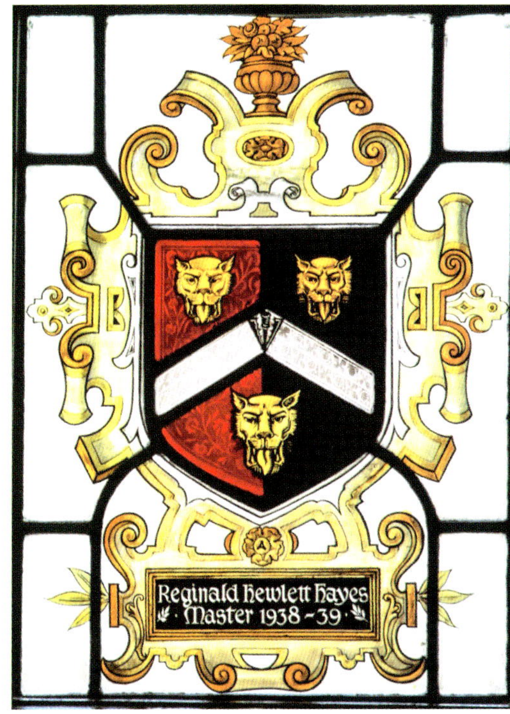

Per pale Gules and Sable, on a Chevron Argent between three Leopard's Faces Or a Pheon of the second

Crest (not shown): *On a wreath of the colours, a Demi-Lion rampant Or, holding in its paws a Flagstaff, therefrom a Pennon gules, and charged on the shoulder with a Pheon Sable*

Motto (not shown): *Renovate Animos* [9]

BORN Dublin 12 Apr 1869; *s* of William Hayes and Kate Hewlett; *unmarried*; *ob.* 11 Jan 1951.

EDUC U Dublin and Guy's Hosp Medical Sch.

QUALIFICATIONS LSA 1895; LRCP MRCS 1895.

CAREER Clin Asst Evelina Hosp and Soho Hosp for Women (1910); Asst Anaesthetist Royal Ear Hosp (1910); Res Obstetrician Guy's Hosp (1910–30)-a1935; Clin Asst Westminster Ophthalmic Hosp (1915–42); Dresser Eye Wards Guy's Hosp (1935)–(1942).

SOCIETY Joined as a Licentiate. Yeoman 1895; Liveryman 1906; elected to the Court 1931 *vice* Frederick Gordon Brown. Junior Warden 1936–37, Senior Warden 1937–38, Master 1938–39.

Presented the William Kent pine mantel in the Parlour from West Harling Hall near Thetford in Norfolk which was demolished in 1932, four silver salt cellars, lighting for the William of Orange picture, an eighteenth-century medical chest, an eighteenth-century pill tile and his stained glass Arms panel; he also left a bequest of £20,000 which was partially used to buy candelabra for dinners.

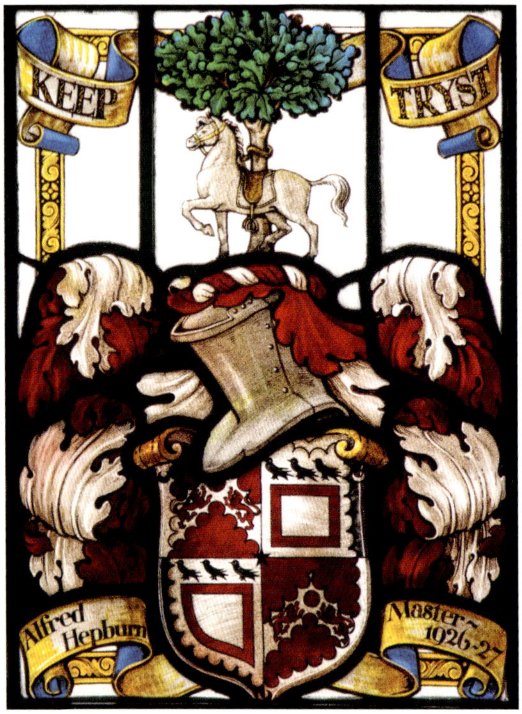

Quarterly: 1st & 4th; Gules, on a Chevron engrailed Argent, a Rose between two Lions counter-combatant of the first (Hepburn); 2nd & 3rd; Argent, an Orle Gules, in chief three Martlets Sable (Rutherford): overall a Bordure wavy quarterly Argent and Sable, on the chief point a Mullet Sable; And for the Crest upon a helm mantled Gules doubled Argent, on a wreath of the colours, a Horse furnished and tied to a Tree proper

Dr Alfred HEPBURN, MRCS, LSA

The Arms are recorded at the Court of the Lord Lyon King of Arms in Edinburgh. The original Hepburn of Monkrig Arms, without the engrailing of the chevron, date to 1672 but Lyon acknowledges they were in use in the fourteenth century.

These Hepburn Arms were rematriculated to include the Rutherford quartering at the Lyon Court on 30 Sep 1919,[10] for Edward Hepburn of Monkridge, Kent, who, as a third son, used the mullet as a cadency mark.

Dr Hepburn was a son of Edward's great uncle (i.e. a first cousin once removed of Edward but only seven years older than him) so not being descended from Edward it is unclear why these Arms were used.

The stained glass panel was made by Francis Spear in 1931 and was installed in window W3-2 in 1931, showing the full Arms with motto and was the first panel to dispense with a cartouche. From Sep 1941 to Jan 1946 all stained glass was removed from the Hall during hostilities and on return in 1946 these Arms were returned to window W3-2.

BORN 1856; 6th *s* of Joseph Gutteridge Hepburn and Emma Smith; *m* 1904 Rosalie Thurston, one dau; *ob.* 1 Aug 1931

EDUC St Bartholomew's Hosp Medical Coll.

QUALIFICATIONS LSA 1877; MRCS 1878.

CAREER Resident Medical Officer National Sanatorium for Consumption and Diseases of the Chest Bournemouth; Clinical Asst Hosp for Women, Soho Square; Surgeon Eastern Telegraph steamship *Chiltern*, which was in service laying cable between 1872–1903.

SOCIETY Yeoman 1880; Liveryman 1890; elected to the Court 1918 *vice* Martindale Ward. Examinations Cttee 1924–29. Junior Warden 1924–25, Senior Warden 1925–26, Master 1926–27. As Senior Warden he put forward proposals which led to the institution of the MMSA in 1928.

It is likely that he commissioned and presented his stained glass Arms panel, although why the cartouche was dispensed with is less clear. Possibly Francis Spear, having just completed the magnificent Apothecary window for the south wall of the Hall, wished to design another spectacular work unconstrained by a cartouche. A few years later, the Honorary Freemen were invited to participate in the glazing scheme and two that accepted were peers with supporters so this continued a general move away from the cartouches and, in fact, they were used for only eight more Arms, the last time being in 1979.

Dr David Treharne Dillon HUGHES, MA, BSc, BM BCh, FRCP

The Arms were designed by Theobald Mathew, Windsor Herald, in 1993 and are recorded at the College of Arms in Volume 60, Folio 160.

The stained glass panel was made by Goddard & Gibbs of London and was installed in window W3-6 in 1994, showing the full Arms and motto without a cartouche.

The colours of the field come from the Society's Arms as does the unicorn crest. The latter is also associated with the Wellcome Foundation. The oars represent his interest in rowing and the masks his interest in the theatre.

The goats and the motto come from the Treherne family.

The motto translates as *Seize the day.*

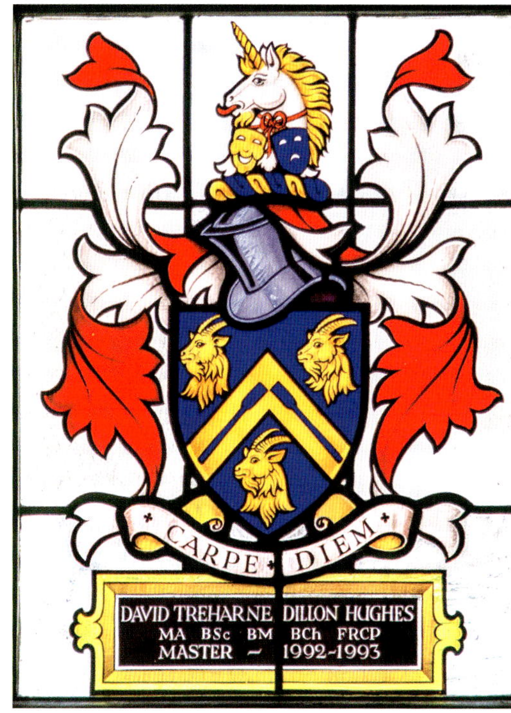

Azure, upon a Chevron between three Goat's Heads erased Or, two Oars the Blades upwards Azure; And for the Crest upon a Helm mantled Gules doubled Argent, on a Wreath Or and Azure, a Unicorn's Head erased Argent, armed and crined Or, gorged by a Ribbon bowed Gules pendant therefrom a Mask of Comedy and a like Mask of Tragedy Azure

Motto: *Carpe Diem*

BORN Cardiff 31 Oct 1931; *s* of Maj Gen W. D. Hughes and Elizabeth Thomas; *m* 1959 Gloria Bailey, one son, two daus.
EDUC Trinity College Oxford (BA, BSc, MA, BM BCh); London Hosp Medical College.
QUALIFICATIONS BA 1952; BSc 1954; MA 1957; BM BCh 1957; MRCP Lond 1959; FRCP Lond 1971.
SERVICES Captain RAMC 1961–62.
CAREER Consultant Physician the London Hosp 1970–96; Senior Lecturer London Hosp Medical School 1969; Clin Director Respiratory Medicine Royal Hospitals Trust 1994–96; Head Dept Clin Investigation Wellcome Research Laboratories 1978–93.
HON APPTS General Medical Council 1993–96, Clin Dir Coalminers' Medical Assesst Process for DTI 1999–2010, President Hunterian Soc 1982–83.
SOCIETY Proposed for the Society by Dr AMA Moore (Master 1961–62). Yeoman 1958; Liveryman 1962; elected to the Court 1981 *vice* Sir Ronald Bodley Scott. Gideon de Launce Lecturer 1986. Junior Warden 1990–91, Senior Warden 1991–92, Master 1992–93. United Examining Board 1993–2005; Past Master Emeritus 2007.
FAMILY LIVERYMEN (son) David Edward Treharne Hughes, (dau) Dr Amanda Louise Elizabeth Hughes, (dau) Dr Carly Anna Hughes.
Presented various books for the Library, the picture lights over the portrait of William of Orange, a silver and gilt dish, his miniature portrait and his stained glass Arms panel.

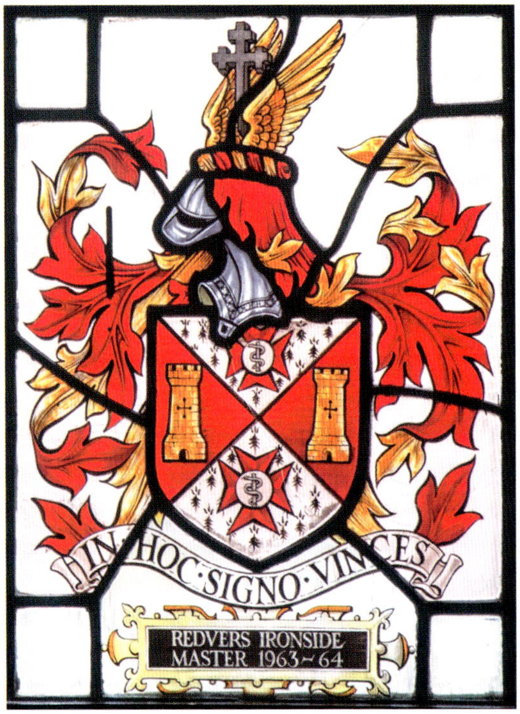

Dr Redvers Nowell IRONSIDE, OStJ, MB ChB, FRCP

The Arms were designed by John Brooke-Little, Bluemantle Pursuivant, in 1962 and are recorded at the College of Arms in Volume Gr 124, Folio 258.

The stained glass panel was made by Carl Edwards and was installed in window W3-14 *c.*1965, showing the full Arms and motto without a cartouche.

The Maltese crosses and ermine field are from the Arms of Charing Cross Hospital and the towers are from the Arms of the City of Aberdeen.

The grant was made to Dr Ironside and his descendants and to his brother, William Dalton Ironside of Biddenden, and his descendants.

The motto translates as *Under this sign you shall conquer.*

Per saltire Ermine and Gules, in pale two Maltese Crosses of the second each surmounted of a Plate charged with a Rod of Asclepius proper and in fess two Towers Or; And for the Crest upon a Helm, mantled Gules and Or, on a Wreath of the colours, a Cross Crosslet fitchée Argent between two Wings Or

Motto: *In Hoc Signo Vinces*

BORN 23 Dec 1899; *s* of William Dalton Ironside and Emma Storrier Yates; *unmarried*; *ob.* 18 Jul 1968.

EDUC U Aberdeen Med Sch (MB ChB).

QUALIFICATIONS MB ChB 1922; MRCP Lond 1925; FRCP Lond 1936.

SERVICES Royal Arty 1917–18; RAF(VR) 1939–45, Sqn Ldr 1940, Air Cdre 1944; Cons Neurologist to the RAF.

CAREER Cons Neurologist: West London Hosp 1926–63; Hosp of St John & St Elizabeth 1927–55; Maida Vale Hosp 1935–65; Charing Cross Hosp 1959–65.

HON APPTS Board of Governors National Hosps for Nervous Diseases 1955–58 and 1962–63.

SOCIETY Yeoman 1929; Liveryman 1930; elected to the Court 1955 *vice* Duncan Campbell Fitzwilliams. Junior Warden 1961–62, Senior Warden 1962–63, Master 1963–64. Catalogued the Society's collection of jars and pill tiles.

HONOURS AND AWARDS OStJ 1932.

Presented the Tabriz carpet in the Parlour, the portrait of Gideon de Laune on the landing, the Parlour pine doors, several pill tiles, the cost of restoring the picture frames in the Parlour, a silver-plated coffee pot and milk jug, his miniature portrait and his stained glass Arms panel. He also left bequests of £500 to the Sustentation Fund and £2,000 to the Restoration Reserve Fund.

Mr Ian MacGilchrist JACKSON, BA, MB BChir, FRCS, FRCOG

The Arms were designed by Colin Cole, Windsor Herald, in 1978 and are recorded at the College of Arms in Volume 141, Folio 105.

The stained glass panel was possibly made by Carl Edwards and was installed in window W3-9 in 1979, showing the shield in Cartouche B. This was the last window to use the cartouche surround.

The field and unicorn are for the Society and the pomegranates are symbols of fertility and regeneration suitable for an obstetrician, once called accoucheurs hence the stance of the unicorn. The latter also acknowledges his Scottish origins.

The Crest may be a play on the Royal College of Obstetrics and Gynaecology's crest.

The motto translates as *Courage tempered with kindness.*

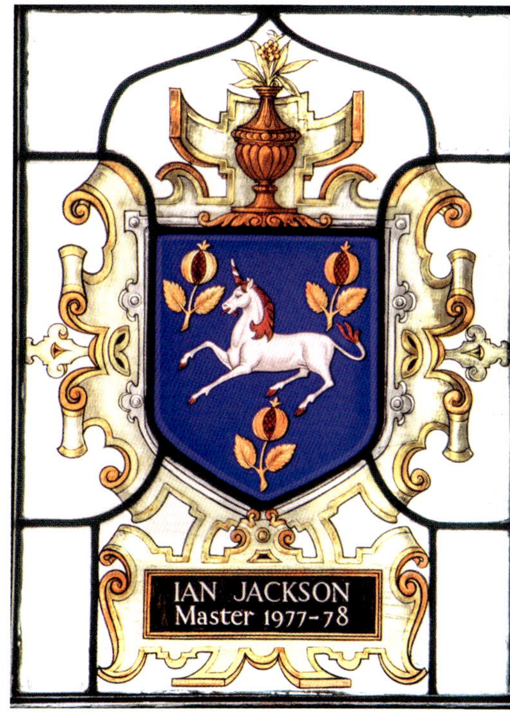

BORN Shanghai 11 Nov 1914; *s* of Dr Ernest David Jackson and Mary MacGillchrist; *m* 1st 1943 Leslie Bellamy, dis 1967, two s, one d; *m* 2nd 1970 Lucy Heitz; *ob.* 24 Jun 2002.
EDUC Trinity Hall, Cambridge (BA, MB BChir); the London Hosp Medical Coll.
QUALIFICATIONS BA 1936; MRCS LRCP 1939; MB BChir 1939; FRCS Eng 1940; MRCOG 1942; FRCOG 1955.
SERVICES RAMC 1943–47: 224 Parachute Field Ambulance; Mobile Surgical Unit 3 Cdo Bde; Consultant in Obs and Gynae to RAF 1964–83.
CAREER Cons Obstetrician and Gynaecologist Middlesex Hosp 1948–79; Cons Gynaecologist Chelsea Hosp for Women 1948–79; King Edward VII Hosp for Officers 1961–84; Royal Masonic Hosp 1963–79; Examiner U London, Us Oxford and Cambridge, Conjoint Bd, Central Midwifery Board, RCOG.
HON APPTS RCOG – Council 1951–70, Hon Secy 1954–61, Chairman Examination Cttee 1962–65; Librarian Royal Society of Medicine 1969–75.
SOCIETY Yeoman 1949; Liveryman 1953; elected to the Court 1966 *vice* Alan Bews. Junior Warden 1975–76, Senior Warden 1976–77, Master 1977–78. Hon Treasurer 1985–89; Assistant Emeritus 1989.
FAMILY LIVERYMEN (nephew) Mr Andrew Malcolm Jackson.
HONOURS AND AWARDS Order of the Star of Africa (Liberia) 1969; Grand Officer of Order of Istiqlal, Jordan 1970.
Presented a modern silver pepper mill with the Society's Arms engraved, his miniature portrait and his stained glass Arms panel.

Azure, a Unicorn couchant Argent, crined, maned and tail tufted Gules, the Horn twisted Argent and Gules between three Pomegranates slipped Or seeded Gules

Crest (not shown): *upon a Helm on a Wreath Argent and Azure two Arms embowed vested Azure crusily Or, the Hands proper supporting a Crescent Ermine, arising therefrom a Sun in splendour Or*
Motto (not shown): *Animus Benignitate Temperatas*

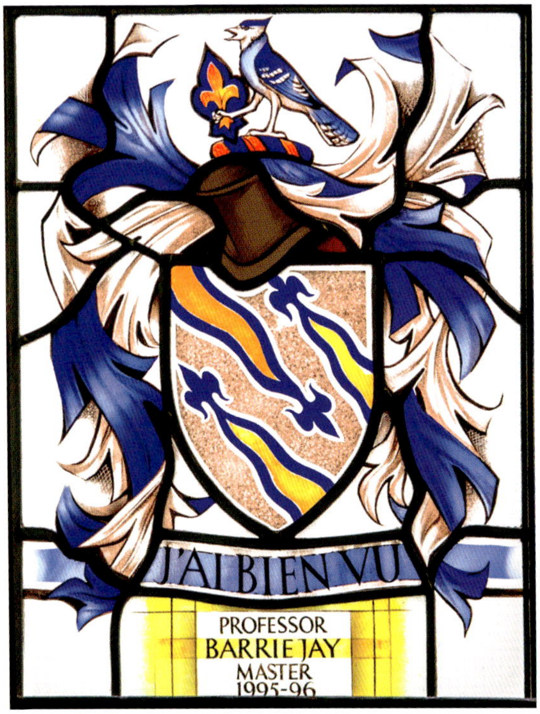

Professor Barrie Samuel JAY, MB BChir, MD, FRCS, DO, FRCOphth

The Arms were designed by Peter Gwynn-Jones, Lancaster Herald, in 1995 and are recorded at the College of Arms in Volume Gr 151, Folio 198.

The stained glass panel was made by Chapel Studio of King's Langley and was installed in window E1-7 in 1997, showing the full Arms and motto without a cartouche.

The wavy piles represent light for an ophthalmologist, golden piles for his mother's maiden name Sterling, and the fleurs-de-lys for his wife's birth in France and his gardening prowess with iris.

The jay is a canting allusion and the North American blue jay is used as English jays are not so distinctive.

The motto translates as *I saw clearly* and is another canting allusion to his name and profession.

Argent, three Piles wavy bendwise, one issuing from the dexter chief, one from the sinister flank and one from the sinister base each terminating in a Fleur-de-Lys Azure and charged with a Pile wavy Or; And for the Crest upon a Helm, mantled Azure doubled Argent, on a Wreath Or and Azure, a Blue Jay calling proper, in the dexter Claw a Fleur-de-Lys Or fimbriated Azure

Motto: *J'Ai Bien Vu*

BORN London 7 May 1929; *s* of Dr Maurice Bernard Jay and Julia Sterling; *m* 1954 Marcelle Ruby Byre, two sons; *ob.* 10 Mar 2007.

EDUC Gonville & Caius Coll Cambridge (BA, MB BChir, MD); University Coll Hosp Medical Sch.

QUALIFICATIONS BA 1949; MB BChir 1952; DO 1959; FRCS Eng 1962; MD 1965; FRCOphth 1988.

CAREER Cons Ophthalmic Surgeon the Royal London Hosp 1965–92; Consultant Surgeon Moorfields Eye Hosp 1969–92; Professor of Clinical Ophthalmology U London 1985–92; Dean Inst Ophthalmology U London 1980–85; Adviser in Ophthalmology to Chief Medical Officer; Examiner RCS 1970–80.

HON APPTS Founding Fellow RCOphth 1988; Council Royal College Surgeons 1983–88; Hon Secretary Academy of Medical Royal Colleges.

SOCIETY Proposed for the Society by Keith Lyle. Yeoman 1962; Liveryman 1966; elected to the Court 1985 *vice* Dr Hugh Sinclair. Junior Warden 1993–94, Senior Warden 1994–95, Master 1995–96. Hon Treasurer 1999–2004; Past Master Emeritus 2004.

CITY AND CIVIC Spectacle Makers' Company: Freeman 1966, Liveryman 1997; Barbers' Company: Freeman 1970, Liveryman 1970.

HONOURS AND AWARDS Hon FRCOphth 1994; Hon FRCPCH 1996; Lifetime Achievement Award European Paediatric Ophthalmological Soc 2004.

Presented various books for the Library, eight cups and saucers for the use of the Private Court, four butter dishes, his miniature portrait and his stained glass Arms panel. Mrs Jay presented his five-volume scrapbook of his Master's year.

Dr James Henry JEFFCOAT, LSA, MRCS

The Arms were designed by George Marshall, Rouge Croix Pursuivant, in 1890 and are recorded at the College of Arms in Volume Gr 65, folio 246.

The stained glass panel was made by James Powell & Sons in 1906 and was installed in window W3-6 in 1906, showing the shield in Cartouche B, as one of the first three panels (the Private Court of 1903–04). From Sep 1941 to Jan 1946 all stained glass was removed from the Hall during hostilities and on return in 1946 these Arms were placed in window W4-5.

The motto translates as *While I live I hope.*

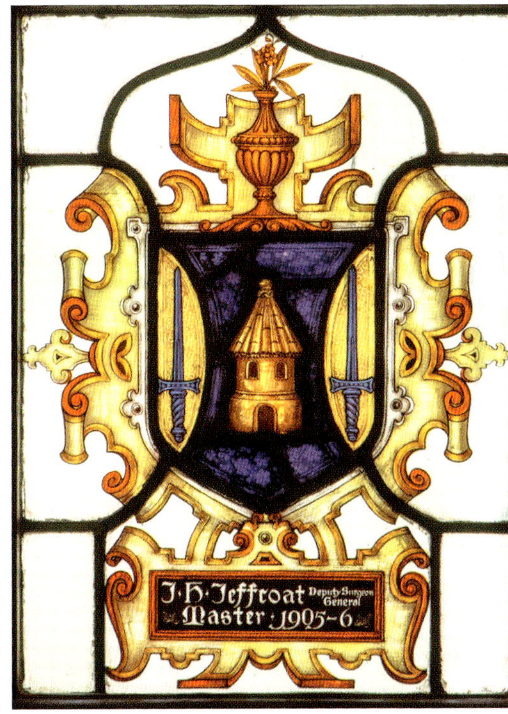

Azure, a Dovecote Or between two Flaunches of the last each charged with a Sword erect of the first

Crest (not shown): *upon a Helm mantled Azure doubled Or, on a Wreath of the colours a Dovecote within Park Pales proper*

Motto (not shown): *Dum Spiro Spero*[11]

BORN Leamington 9 May 1837; *s* of James Jeffcoat and Elizabeth Gale; *m* Anna Margaretha Sophia Hertzog, five sons, one dau; *ob.* 5 Jul 1922.

EDUC St Mary's Hosp Medical Sch.

QUALIFICATIONS LSA 1858; MRCS 1858.

SERVICES Asst Surgeon Royal Arty 1858; Surgeon 1873; Surgeon Major 1873; Afghan War 1878–80; Brigade Surgeon 1884; Hon Deputy Surgeon General 1885 on retirement.

SOCIETY Apprenticed 1853; Yeoman 1862 but given precedence of 1860 by Court; Liveryman 1880; elected to the Court 1895 *vice* Sir George Buchanan; Court of Examiners 1899–1905. Junior Warden 1903–04, Senior Warden 1904–05, Master 1905–06.

FAMILY LIVERYMEN (son) Rev William Frederick Hertzog Jeffcoat, (son) Rev Reginald Jeffcoat, (son) Col Algernon Cautley Jeffcoat.

Between 1902–18 he donated £1,000 to the Widows' Fund and he presented the first three stained glass panels to be installed representing the Private Court of 1903–04 (Jeffcoat, Day, Cooper).

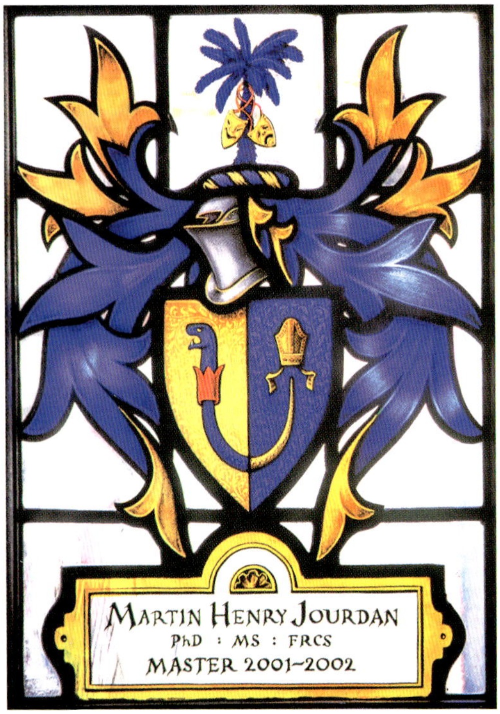

Per pale Or and Azure, a Serpent counter changed engorged with a Coronel Gules; above the Serpent's Tail a Mitre of the first. And for the Crest, upon a Helm mantled Azure doubled Or, on a Wreath of the colours, a Palm Tree Azure hung with the Masques of Comedy and Tragedy Or

Mr Martin Henry JOURDAN, LRCP MRCS, MB BS, PhD, FRCS, MS

The Arms were designed by Hubert Chesshyre, Clarenceaux King of Arms, in 2004 and are recorded at the College of Arms in Volume Gr 168, Folio 66.

The stained glass panel was made by Leonie Seliger of Canterbury in 2004 and was installed in window W1-10 in 2004, showing the full Arms without a cartouche.

The serpent represents medicine and the surmounting coronel is a representation of an ancient device used for blunting or rebating lances in a tournament to indicate his treatment of Crohn's disease and in allusion to the Eastern crowns of Guy's Hospital.

The mitre represents Bishopshalt Grammar School, Hillingdon and his marriage in a cathedral and the palm tree alludes to time spent in Saudi Arabia and the Yemen. The masques of comedy and tragedy symbolise family links with the theatre.

The colours of gold and blue also represent the Society's colours.

BORN 7 Oct 1941; *s* of Henry George Jourdan and Jocelyn Louise Courteney; *m* 1966 May McElwain, two sons, two daus.

EDUC Guy's Hosp Medical Sch (MB BS, PhD).

QUALIFICATIONS LRCP MRCS 1966; MB BS 1970; PhD 1970; FRCS Eng 1974, MS 1980.

CAREER Cons Surgeon Guy's Hosp 1977–2007; Cons Surgeon St Thomas' Hosp 1982–2007; Reader in Surgery U London 1982–2007; Court of Examiners RCS 1987–2000; Chairman Examiners in Surgery U London 1989–91.

SOCIETY Proposed for the Society by Past Master Mr Guy Blackburn. Yeoman 1980; Liveryman 1985; elected to the Court 1988 *vice* Sir Gordon Wolstenholme. Chairman Examinations Cttee 1991–99. Junior Warden 1999–2000, Senior Warden 2000–01, Master 2001–02. Past Master Emeritus 2017.

FAMILY LIVERYMEN (son) Mr Iain Jourdan FRCS, (dau) Ms Anthea Jourdan (Mrs Lord).

Presented various books for the library, two nineteenth-century silver dishes, half the cost of the library steps, 150 steak knives, his miniature portrait and his stained glass Arms panel.

Dr Paul Anthony KNAPMAN, DL, LRCP MRCS, MB BS, FRCP, FRCS, DMJ, Barrister

The Arms were designed by William Hunt, Windsor Herald, in 2009 and are recorded at the College of Arms in Volume 173, Folio 239.

The stained glass panel was made by Richard Scowen of Cornwall and was installed in window W3-1 in 2009, showing the full Arms without a cartouche.

The Knapmans have been a Stannary family near Chagford since the sixteenth century and this is a variant of their Arms. Stannators used to have their own marks and the portcullises on the blocks of tin follow this tradition and represent his time as the Westminster Coroner.

The original Knapman Arms were mentioned in the visitation of Devon of 1620 but as family records were destroyed in Exeter Library and City Hall by enemy action in 1941 no direct connection could be proven and these new Arms had to be differenced. The original Arms in 1620 had no crest and it was decided not to apply for a crest for this grant either.

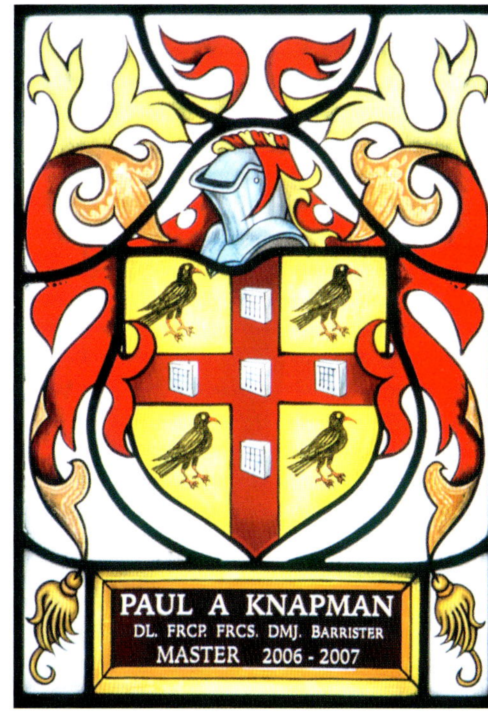

Or, on a Cross Gules, between four Cornish Choughs proper, five Blocks of Tin proper marked with Portcullises; And a Helm mantled Gules doubled Or with a Wreath of the colours

---

BORN 5 Nov 1944; *s* of Frederick Ethelbert Knapman and Myra Smith; *m* 1970 Penelope Cox, one son, three daus.

EDUC St George's Hosp Medical Sch (MB BS), called to the Bar, Gray's Inn.

QUALIFICATIONS LRCP MRCS 1968: MB BS 1968; Barrister 1972; DMJ 1975.

SERVICES Surg Lieut RNVR 1965–70, Hon Col Westminster Dragoons (C&S Sqn), the Royal Yeomanry 2016–d.

CAREER Dep Coroner for Inner West London 1975–80; HM Coroner for Westminster (Inner West London) 1980–2011; Hon Lecturer Med Jurisprudence St George's Hosp Medical Sch 1978–2004; Hon Clinical Teacher (Forensic Medicine) Royal Free and University Coll Medical Sch 1981–2004; Hon Clinical Senior Lecturer Imperial Coll Sch Medicine 1987–2006.

SOCIETY Proposed for the Society by Dr P. C. Edmondson and Dr H. R. Petty. Yeoman 1980; Liveryman 1986; elected to the Court 1993 *vice* Dr F. G. Neild. Junior Warden 2004–05, Senior Warden 2005–06, Master 2006–07. Society Representative on Chelsea Physic Garden Advisory Cttee 2007–16.

CITY AND CIVIC Deputy Lieutenant for Greater London 2008–d and Representative Deputy Lieutenant for Westminster (Greater London Lieutenancy) 2013–d.

HONOURS AND AWARDS FRCS Eng (Hon Caus) 1995; FRCP Lond (Hon Caus) 1997.

Presented his miniature portrait and his stained glass Arms panel.

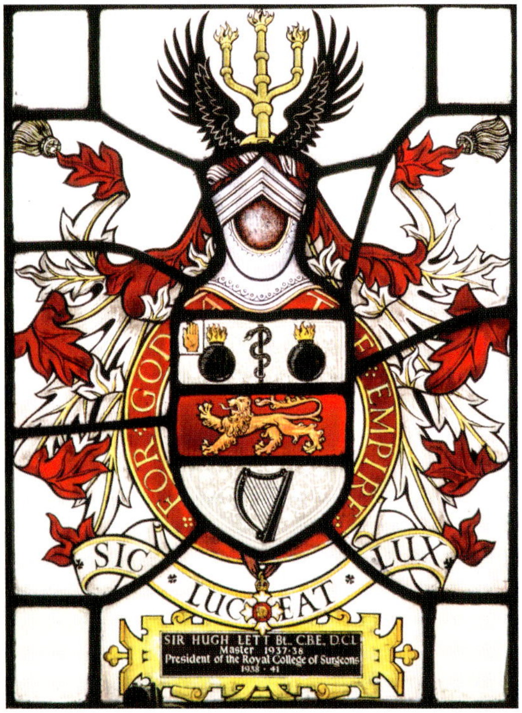

Sir Hugh LETT, Bt of Walmer, KCVO, CBE, LRCP MRCS, MB ChB, FRCS

The Arms were designed by Alfred Butler, Windsor Herald, in 1940 and are recorded at the College of Arms in Volume 106, Folio 124.

The stained glass panel was made by James Powell & Sons in 1943 and was installed in window W3-8 in 1946, showing the full Arms surrounded by the insignia of the Most Excellent Order of the British Empire and motto without a cartouche.

It is likely that the red and silver of the field and the lion are derived from the Royal College of Surgeons' Arms, the rod of Asclepius is for medicine and the red hand of Ulster signifies his baronetcy. It is not clear why the harp, grenades or crest were chosen, although the latter may reflect the motto.

The grant is made to Sir Hugh and the other descendants of his father Richard Alfred Lett as he had no sons to inherit the Arms.

The motto translates as *Let the light shine forth.*

Argent, on a Fess Gules between, in chief a Rod of Asclepius between two Grenades Sable fired proper and in base a Harp of the third, a Lion passant Or; And for the Crest upon a Knight's Helm mantled Gules doubled Argent, on a Wreath of the colours, an Antique Lamp Or inflamed proper between two Wings Sable

Motto: *Sic Luceat Lux*

BORN Waddingham 17 Apr 1876; *s* of Dr Richard Alfred Lett and Bithiah Appleford; *m* 1906 Helen, dau of Sir Buckston Browne, three daus; *ob.* 19 Jul 1964.

EDUC U Leeds Medical Sch (MB ChB); London Hosp Medical Coll.

QUALIFICATIONS MB ChB 1899; LRCP MRCS 1901; FRCS Eng 1902.

SERVICES Major RAMC 1914–16; Anglo-American Hosp Wimereuse-Furnes 1914–15; Belgian Hosp Veurne 1915.

CAREER Lecturer in Anatomy U London 1909–12; Cons Surgeon to London Hosp 1915–34.

HON APPTS President Hunterian Soc 1917; Royal College of Surgeons – Court of Examiners 1923–25, Council 1927–33, President 1938–41, Chairman of Trustees 1955–59; Hon Sec King Edward's Hosp Fund 1941–47; President British Medical Assoc 1946–48.

SOCIETY Yeoman 1911; Court of Examiners 1913–15 and 1918–19; Liveryman 1921; elected to the Court 1931 *vice* George Amsden. Junior Warden 1935–36, Senior Warden 1936–37, Master 1937–38. Examination Cttee 1938–44; Sustentation Cttee 1947–50. Retired from the Court in 1952.

HONOURS AND AWARDS CBE 1920; Hon DCL U Durham 1940; Bart 1941; KCVO 1947; Hon DSc U Cambridge 1948.

Between 1935–37 he donated 20 guineas to the Widows' Fund and left a significant legacy to the Restoration Reserve Fund. Presented his portrait on the landing by Sir James Gunn in 1948, a silver rose bowl made in 1899, his miniature portrait and his stained glass Arms panel.

Professor Brian LIVESLEY, JP, KStJ, MD, FRCP, MB ChB, DHMSA

The Arms were designed by Peter Gwynne-Jones, Garter King of Arms, in 2007 and are recorded at the College of Arms in Volume 161, Folio 223.

The stained glass panel was made by Mel Howse of Chichester and was installed in window W2-4 in 2007, showing the full Arms and motto without a cartouche.

The owl represents Leeds University and learning in general. The quill represents authorship and the acorns research ideas planted for future growth. The Maltese crosses represent the Order of St John with the circlet for his time as Director General. The unicorn crest is for the Society and the roses on each shoulder, visible and invisible, living and departed, represent his two Lancastrian wives.

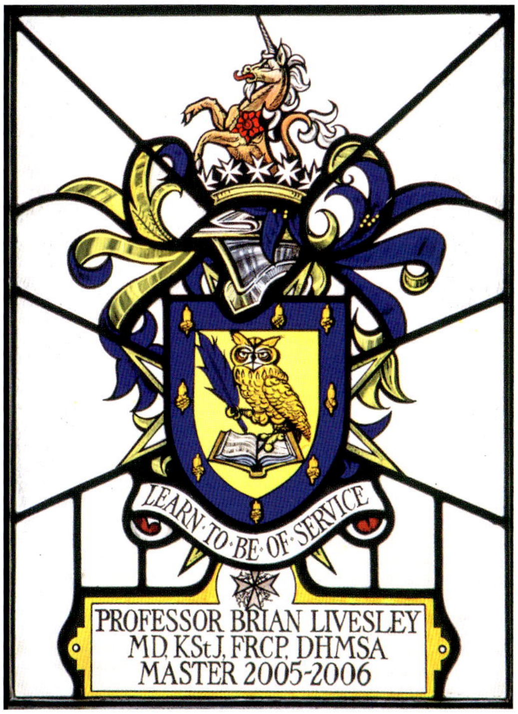

Or, upon an open Book in base an Owl statant guardant proper, holding in the dexter Claw a Quill Pen Azure; all within a bordure also Azure charged with nine Acorns Gold; And for the Crest, upon a Helm mantled Azure doubled Or, out of a Circlet Or set with eight Maltese Crosses Argent, a Demi-Unicorn Or, armed, crined and unguled Argent charged on each shoulder with a Rose Gules, one manifest

Motto: *Learn to be of Service*

BORN 31 Aug 1936; *s* of Thomas Livesley and Stella Simons; *m* 1st 1963 Beryl Hulme (*ob.* 1966), one son; *m* 2nd 1969 Valerie Nuttall, two daus.

EDUC U Leeds Medical Sch (MB ChB 1960; U London (MD 1979).

QUALIFICATIONS MB ChB 1960; MRCP UK 1971; DHMSA 1973; MD 1979; FRCP Lond 1989.

CAREER Cons Phys Geriatric Med Lambeth, Southwark & Lewisham HA 1973–87; Clin Exr in Med U London 1980–94; Exr for Dip Geriatric Med RCP 1987–93; U Professor in the Care of the Elderly London 1988–2001; External Exr Royal Free & UC Med Sch 1998–2001; Emeritus Prof Imperial Coll London 2003–d; Consultant Forensic Physician 2001–11.

HON APPTS St John Ambulance – Asst Dir-Gen 1993–94, Dir-Gen 1994–96.

SOCIETY Osler Lecturer 1975 and proposed for the Society by Dr Douglas Whittet. Yeoman 1975; Liveryman 1980; LMSSA Examiner in Medicine 1987–2001; elected to the Court 1990 *vice* Dr Geoffrey Cashell. Chairman Futures Cttee 1999–2004, Chairman Academic Cttee 2000–03; Gideon de Laune Lecturer 2001 and 2016. Junior Warden 2003–04, Senior Warden 2004–05, Master 2005–06. John Keats Memorial Lecturer 2009; Past Master Emeritus 2016.

CITY AND CIVIC JP South East London 1983–96.

HONOURS AND AWARDS KStJ 1994.

Presented various books for the Library, his miniature portrait and his stained glass Arms panel.

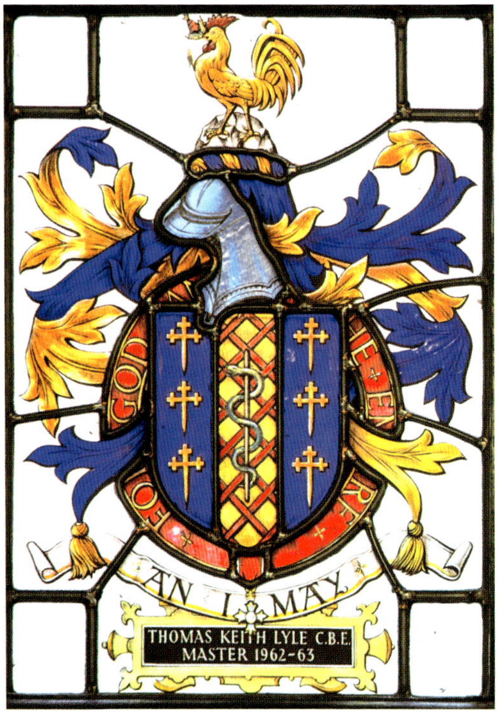

Azure, on a Pale Or fretty Gules, between six Cross Crosslets fitchee Or, a Rod of Asclepius proper; And for the Crest upon a Helm, mantled Azure doubled Or, on a Wreath of the colours upon a Rock proper, a Cock Or combed, wattled and jelloped Gules holding in its Beak a sprig of Cornish Heath proper

Motto: *An I May*

Mr Thomas Keith Selfe LYLE, CBE, LMSSA, LRCP MRCS, MB BChir, MD, MChir,FRCP, FRCS

The Arms were designed by Walter Verco, Norroy and Ulster King of Arms, in 1971 and are recorded at the College of Arms in Volume Gr 134, Folio 165. The grant was made to descendants of his late father Herbert Willoughby Lyle.

The stained glass panel was made by Carl Edwards and was installed in window E2-5 *c*.1972, showing the full Arms surrounded by the insignia of the Most Excellent Order of the British Empire and motto without a cartouche.

This is a variant of the Scots Lords Lyle's Arms (extinct in the 4th Lord c.1551),[12] which is quarterly; Azure a Bend between six Cross crosslets fitchee Or (Earldom of Mar) and Gules, fretty Or (Lyle); the crest is a Cock Or, crested Gules and the motto is the same.

Asclepius' rod indicates medicine and presumably the family has Cornish heritage but a direct connection with an extinct sixteenth-century Scottish family seems unlikely.

BORN Bromley 26 Dec 1903; *s* of Herbert Willoughby Lyle FRCS and Elizabeth Ada Selfe; *m* 1949 Jane Maxwell, one son, three daus; *ob.* 9 May 1987.

EDUC Sidney Sussex Coll Cambridge (MB BChir, MChir); King's Col Hosp Medical Sch.

QUALIFICATIONS LMSSA 1928; LRCP MRCS 1928; MB BChir 1930; MRCP Lond 1930; FRCS Eng 1932; MChir 1933; MD 1935; FRCP Lond 1963.

SERVICES RAFVR Medical Branch 1939–46; Temp Air Cdre 1945–46; Cons in Ophthalmology to the RAF 1948.

CAREER Cons Ophthalmic Surgeon King's College Hosp 1936–69; the National Hosp Queen Square 1936–69; Moorfields Eye Hosp 1936–69; Dir Orthoptic Dept Moorfields 1947–69; Dean, Inst of Ophthalmology 1959–67.

HON APPTS Royal Col Surgeons – Court of Examiners, Council; Pres British Orthoptic Bd.

SOCIETY Yeoman 1929; Liveryman 1933; elected to the Court 1954 *vice* John Francis Carter Braine. Junior Warden 1960–61, Senior Warden 1961–62, Master 1962–63. Assistant Emeritus 1985.

CITY AND CIVIC Order of St John – Deputy Hospitaller 1960–69; Hospitaller 1969–81; Bailiff Grand Cross 1981.

HONOURS AND AWARDS CBE 1949; CStJ 1956; KStJ 1960; Kt of the Order of the Holy Sepulchre 1970; GStJ 1981.

Presented various books for the Library, his miniature portrait and his stained glass Arms panel.

Professor Charles Gerard MACKWORTH-YOUNG CVO, MA, MB BChir, MD, FRCP

The Arms were granted in 1813 to his great-great-great grandfather Sir Samuel Young Bt (1813) of Formosa Place and are recorded at the College of Arms in Volume Gr 27, Folio 374.

The stained glass panel was made by Leonie Seliger of Canterbury and was installed in window E2-2 in 2019, showing the full Arms and motto without a cartouche.

The Younges of Dorset have similar Arms: *per fess Sable and Argent, three Lions rampant, guardant counterchanged.*[13] Their crest was a Sea Unicorn Argent, armed, finned and horned Gules.

Sir Samuel was the only son of Sir George Young, Admiral of the White, 1732–1810, which accounts for the naval allusions of the anchors and naval crown.

In 1995 Thomas Woodcock, Somerset Herald, designed a grant of supporters (Vol. Gr 161, Fol. 93) to Prof Mackworth-Young's father Sir Robin Mackworth-Young for his lifetime by virtue of his GCVO.

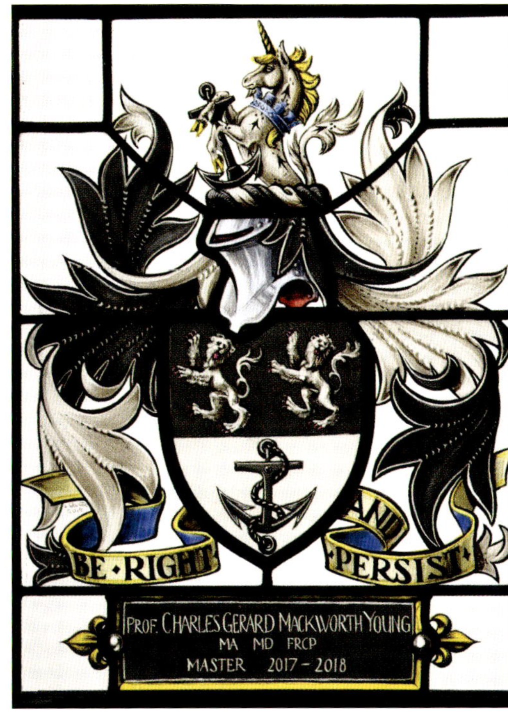

Per fess Sable and Argent, in chief two Lions rampant guardant and, in base, an Anchor erect with a cable, all counterchanged; And for the Crest upon a Helm, mantled Sable doubled Argent, on a Wreath of the colours a demi-Unicorn couped Ermine, armed, maned and hoofed Or, gorged with a Naval Crown Azure supporting an Anchor erect Sable

Motto: *Be Right and Persist*

BORN 6 Jul 1954; *s* of Sir Robin Mackworth-Young and Rosemary Aue; *m* 1983 Lady Iona Lindsay, one son, two dau.

EDUC Magdalene Coll Cambridge (MA, MB BChir, MD); St Bartholomew's Hosp Medical Coll.

QUALIFICATIONS BA 1975; MB BChir 1978; MA 1979; MRCP UK 1980; MD 1987; FRCP Lond 1995.

CAREER Cons Phys Rheumatology Charing Cross Hosp 1990, Chelsea and Westminster Hosp 1992–2016, King Edward VII Hosp for Officers 1992 (Medical Dir 2006–18); Imperial College Sch Med: Hon Sen Lect 1994–2017, Prof Rheumatology 2017–d; Hammersmith Hospitals NHS Trust, Chief of Service for Clinical Medicine 1998–2008.

HON APPTS RCP Specialist Advisory Cttee for Rheumatology 2006–10, Chairman British Society of Rheumatology Education and Training Cttee 2007–10, Chairman National Specialist Certificate Examination in Rheumatology 2010–12, Specially Appointed Commissioner Royal Hospital Chelsea 2018–d.

SOCIETY Proposed for the Society by Dr Julia Neild and Dr John Glynn. Yeoman 1992; Liveryman 1996; elected to the Court 2003 *vice* WFW Southwood. Chairman of the Examinations Committee 2009–12, Chairman of the Anniversary Committee 2009–17. Junior Warden 2015–16, Senior Warden 2016–17, Master 2017–18.

CITY AND CIVIC Company of Goldsmiths: Liveryman 2003, Court of Assistants 2011.

HONOURS AND AWARDS CVO 2020.

Presented his miniature portrait and his stained glass Arms panel.

Sir Arthur Salusbury MacNALTY, KCB, BA, LRCP MRCS, BM BCh, DPH, FRCP, FRCS

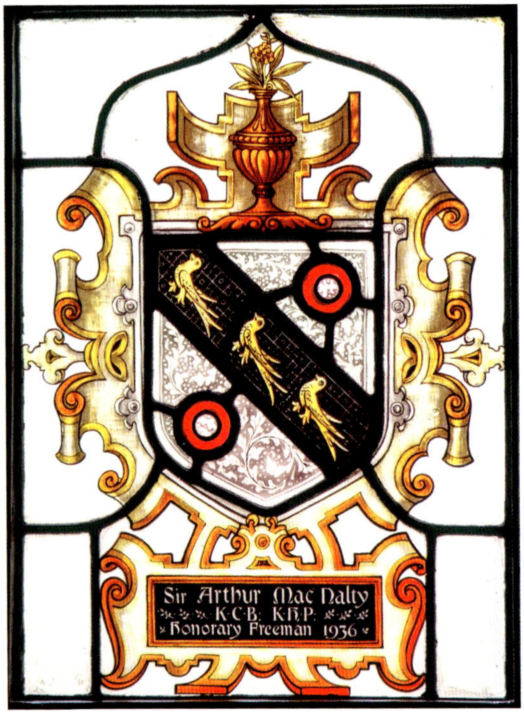

Argent, on a Bend Sable, between two Annulets Gules, three Martlets Or

The stained glass panel was made by Christopher Powell of James Powell & Sons in 1938 and was installed in window W4-5 in 1938, showing the shield in Cartouche B. From Sep 1941 to Jan 1946, all stained glass was removed from the Hall during hostilities and on return in 1946 these Arms were placed in window W4-11.

There is no record of the grant of these Arms to Sir Arthur or to any other MacNalty.

BORN Glenridding 20 Oct 1880; *s* of Dr Francis Charles MacNalty and Hester Emma Frances Gardner; *m* 1913 Dorothea de Wesslow, two daus; *ob.* 17 Apr 1969.

EDUC Corpus Christi Coll Oxford (BA, BM BCh, DM); University Coll Hosp Medical Sch.

QUALIFICATIONS BA 1904; LRCP MRCS 1907; BM BCh 1909; DM 1911; MRCP 1925; DPH 1927; FRCP Lond 1930; FRCS Eng 1939.

CAREER Brompton Hosp: RMO 1908–11 Dep Asst Physician 1911–13; Local Govt Board Medical Inspector 1913–19; Ministry of Health: Medical Officer 1919–32, Senior Medical Officer 1932–34, Chief Medical Officer 1935–41; Secy Tuberculosis Cttee Medical Research Council 1920–32; 1939–45 Chairman Cttees on Hospital and Nursing Provision; 1941 Editor in Chief Official Medical History of World War II; Examiner U Oxford, Birmingham, London.

HON APPTS Council Royal College of Physicians 1937–39; General Medical Council –1943; Life Governor Imperial Cancer Research.

SOCIETY Hon Freeman 1936; Monckton Copeman Lecturer 1967. Hon Fellow Faculty of the History of Medicine and Pharmacy.

CITY AND CIVIC Hon Freeman Barbers' Company 1954.

HONOURS AND AWARDS KCB 1936; KHP 1937–46; Hon FRS Edin 1949; Hon FRSM 1959; Hon FRSH; Hon FRIPHH.

Dr Gordon Barrett MITCHELL-HEGGS, OBE, ERD, TD, MD, FRCP

The Arms were designed by Archibald Russell, Lancaster Herald, in 1948 and are recorded at the College of Arms in Volume Gr 110, Folio 119. The grant was made to the descendants of his late father Francis Raymond Mitchell-Heggs.

The stained glass panel was made by Lawrence Lee and was installed in window E2-11 in 1975 showing the full Arms and motto without a cartouche. Suspended from the shield is the OBE medal.

The sickles reflect hedgers from which Heggs is derived and the caduceus is for medicine. The scallops are for pilgrims or those who help people.

These Arms are a variant of Mitchell of Monmouth: *Sable, a Chevron between three Escallops Or* and Mitchell of Dorset & York: *Sable, a Chevron Or between three Escallops Argent*.[14]

The motto is the Society's motto.

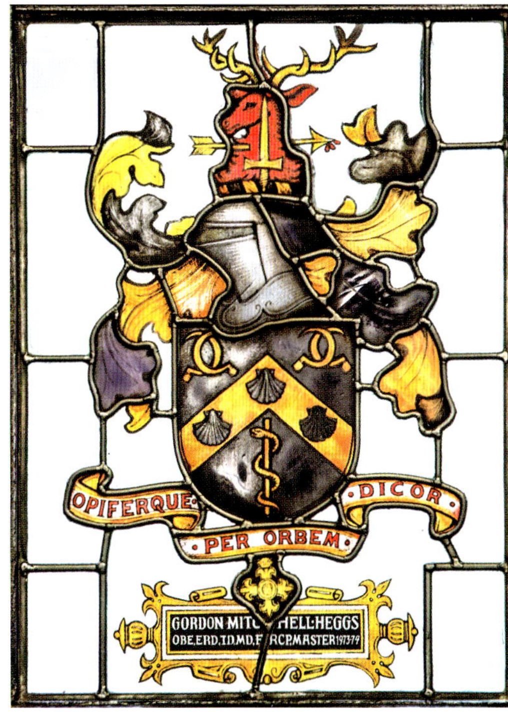

Sable, on a Chevron, between in chief two pairs of Sickles interlaced and in base a Rod of Asclepius Or, three Escallops of the field; And for the Crest upon a Helm, mantled Sable doubled Or, on a Wreath of the colours, a Stag's Head erased Gules, attired and pierced through the neck with an Arrow in fess Or flighted Argent embrued proper, and charged with a Sword erect Or

Motto: *Opiferque per Orbem Dicor*

BORN West Bromwich 10 Jun 1904; *s* of Dr Francis Raymond Mitchell Heggs LSA and Maud Ethel Sansome; *m* 1937 Nora Margaret Finch, one son; *ob.* 15 Dec 1975. 1939 assumed name of Mitchell-Heggs by deed poll.

EDUC Kitchener Scholar St Mary's Hosp Medical Sch (MB BS).

QUALIFICATIONS LRCP MRCS 1927; MB BS 1929; MD 1932; MRCP Lond 1933; FRCP Lond 1944.

SERVICES RAMC 1937–45; CO 17 (London) General Hosp, later Hon Col 1955; Hon Consultant Dermatologist to the Army 1964.

CAREER Medical Superintendent and Dermatologist St Mary's Hosp 1934–; St John's Hosp for Diseases of the Skin 1945–69; Dean of St Mary's Medical School 1960–67.

HON APPTS International Cttee of Dermatology; President British Assoc of Dermatologists 1968–69; President Hunterian Soc.

SOCIETY Yeoman 1938; Liveryman 1943; elected to the Court 1963 *vice* Thomas Bramley Layton. Junior Warden 1971–72, Senior Warden 1972–73, Master 1973–74.

FAMILY LIVERYMEN (nep) Dr Peter Francis Mitchell-Heggs; (niece-in-l) Dr Nita Ann Mitchell-Heggs.

HONOURS AND AWARDS OBE 1944; ERD; TD.

Presented his miniature portrait and his stained glass Arms panel.

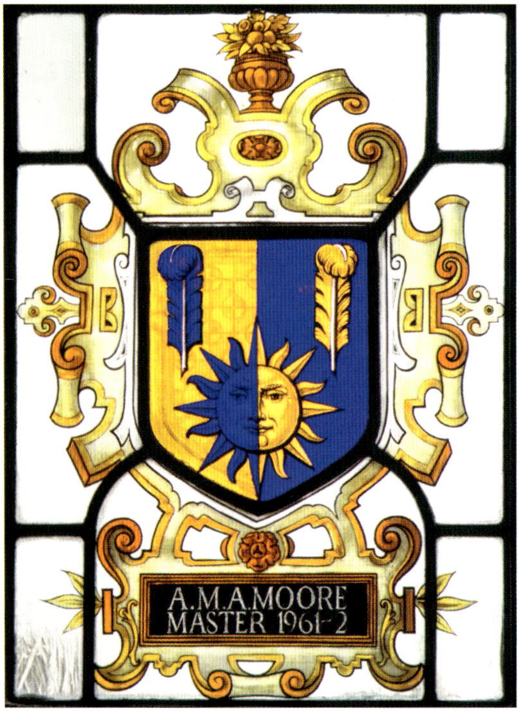

Per pale Or and Azure, a Sun in splendour and in chief two Ostrich Feathers counterchanged, the Quills argent

Crest (not shown): *upon a Helm, mantled Sable doubled Or, on a Wreath of the colours, a Moor's Head proper between two Wings Or each charged with a Shamrock Leaf slipped Vert*

Mr Archie Murrell Acheson MOORE, CStJ, LRCP MRCS, FDS RCS, FRCS, FICS

The Arms were designed by John Brooke-Little, Richmond Herald, in 1967 and are recorded at the College of Arms in Volume 130, Folio 258.

The stained glass panel was probably made by Carl Edwards and it was installed in window W3-7 in 1967, showing the shield in Cartouche A.

The colours of the field represent the Society, the sun is for Apollo and the ostrich feathers are for the Royal London Hospital.

The Moor's head in the Crest is a canting allusion and the shamrocks are for his Irish heritage.

BORN Pretoria 14 Aug 1904; *s* of Archie Moore; *m* Marjorie Aitken, one son, two daus; *ob.* 16 Apr 1979.

EDUC London Hosp Medical Coll.

QUALIFICATIONS LRCP MRCS 1927; FRCS Eng 1930; FDS RCS.

CAREER Surgeon to the London Hosp 1951–68; Senior Surgeon Poplar Hosp; Orthopaedic Surgeon King George Hosp Ilford; Cons Surgeon St Luke's Hosp for the Clergy; Hon Cons Surgeon Dr Barnado's Homes; Hon Cons Surgeon Arthur Stanley Inst for Rheumatism; Chairman Academic Board, London Hosp Medical Coll; MB BS examiner U London and Durham; FRCS examiner; FDS examiner.

HON APPTS President Board of Medical Auxiliaries; British Medical Assoc – Treasurer 1948–54, Vice President 1954.

SOCIETY Yeoman 1931; Liveryman 1934; elected to the Court 1952 *vice* Eric Morse Townsend. Junior Warden 1959–60, Senior Warden 1960–61, Master 1961–62. Hon Treasurer 1963–75.

FAMILY LIVERYMEN (son) Andrew Lionel Archibald Moore; (grandson) Theo Harry Moore; (grandson) Thomas Lionel Moore.

CITY AND CIVIC Barbers' Company: Freeman 1960, Liveryman 1960.

HONOURS AND AWARDS Hon FICS; OStJ 1963, CStJ 1968.

Presented a Lambeth delft blue and white heart shaped pill slab of *c.*1700, his miniature portrait and his stained glass Arms panel.

Dr John Christopher MOORE-GILLON, MA, MB BChir, LLB, MD, FRCP

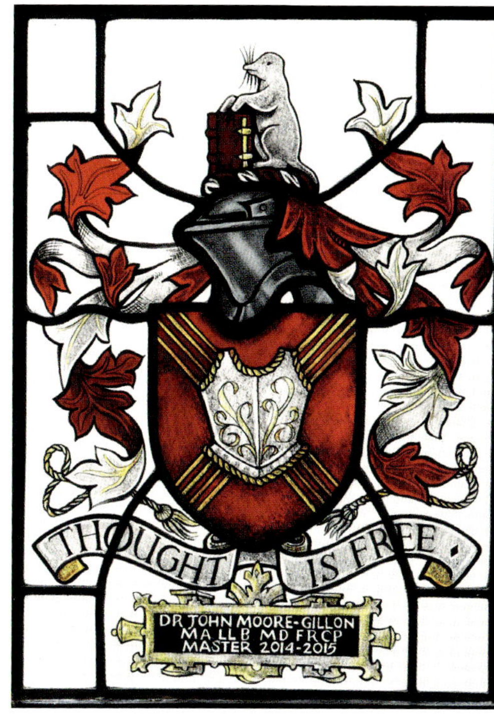

The Arms were designed by Patric Dickinson, Richmond Herald, in 2006 and are recorded at the College of Arms in Volume Gr 172, Folio 34.

The stained glass panel was made by Caroline Benyon and was installed in window E1-15 in 2019, showing the full Arms and motto without a cartouche.

The charge is described in the blazon as a breastplate and refers to his speciality. The Greek for breastplate was θώραξ – thorax, which originally meant a breastplate and not the part of the body which it covered. The four violin strings represent his wife and three children, all of whom are musical.

In the crest the mole derives from a pet name for the children when they were very small and the book is a reference to his bibliophilia.

The motto can be read in two ways: that it costs nothing to think; and also that one's thoughts are essentially unconstrained.

Gules four Violin Strings in bend and four Violin Strings in bend sinister throughout Or overall a Breastplate Argent garnished Or; And for the Crest upon a helm, mantled Gules doubled Argent, on a Wreath of the colours, a Mole Sejant erect Sable supporting with the Forefeet a closed Book Gules edged and clasped Or

Motto: *Thought Is Free*

BORN London 2 Jan 1953; *s* of John Alec Moore-Gillon and Daphne Smith; *m* 1980 Victoria Kirby, one son, two daus.

EDUC St Catherine's Coll Cambridge (BA, MA, MB BChir); St Thomas's Hosp Medical Sch; U London (MD, LLB).

QUALIFICATIONS BA 1973; MB BChir 1976; MA 1977; MRCP UK 1978; MD 1987; FRCP Lond 1992; LLB 2003.

CAREER Senior Lect & Hon Cons Physician Medical Coll of Barts Hosp 1988–92; Cons Physician Barts Hosp 1992–2010; Royal Lond Hosp 1998–2010; Cons Physician King Edward VII's Hosp 2001–d; Cons Physician Emeritus Barts Hosp 2010–d.

HON APPTS President British Lung Foundation 2001–07.

SOCIETY Proposed for the Society by Dr Christopher Cooper and Dr Nicholas Sheldon. Yeoman 1983; Liveryman 1990; elected to the Court 1999 *vice* Prof Tony Glenister. Junior Warden 2012–13, Senior Warden 2013–14, Master 2014–15.

FAMILY LIVERYMEN (wife) Mrs Victoria Moore-Gillon FRCS.

Presented several books for the Library, the electric baby-grand clavinova (with Past Master Dr R. N. Palmer), his miniature portrait and his stained glass Arms panel.

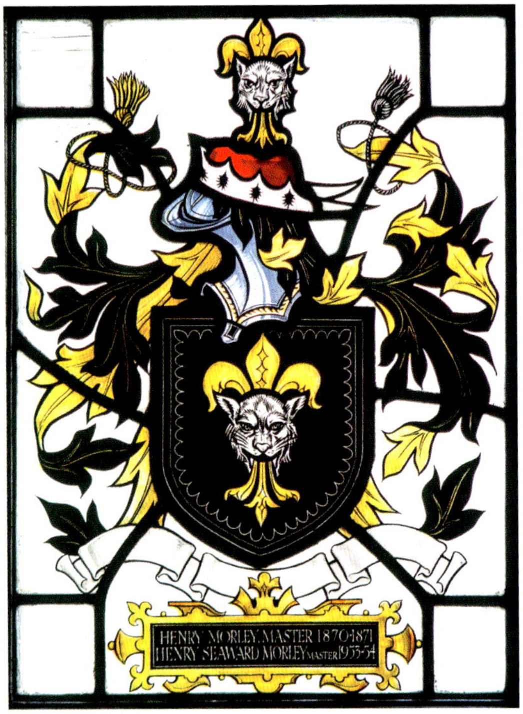
HENRY MORLEY. MASTER 1870-1871
HENRY SEAWARD MORLEY MASTER 1953-54

Sable, a Leopard's Head Argent jessant-de-lys Or. And for the Crest upon a Helm, mantled Sable doubled Or, on a Chapeau Gules turned up Ermine a Leopard's Head Argent jessant-de-lys Or

The stained glass panel was made by Carl Edwards *c*.1955 and was installed in window W1-2 *c*.1955, showing the full Arms without a cartouche.

The engrailed etching around the shield is the glass maker's foible.

Dr Henry MORLEY, MRCS, MS
Dr Henry Seaward MORLEY, LRCP MRCS MB BS, MD, FRCP

The leopard's face jessant-de-lys was originally granted to Morley of Morley, Co Lancashire *temp* Edward III.[15] Arms are recorded at the College of Arms for Morley of Newton-super-Ouse as *Sable, a Lion's head jessant-de-lys Argent* in Volume C40, Folio 134, dated 13 Sep 1665. Possibly this reversed the colours of the senior line.

The Arms illustrated, with the differenced fleur-de-lys, descend from Morley of Halnaker, Co Sussex *temp* James I, and the Drs Henry Morley probably descend from a younger brother of Sir John Morley of Halnaker whose son died without surviving male issue in 1701.

HM: BORN Lichfield 19 Sep 1793; *s* of William Morley and Alice Abbott; *m* 1st 1815 Ann Hicks, two sons; *m* 2nd 1827 Elizabeth Bond, one dau; *ob.* 29 Dec 1877.

EDUC Guy's Hosp Medical Sch (MS).

QUALIFICATIONS MRCS 1815; MS 1818.

CAREER GP in Hatton Garden and Kennington; 1843 retired to Midhurst due to ill health which then improved.

SOCIETY Yeoman 1818; Liveryman 1843; Court of Examiners 1841; elected to the Court 1862. Junior Warden 1868–69, Senior Warden 1869–70, Master 1870–71.

HSM: BORN 16 Mar 1897; *s* of Henry Forster Morley and Ida Rose Tayler; *m* 1934 Alison Hill, two sons, *ob.* 5 Jul 1960.

EDUC University Col Hosp Medical Sch (MB BS); U of London (MD).

QUALIFICATIONS LRCP MRCS 1924; MB BS 1925; MD 1929; MRCP Lond 1929; FRCP Lond 1948.

SERVICES Lieut Royal Field Arty 1915–19.

HON APPTS Crown Representative General Medical Council 1952–60.

CAREER Senior Physician, Royal West Sussex Hosp 1932–60; Physician Haslemere Hosp 1944–60; Cons Physician Graylingwell Hosp 1945–60; Physician St Richard's Hosp 1954–60.

SOCIETY Yeoman 1919; Liveryman 1926; elected to the Court 1943 *vice* Dr Russell Edwards Palmer. Examination Cttee 1947–52. Briefly Junior Warden 1952 until elected Senior Warden on the death of Dr Eric Morse Townsend shortly after taking office; Senior Warden 1952–53, Master 1953–54.

FAMILY LIVERYMEN *(of HSM)* (gt grandfather) Henry Morley, Master 1870–71; (grandfather) Henry Morley, Senior Warden 1893–94, whose portrait painted by Ida Morley is on the landing; (father) Henry Forster Morley; (son) John Henry Morley; (son) Timothy Rowland Morley; (grandson) Rupert Oliver Henry Morley; (grandson) David Mark Rowland Morley.

HM between 1862–77 donated 175 guineas to the Widows' Fund and 10 guineas to the Distressed Members Fund; **HSM** presented a silver Armada dish in 1962, his miniature portrait and his stained glass Arms panel.

Colonel Frederic (Eric) Guy NEILD, LRCP MRCS, DPH, DIH, MFCM, MFOM

The Arms were designed by Theobald Mathew, Windsor Herald in 1991 and are recorded at the College of Arms in Volume 156, Folio 317.

The stained glass panel was made in 1991, possibly by Messrs Goddard & Gibbs and was installed in window W4-7 in 1991, showing the full Arms and motto without a cartouche.

The colours of the field and bend are the RAMC colours. The parachute and kukris represent his service with a Gurkha parachute battalion and the three arrows are for his three children. Hygeia represents public health and hygiene, and his work as an occupational physician.

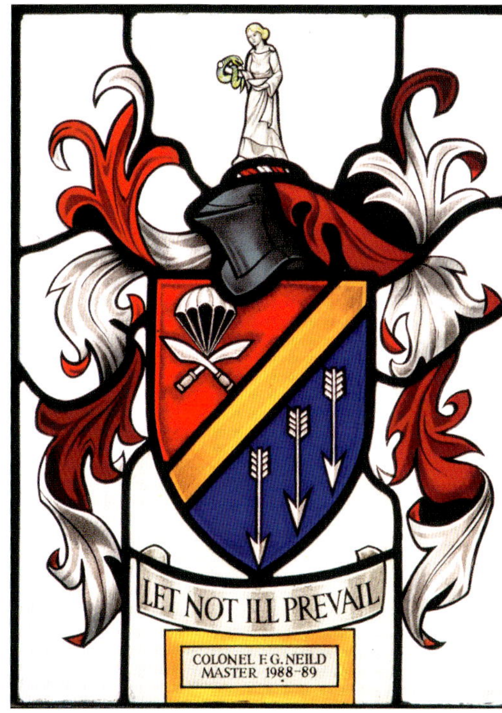

Per bend sinister Gules and Azure, a Bend sinister Or between in chief a Parachute ensigning two crossed Kukris in saltire and in base three Arrows barbs downwards Argent; And for the Crest upon a Helm mantled Gules doubled Argent, on a Wreath of the colours a representation of the Goddess Hygeia proper

Motto: *Let Not Ill Prevail*

BORN Shanghai 1 Jan 1917; *s* of Dr Frederic Miller Neild and Susan Elizabeth Pruen; *m* 1947 Marjorie Hume, one son, two daus; *ob.* 7 Aug 1999.
EDUC St Thomas's Hosp Medical Sch (DIH); U London (DPH).
QUALIFICATIONS LRCP MRCS 1940; DPH 1953; DIH 1954; MFCM 1972; MFOM 1979.
SERVICES RAMC 1941–1971; RMO 50th Indian Parachute Bn 1941–42; RMO 153 Gurkha Parachute Bn 1942–45; HQ Berlin 1949–51; HQ Cyprus 1954–57; seconded Nigerian Army 1960–63; Col 1964.
CAREER Chief Medical Offr UN Peacekeeping Force in Cyprus 1966–67; Dept Health & Safety Executive 1971–81; International Commission on Occupational Health.
SOCIETY Proposed for the Society by Dr John Mennell and Prof Alistair Dudgeon. Yeoman 1954; Liveryman 1958; elected to the Court 1978 *vice* Sir Brian Windeyer. Hon Editor 1979–86. Junior Warden 1986–87, Senior Warden 1987–88, Master 1988–89. Assistant Emeritus 1992.
FAMILY LIVERYMEN (son) Dr Guy Hume Neild; (dau) Assistant Dr Julia Elizabeth Neild (Lady Walport); (dau) Dr Valerie Susan Neild (Mrs C. J. Lamb).
Presented various maps and prints for the Library, the Rhinebeck panel prints, leather covers for the Private Court year books, a set of E Type Eye tests, his miniature portrait and his stained glass Arms panel. He also created, with Past Master Prof Dudgeon, a bound record of the refurbishment of the Hall 1980–87.

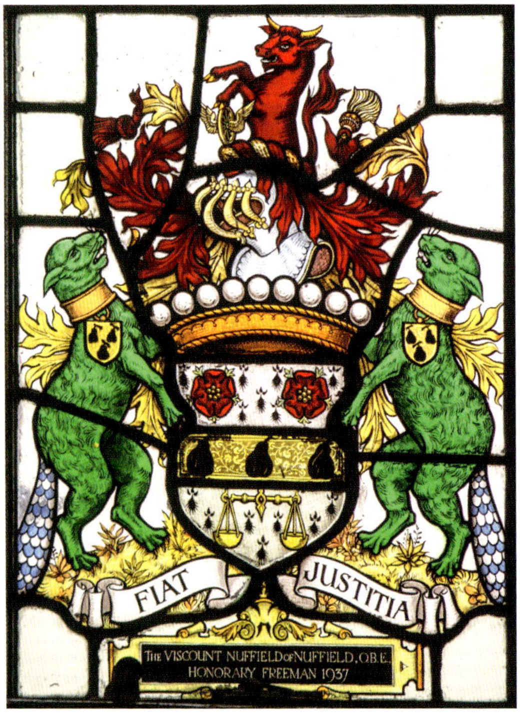
FIAT
JUSTITIA
THE VISCOUNT NUFFIELD OF NUFFIELD, O.B.E.
HONORARY FREEMAN 1937

Ermine, on a fess Or, between in chief two Roses Gules, barbed & seeded proper, and in base a Balance Or, three Pears Sable; And for the Crest upon a peer's Helm, ensigned by the coronet of a Viscount, mantled Gules doubled Or, on a Wreath of the colours, a demi Bull Gules armed and unguled Or resting the sinister Hoof on a Winged Wheel of the last; For supporters on either side a Beaver Vert the tail scaly Argent & Azure gorged with a Collar pendant therefrom an Escutcheon Or charged with three Pears slipped Sable

The stained glass panel was made by James Powell & Sons in 1938 and was installed in window W3-8 in 1938, showing the full Arms, supporters and motto, without a cartouche. From Sep 1941 to Jan 1946, all stained glass was removed from the Hall during hostilities and on return in 1946 these Arms were placed in window W1-8.

The roses probably represent England and the pears are taken from the Arms of the City of Worcester, where Lord Nuffield was born. The scales complement the motto *Fiat Justitia* (*Let justice be done*).

The bull in the crest is taken from the Arms of the City of Oxford, and the winged wheel that it holds represents the motor industry. The beavers are also taken from the Arms of the City of Oxford.

the Rt Hon William Richard MORRIS, Viscount NUFFIELD of Nuffield, Bt, GBE, CH, FRS

The Arms were designed by Alfred Butler, Portcullis Pursuivant, granted in 1929 and are recorded at the College of Arms in Volume Gr 96, Folio 197. On his ennoblement in 1934, Butler, by now Windsor Herald, designed supporters which are recorded in Volume Gr 101, Folio 74.

BORN Worcester Oct 1877; *s* of Frederick Morris and Emily Pether; *m* 1903 Elizabeth Anstey; *no children*; *ob.* 22 Aug 1963

CAREER Chairman Morris Motors Ltd 1910–1952, Director British Motor Corporation 1952. Philanthropist with significant funding to the Sea Cadet Corps, Birmingham University, the Nuffield Foundation, Nuffield College Oxford.

Medical philanthropy:

– 1924 donation of £90,000 to the Radcliffe Infirmary Oxford to develop the Nuffield Maternity Home, a nurses' home, kitchens, operating theatre and wards; this led to the Nuffield Institute for Medical Research in the Radcliffe Observatory.

– 1931 donation of £70,000 to the Wingfield (Morris Orthopaedic) Hospital allowing it to be rebuilt in 1933 to provide new nurses' quarters, seven new wards and a massage department.

– 1937 the first Professor of orthopaedics in Britain appointed as the Nuffield Professor of Orthopaedic Surgery and led to the scheme for the Nuffield Orthopaedic Centre in 1949. The NOC NHS Trust is a main centre for rheumatology and metabolic bone disease.

– Shortly before the war, Lord Nuffield dedicated factory space to manufacturing 'iron lungs' and donated over 5,000 to hospitals in the UK. In the same period, he also financed a new bed block at Guy's Hospital.

– 1936–37 £2 million to establish Oxford's Postgraduate Medical School, followed by £200,000 for the buildings. The medical school became a clinical school for the training of medical students, which is still in existence. His endowments provided three medical chairs, a chair in anaesthetics and later a chair of plastic surgery, a new fifty-bed department for the Nuffield Professor of Clinical Medicine plus adjacent laboratories, and twin theatres and lab space for the Nuffield Professor of Surgery.

– 1939 endowment of £1,200,000 to form the Nuffield Provincial Hospitals Trust, and this led to post-war support in the founding of BUPA and the establishment of the Nuffield Hospitals.

CITY & CIVIC Hon Freeman of the Master Mariners' Company 1941, Hon Freeman of the Grocers' Company 1955.

HONOURS & AWARDS CBE 1918, Baronet 1929, Baron Nuffield 1934, Viscount Nuffield 1938, FRS 1939, GBE 1941, CH 1958.

SOCIETY Elected an Honorary Freeman of the Society in 1937 for his medical philanthropy.

Mr Samuel OSBORN, JP, DL, LSA, FRCS

The stained glass panel was made *c.*1920, probably by W. B. Simpson & Sons, and installed in window W3-14 between 1920 and 1922, showing the shield in Cartouche B. From Sep 1941 to Jan 1946 all stained glass was removed from the Hall during hostilities and on return in 1946 these Arms were placed in window W4-13.

These Arms appear to be a variant of Osborne of Debenham Co Suffolk (*Sable, a Griffin segreant between ten Billets Or*) but no direct connection has been established to this family.[16]

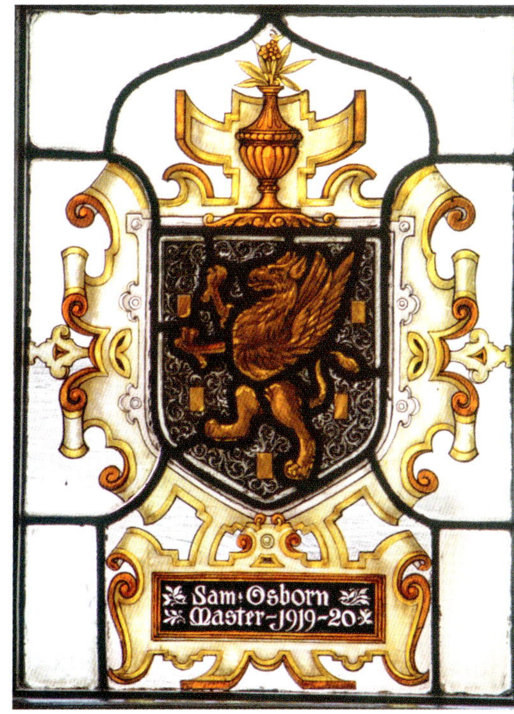

Sable, a Griffin sergreant between five Billets, 2, 2 and 1, Or

Crest (not shown): *upon a Helm on a Wreath of the colours, a Unicorn passant Or, ducally gorged, ringed, lined, armed and crined Sable*

BORN London 15 Apr 1848; *s* of Samuel Osborn FRCS and Matilda Mayhew; *m* 1884 Elizabeth Boyd, one son, one dau; *ob.* 16 Apr 1936.
EDUC St Thomas's Hosp Medical Sch.
QUALIFICATIONS LSA 1870; MRCS Eng 1871; FRCS Eng 1876.
SERVICES Surgeon Royal Naval Artillery Volunteers 1876; Lord Methuen's Column South Africa 1899.
CAREER Surgeon to the Hospital for Women, Soho Square; Surgeon to Surgical Appliance Assoc 1880–1922; Greco-Turkish war 1897; Perm Secy International Red Cross Soc 1901; Surgeon to Red Crescent Balkan War 1912; set up a private hospital in Belgium 1914; Chief Surgeon to the metropolitan corps of the St John Ambulance Brigade.
HON APPTS Society Representative on the General Medical Council 1924–29.
SOCIETY Yeoman 1870; Liveryman 1886; elected to the Court 1908 *vice* John Winter. Junior Warden 1917–18, Senior Warden 1918–19, Master 1919–20.
CITY AND CIVIC Liveryman Haberdashers' Company, Master 1910–11; HM Lieutenant City of London; JP for Buckinghamshire 1893.
HONOURS AND AWARDS Greek Officier de l'Ordre Royal du Sauveur 1897; KStJ 1900; Belgian Croix de Chevalier de l'Ordre de la Couronne 1918; Japanese Royal Red Cross decoration.

In 1898 he gave 10 guineas to the Distressed members' Fund and in 1900 10 guineas to the Widows' Fund. Presented the Standing Salt – a copy of one given to him by the Haberdashers for his Mastership – and the modern Master's jewel.

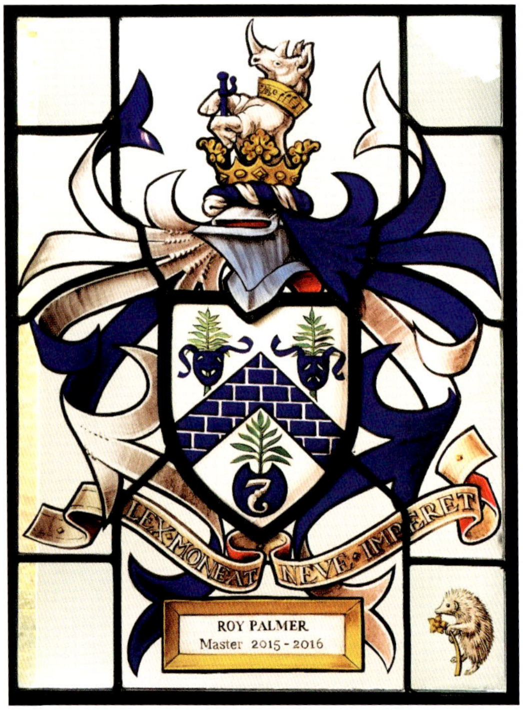

Dr Roy Newberry PALMER, MRCS LRCP, MB BS, DObstRCOG, LLB, FFFLM

The Arms were designed by Thomas Woodcock, Garter King of Arms, in 2011 and are recorded at the College of Arms in Volume Gr 176, Folio 324.

The stained glass panel was made by Leonie Seliger of Canterbury and was installed in window E1-13 in 2016 showing the full Arms and motto without a cartouche.

The bricked chevron from his father's and grandfather's activities, the palms a canting allusion to the surname, the masks reflecting a love of opera and the theatre and the fleam and barber's bowl for the Barbers' Company.

In the crest the crown is a reference to crowner or coroner, the rhinoceros to the Society, the musical notation to reflect a love of music and a musical daughter. The staff is another canting reference.

The motto translates as *Laws are for the guidance of the wise.*

Also shown at the bottom right is Dr Palmer's badge which is a hedgehog holding a cinquefoil flower.

Argent, a Chevron Azure masoned Argent between, in chief two Palm Fronds slipped Vert each surmounted by an untied Mask Azure that on the dexter of comedy and that on the sinister of tragedy and in base a like Palm Frond the stalk surmounted by a Barber's Bowl Azure thereon a Fleam Argent; And for the Crest upon a Helm, mantled Azure doubled Argent, on a wreath of the colours, issuing from a Coronet Or a demi Rhinoceros Argent gorged with a Collar Or thereon bar lines with a base clef and musical notes Sable and supporting between the forelegs a Palmer's Staff Azure

Motto: *Lex Moneat Neve Imperet*

BORN Peterborough 2 Aug 1944; *s* of George Joseph Palmer and Muriel Joyce Clarke; *m* 1967 Celia Mountford, two daus.

EDUC London Hosp Medical Coll (MB BS); U London (LLB); Hon Soc of Middle Temple.

QUALIFICATIONS MRCS LRCP 1967; MB BS 1968; DObstRCOG 1970; LLB 1974; Barrister 1977; FFFLM 2005.

CAREER GP Sawbridgeworth 1970–73; Medical Protection Soc: Asst Secy 1973–85; Dep Secy 1985–89; Secy & Medical Dir 1989–98; Dep Coroner Greater London West 2000–01; Coroner Greater London South 2001–14; Dep Coroner City of London 2002–13, Asst Coroner City of London 2013–d.

HON APPTS President Medico-Legal Soc 2000–02; Governor Expert Witness Inst 2000–06; President British Academy of Forensic Sciences 2009–11; President Medical Soc of London 2012.

SOCIETY Proposed for the Society by the Master, Mr Michael Pugh. Yeoman 1998; Liveryman 2002; Chairman of the Livery Cttee and *ex officio* Court Assistant 2007–09; elected to the Court 2009 *vice* Mrs Enid Taylor. Junior Warden 2013–14, Senior Warden 2014–15, Master 2015–16.

FAMILY LIVERYMEN (wife) Dr Celia Palmer.

CITY AND CIVIC Hon Warden Queen's Chapel of the Savoy 1987–2011; Barbers' Company: Freeman 2008, Liveryman 2012.

HONOURS AND AWARDS Hon FRCPath 2013.

Presented various books for the Library, the electric baby-grand clavinova (with Past Master Dr JC Moore-Gillon), his miniature portrait and his stained glass Arms panel.

Mr Andrew Martin Ingledew PARIS, OStJ, LRCP MRCS, MB BS, DObstRCOG, FRCS

The Arms were designed by Timothy Duke, Chester Herald, in 2009 and are recorded at the College of Arms in Volume Gr 174, Folio 144.

The stained glass panel was made by Richard Scowen of Cornwall in 2010 and was installed in window W1-7 in 2010, showing the full Arms and motto without a cartouche.

The field is for his lifelong predilection with the colour green, the unicorn horns for the Society of Apothecaries, the ostrich feathers for the Royal London Hospital and the martlets for his home county of Sussex.

The fleam on the crest represents surgery and the bee with its sting extended is for his enduring interest in bees and the advantages this has brought him.

The motto translates as *Expertise and timing*.

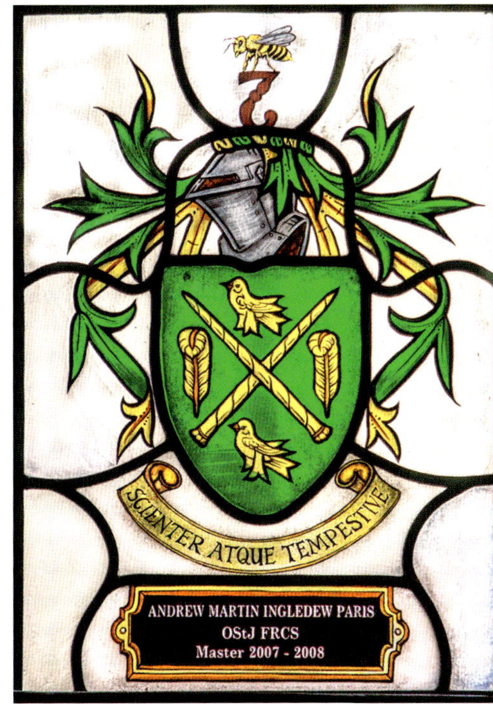

Vert, two Unicorn Horns in saltire between two Martlets in pale and two Quills in fess palewise Or. And for the Crest upon a Helm, mantled Vert doubled Or, on a Wreath of the colours, a Fleam Gules surmounted by a Bee proper

Motto: *Scienter Atque Tempestive*

BORN 27 Nov 1940; *s* of Vernon Patrick Paris and Heather Constance Ingledew Dear; *m* 1975 Susan Jenkins.

EDUC London Hosp Medical Coll (MB BS).

QUALIFICATIONS LRCP MRCS 1964; MB BS 1964; DObstRCOG 1967; FRCS Eng 1971.

CAREER Cons Urological Surgeon Royal London Hosp 1976–2005; Cons Urological Surgeon Barts Hosp 1994–2005; Clin Dir of Surgery & Urology Royal London Hosp then Barts & the London NHS Trust 1979–2002; Emeritus Surgeon the Royal London Hosp and St Bartholomew's Hosp 2005-d; Cons Paed Urolog Surg Newham General Hosp 1979–90; Examiner Dental Surgery RCS 1983–89; Hon Urological Surgeon, Italian Hosp London 1979–90.

HON APPTS Founder Mem St John Ambulance Air Wing, Hon Surgeon 1971–d; Chairman Marie Celeste Samaritan Soc 1996–d.

SOCIETY Proposed for the Society by Past Master Mr AMA Moore. Yeoman 1967; Liveryman 1972; Chairman of the Livery Cttee 1992–94; elected to the Court 1994 *vice* Dr Michael Linnett. Junior Warden 2005–06, Senior Warden 2006–07, Master 2007–08. Past Master Emeritus 2019.

HONOURS AND AWARDS OStJ 1985.

Presented a new frame for Past Master W. F. W. Southwood's miniature, his own miniature portrait and his stained glass Arms panel.

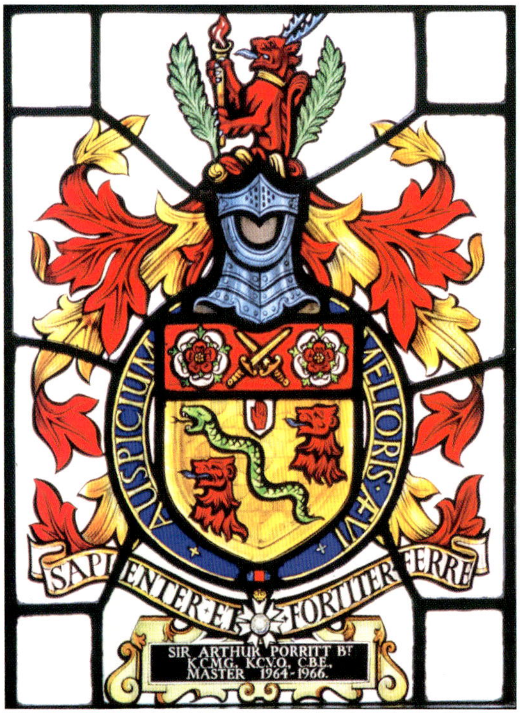

Or, a Serpent in bend Vert between two Lion's heads erased Gules, on a chief of the last two Swords points upwards in saltire of the first between as many Roses Argent both surmounted by another Gules, barbed and seeded proper; And for the Crest upon a Knight's Helm mantled Gules and Or on a Wreath of the colours, a demi-heraldic Antelope Gules, armed Azure, collared Or holding a Torch of the last enflamed proper between two Fern Fronds Vert

Motto: *Sapienter et Fortiter Ferre*

the Rt Hon Arthur Espie Porritt, Baron PORRITT of Wanganui and Hampstead, Bt, GCMG, GCVO, KStJ, CBE, MA, MCh, FRCS

The Arms were designed by Sir John Heaton-Armstrong, Chester Herald, in 1951 and are recorded at the College of Arms in Volume 113, Folio 223.

The stained glass panel was made by Carl Edwards *c.*1967 and was installed in window W4-14 *c.*1967, showing the full Arms surrounded by the insignia of the Most Distinguished Order of St Michael and St George and motto without a cartouche.

In 1970 as a Knight Grand Cross he was granted supporters by Sir Anthony Wagner, Garter King of Arms (recorded in Volume 113, Folio 314), viz. an Eagle proper (dexter) and a Tui Bird proper (Sinister) and from 1973 he would be entitled to a peer's helm.

The motto translates as *To bear bravely and wisely.*

BORN Wanganui 10 Aug 1900; *s* of Ernest Edward Porritt FRCS and Ivy Elizabeth Mackenzie; *m* 1st 1926, Mary Frances Wynne *diss* 1946, *m* 2nd 1946 Kathleen (Kay) Peck, two sons, one dau; *ob.* 1 Jan 1994.

EDUC Otago Medical Sch; Rhodes Scholar Magdalen Coll Oxford (BA, MA, BM BCh, MCh); St Mary's Hosp Medical Sch.

QUALIFICATIONS BA 1926; MRCS LRCP 1928; BM BCh 1928; FRCS Eng 1930; MA 1932; MCh 1932.

SERVICES RAMC 1940–45, temp Lt Col 1943, acting Col 1943, local Brigadier 1943–45, Lt Col 1945; RAMC(V) 1945–56; Cons Surgeon to the Army.

CAREER New Zealand Olympic Team 1924 (Bronze Medal) and 1928 (Captain); Surgeon St Mary's Hosp, Hosp of St John & St Elizabeth, King Edward VII Hosp for Officers, Royal Masonic Hosp; Surgeon in Ordinary to the Duke of York's Household; Surgeon to King George VI 1946–52; Hon Col 57 (Middlesex) Gen Hosp 1950–56; Serjeant Surgeon to The Queen 1952–67; Governor General of New Zealand 1967–72.

HON APPTS President RCS 1960–63; President BMA 1960–61; President RSM 1966–67.

SOCIETY Yeoman 1938; Liveryman 1944; elected to the Court 1954 *vice* Frank Dutch Howitt. Examination Cttee 1955. Junior Warden 1963 becoming Senior Warden 1963–64 on the death of Lord Evans on 26 Oct 1963, Master 1964–65 and 1965–66. As Immediate Past Master, he resumed the Mastership on the death of the Master, Alan Brews on 25 Dec 1965 and completed the year to August, 1966. He resigned from the Court in 1969.

FAMILY LIVERYMEN (son) Sir Jonathan Porritt Bt.

HONOURS AND AWARDS OBE 1943; CBE 1945; USA Legion of Merit 1947; Hon LLD U St Andrews; Hon LLD U Otago; Hon LLD U Birmingham; Hon DSc U Oxford; Hon MD U Bristol; Hon FRCS Edin; Hon FRCS Glas; Hon FRCSI; Hon FRACS; Hon FACS; KCMG 1950; KCVO 1957; Bart 1963; KStJ 1957; GCMG 1967; GCVO 1970; Life Barony 1973.

Mr Michael Arthur PUGH, AE, MB BS, FRCS, FRCOG

The Arms were designed by Hubert Chessyre, Norroy and Ulster King of Arms, in 1997 and are recorded at the College of Arms in Volume 164, Folio 204.

The stained glass panel in a modern style was made by Stella Timmins of London in 1997 and was installed in window W4-4 in 1997, showing the full Arms and motto without a cartouche.

The division of the field echoes the Arms of St Bartholomew's Hospital and the colours are from the Middlesex Hospital and the City of Manchester. The seaxes are also from the Middlesex and possibly also allude to surgery. The lozenge in heraldry represents ladies and refers to obstetrics and gynaecology, with barry wavy for the spring of eternal youth.

The dragon is for Wales and the red also suggests Lancaster and the City of London. The lion alludes to Westminster Abbey. The cross ansata is also from the Middlesex Hospital.

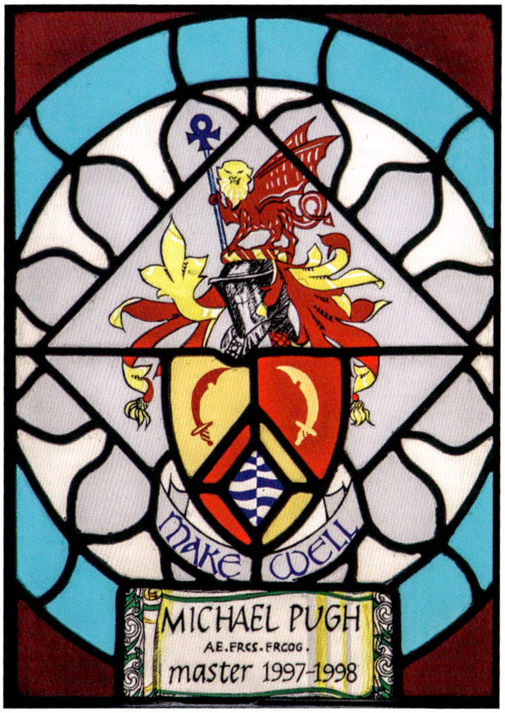

Per pale and per chevron Or and Gules in chief two Seaxes hilts downwards Blades curving inwards counterchanged, in base a Lozenge barry wavy Argent and Azure counter-changed; And for the Crest upon a helm mantled Gules doubled Or, on a wreath of the colours, a Dragon passant also Gules with a Lion's Head guardant Or and supporting with the dexter Foreclaws a Rod terminating in a Cross ansata Azure

Motto: *Make Well*

BORN Manchester, 6 Oct 1929; *s* of Arthur Pugh and Norah Rees; m 1965 Jennifer Murray, one son, one dau; ob. 10 June 2018.

EDUC St Bartholomew's Hosp Medical Coll (MB BS).

QUALIFICATIONS MB BS 1953; MRCOG 1959; FRCS Eng 1962; FRCOG 1971.

SERVICES RAF Medical Branch, Flight Lt 1954–56, Royal Auxiliary Air Force, Sqn Ldr 1957–65.

CAREER Consultant Gynaecologist and Obstetrician Whittington Hosp, United Hosp, Elizabeth Garrett Anderson Hosp for Women and Middlesex and University Coll Hosps; Consultant Obstetrician Royal Northern Hospital; examiner for U London, Royal Coll O and G, Conjoint Board.

HON APPTS President Medical Society of London; Medical Protection Society Council.

SOCIETY Proposed for the Society by Morris Sheridan and Robin Venn. Yeoman 1969; Liveryman 1974; LMSSA Examiner 1978–85; elected to the Court 1987 *vice* Mr Guy Blackburn. Examinations Cttee 1987–2004, Sustentation Cttee (Chairman 2000) 1995–2004. Junior Warden 1995–96, Senior Warden 1996–97, Master 1997–98. United Examining Board 1997–97; Christ's Hospital Donation Governor 2000–04; Past Master Emeritus 2004.

FAMILY LIVERYMEN (wife) Dr Jennifer Leslie Pugh; (dau) Dr Emma Caroline Pugh.

HONOURS AND AWARDS AE.

Presented various books for the Library, fourteen pepper mills for use at dinners, the painting of an Apothecary's Rose, the Axminster blue-patterned carpet in the Cloakroom, his miniature portrait, his stained glass Arms panel and the quater-centennial Loving Cup in memory of his wife Jennifer.

the Rt Hon John Samuel Richardson, Baron RICHARDSON of Lee, Bt, LVO, CStJ, MA, MB BChir, MD, FRCP, FRCP Ed

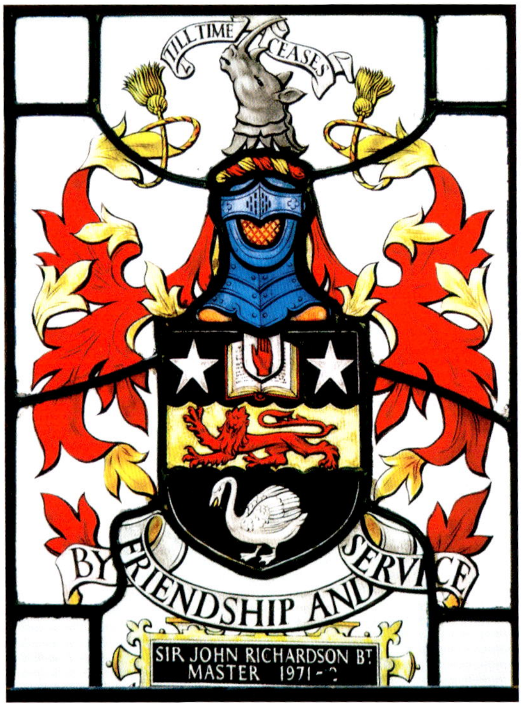

The scroll behind the crest, *'Til time ceases,* is the response to the Society's toast.

Sable, on a Fess engrailed Or, between in chief an Open Book proper, bound Gules edged Or between two Mullets and in base a Swan Argent, a Lion passant guardant also Gules; And for the Crest upon a Knight's Helm, mantled Gules doubled Or, on a Wreath of the colours, the Head of a Rhinoceros erased Sable, behind the head a scroll Argent inscribed with the words 'Till Times Ceases' in letters Gules

Motto: *By Friendship and Service*

The Arms were designed by Colin Cole, Portcullis Pursuivant, in 1960 and are recorded at the College of Arms in Volume Gr 123, Folio 198. As he had no sons, the grant was made to the descendants of his father John Watson Richardson deceased.

The stained glass panel was made by Carl Edwards in 1975 and was installed in window E1-8 in 1975, showing the full Arms and motto without a cartouche.

Following elevation to the peerage a further design by Sir Colin Cole, now Garter King of Arms, was granted in 1980 and recorded in Volume 43, Folio 101, viz. two supporters were added: two horses reguardant, the dexter a grey with saddlecloth of the Metropolitan Police Force, the sinister also a grey with the saddlecloth of the Royal Army Medical Corps, both saddled bridled with headstall, horsehair plume and breast girth, all with silver buckles and bosses proper.

BORN Sheffield 16 Jun 1910; *s* of John Watson Richardson and Elizabeth Blakeney Roberts; *m* 1933 Sybil Angela Stephanie Trist, two daus; *ob.* 15 Aug 2004.

EDUC Trinity Coll Cambridge (MA, MB BChir); St Thomas's Hosp Medical Sch.

QUALIFICATIONS MB BChir 1936; MRCP 1937; MA 1940; MD 1940; FRCP Lond 1948; FRCP Edin 1975.

SERVICES RAMC Temp Major 1939, Temp Lt Col 1942; Consultant Emeritus to the Army.

CAREER Consulting Physician St Thomas' Hosp 1947–75; King Edward VII Hosp for Officers; Cons Physician Metropolitan Police 1957–80; Examiner Us Cambridge, London, Manchester, NUI, RCP Lond & Edin, Conjoint Board; Chairman Joint Consultants Cttee 1967–72; consultant to Hon Freeman Harold MacMillan.

HON APPTS Royal Society of Medicine: Hon Librarian 1957–63, President 1969–71; Vice Pres Medical Soc London 1961–63; President Internat Soc Internal Medicine 1966–70; President British Medical Association 1970–71; President General Medical Council 1973–80.

SOCIETY Yeoman 1949; Liveryman 1953; elected to the Court 1960 *vice* Sir Wilson Jamieson. Junior Warden 1969–70, Senior Warden 1970–71, Master 1971–72. Assistant Emeritus 1985.

CITY AND CIVIC Hon Bencher Gray's Inn 1974.

HONOURS AND AWARDS MVO 4th class (now LVO) 1943; Kt Bachelor 1960; Baronet 1963; CStJ 1970; Hon FPS 1974; Hon FRCPI 1975; Hon DSc NUI 1975; Hon FFCM 1977; Life Peerage 1979; Hon Fellow Trinity Coll Cambridge 1979; Hon FRCPsych 1979; Hon FRCS Eng 1980; Hon FRCPS Glas 1980; Hon DCL U Newcastle 1980; Hon FRCP Edin 1981; Hon LLD U Nottingham 1981; Hon DSc U Hull 1981; Hon LLD U Liverpool 1983.

Presented various books for the Library, a large albarello, the oak bible box dated 1626, a large silver tray with his and the Society's Arms engraved, a leech jar, his miniature portrait and his stained glass Arms panel.

Mr William Stewart SHAND, MA, LRCP MRCS, MB BChir, MD, FRCS, FRCS Ed

The Arms were designed by Henry Paston-Bedingfeld, York Herald, in 2007 and are recorded at the College of Arms in Volume 172, Folio 12.

The stained glass panel was made by Richard Scowen of Cornwall and was installed in window W2-9 in 2007, showing the full Arms and motto without a cartouche.

The name Shand is associated with a number of armorial bearings recorded in Lord Lyon's office, most of which are a variant of *Azure a boar's head couped Argent with three mullets on the chief and a dove for crest.*

The boar passant represents a significant variation together with the three fleurs-de-lys for Mrs Caroline Shand whose father was French.

The fleams on the crest indicate the profession of surgery and the connection with the Barbers' Company.

The motto translates as *With valour my leader and good fortune my companion.*

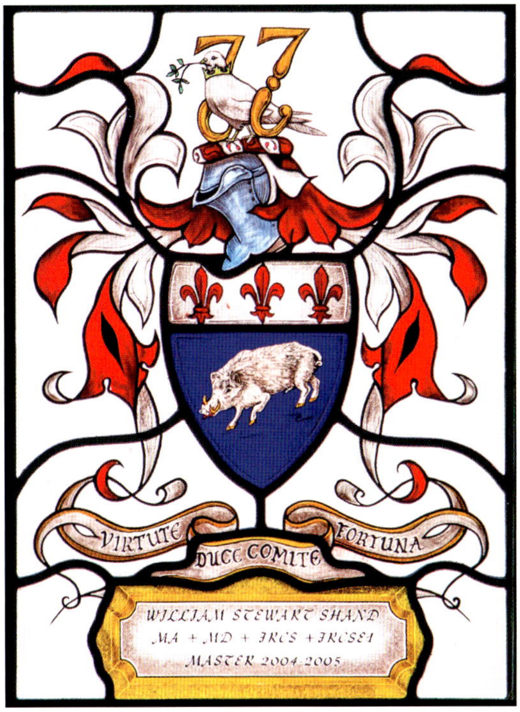

Azure, a Boar passant, on a Chief Argent three Fleurs-de-Lys Gules; And for the Crest upon a Helm mantled Gules doubled Argent, on a Wreath of the colours, a Dove Argent gorged with an ancient Crown Or, holding in the Beak a Sprig of Olive proper, all between two Fleams Or

Motto: *Virtute Duce Comite Fortuna*

BORN Derby 12 Oct 1936; *s* of William Paterson Shand and Annabella Kirkland Stewart Waddell; *m* 1972 Anne Caroline Dashwood Mansell (née Charvet), two sons, one step-son, two step-daus.

EDUC St John's Coll Cambridge (BA, MA, MB BChir, MD); St Bartholomew's Hosp Medical Coll.

QUALIFICATIONS BA 1958 MA 1962; LRCP MRCS 1962; MB BChir 1962; MD 1970; FRCS Eng 1970; FRCS Edin 1970.

CAREER Cons Surgeon St Bartholomew's, Hackney and Homerton Hosps 1973–96; King Edward VII Hosp for Officers 1995–97; Hon Cons Surgeon St Luke's Hosp for the Clergy 1982–97; Court of Exrs RCS Eng 1985–91; Visiting Cons Surg St Mark's Hosp for the Diseases of the Colon & Rectum 1986–96; Board of Exrs RCS Edin 1986–96; Exr U London 1990–96; U Liverpool 1991–96; Hon Consulting Surgeon Barts and the Royal London Hosps 1997–d.

SOCIETY Proposed for the Society by Mr John Chalstrey and Past Master Henry Thompson. Yeoman 1975; Liveryman 1979; elected to the Court 1990 *vice* Ian McGilchrist Jackson. Soc Rep Brit Postgrad Med Fed 1991–96. Junior Warden 2002–03, Senior Warden 2003–04, Master 2004–05. Monckton Copeman Lecturer 2005; Past Master Emeritus 2016.

CITY AND CIVIC Company of Barbers: Freeman 1980, Liveryman 1981, Court of Assistants 1992, Master 2001–02: Governor Sutton's Hosp in Charterhouse 1989–2009. Presented framed certificates of Joseph Dalton LSA, his miniature portrait and his stained glass Arms panel.

Dr Hugh Macdonald SINCLAIR, MA, BSc, LMSSA, BM BCh, FRCP

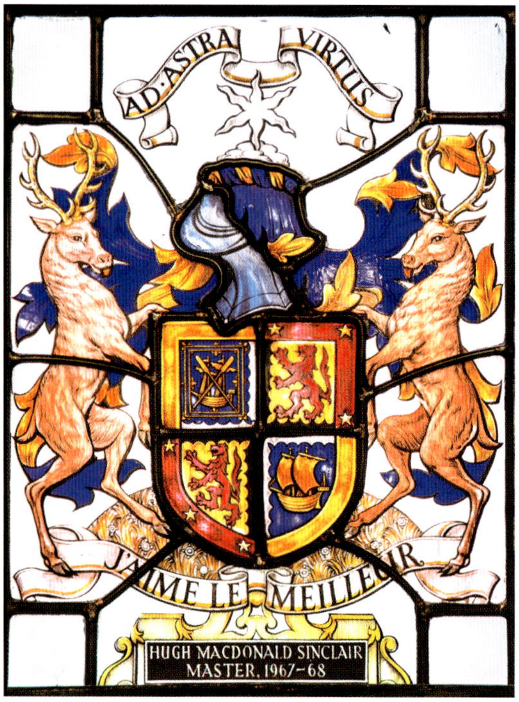

Quarterly – 1st: Azure, a ship at anchor her oars erect in saltire within the royal tressure Or (Earldom of Orkney); 2nd & 3rd: Or a lion rampant Gules (Spar-Nithsdale); 4th: Azure a ship under sail Or (Earldom of Caithness): overall dividing the quarters, a cross engrailed quarterly Argent and Sable (Sinclair), all within a bordure quartered Or and Gules, the last charged with three stars of the first; And for a Crest upon a helm, mantled Azure and Or, on a wreath of the colours, a star of six points waved Argent; for supporters on either side a red deer proper

Mottoes: *Ad Astra Virtus* and *J'Aime le Meilleur*

The Arms, including supporters, were granted by Lord Lyon in 1778 to John Sinclair of Ulbster and recorded at the College of Arms in Volume Scot II, Folio 183 on the grant of his GB baronetcy in 1786. These Arms are now borne by Viscount Thurso.

The stained glass panel was made by Carl Edwards and was installed in window E2-8 *c.*1972, showing the full Arms, supporters and two mottoes without a cartouche.

The Sinclairs of Ulbster descend from the 4th earl of Caithness (4th quarter) whose ancestor was forced by King James III in 1470 to resign the earldom of Orkney (1st quarter) for Caithness. The 2nd and 3rd quarters refer to the 1st earl of Caithness' claim to Nithsdale (also given up in 1470) in right of his Douglas mother. The border represents a minor cadet branch and the red portion with the stars refers to intermarriage with the earls of Sutherland. The almost invisible overall cross is for the name of Sinclair which, interestingly, the main line earls of Caithness and lords Sinclair bear as a pure black cross but the lesser cadets use silver and black.

The mottoes translate as *Virtue knows no bounds* and *I love the best.*

BORN Edinburgh 4 Feb 1910; s of Col Hugh Montgomerie Sinclair and Rosalie Sybil Jackson; *unmarried*; *ob.* 22 Jun 1990.

EDUC Oriel Coll Oxford (BSc, MA, BM BCh, DM); University Coll Hosp Medical Sch.

QUALIFICATIONS BSc 1932; LMSSA 1936; BM BCh 1936; MA 1936; DM 1939; MRCP Lond 1953; FRCP Lond 1964.

CAREER Tutor in Physiology and Biochemistry Magdalen Coll, Oxford 1937–47; Director of the Oxford Nutrition Survey 1940–46; Reader in Human Nutrition and Director of the Laboratories U Oxford 1951–58; Fellow and Lecturer in Physiology and Biochemistry Magdalen Coll Oxford 1956–58; Lecturer in Biological Sciences U Oxford 1968.

SOCIETY Yeoman 1937; Liveryman 1939; elected to the Court 1957 *vice* John Oglethorpe Wakelin Barratt. Sydenham Lecturer 1966. Junior Warden 1965–66, Senior Warden 1966–67, Master 1967–68. Assistant Emeritus 1985.

HONOURS AND AWARDS Dutch Chevalier of the Order of Orange-Nassau 1945; USA Presidential Medal of Freedom with Silver Palm 1946; Hon DSc Baldwin-Wallace Coll 1968.

Presented eleven silver goblets to commemorate the Society's 350th Anniversary and his stained glass Arms panel. He also left a bequest of £500.

Further note on the Arms: Under English heraldic law, Dr Sinclair is entitled to bear these Arms as a legitimate male descendant of the grantee and, although Scottish in origin, these Arms were recorded at the English College of Arms in 1786. There is no authority for the retention of the Supporters, however (cf. Mackworth-Young *supra*).

Mr William Frederick Walter SOUTHWOOD, MA, MD, MChir, FRCS

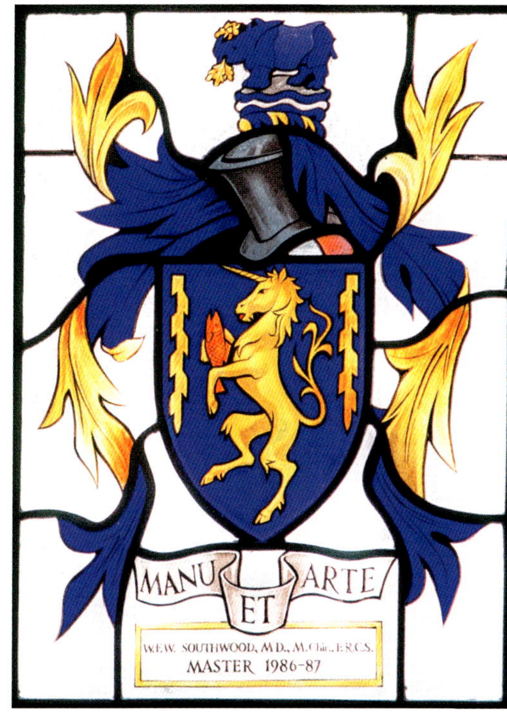

The Arms were designed by Conrad Swan, York Herald, in 1990 and are recorded at the College of Arms in Volume 155, Folio 243.

The stained glass panel-maker is unknown but was possibly Messrs Goddard & Gibbs. The panel was installed in window W3-12 in 1991, showing the full Arms and motto without a cartouche.

The colours of blue and gold are for the Society.

The unicorn and rhinoceros are also derived from the Society's Arms. The posts are a canting allusion to his name and the salmon refers to his interest in fishing. The water barry wavy refers to the sea at Holderness and the fructed oak to his children.

The motto translates as *By hand and dexterity.*

BORN London 8 Jun 1925; *s* of Stuart Walter Southwood BDS and Mildred Mary Southwood; *m* 1965 Margaret Holderness, two sons; *ob.* 27 Apr 2002.

EDUC Trinity Coll Cambridge (BA, MB BChir, MChir, MD); Guy's Hosp Medical Sch.

QUALIFICATIONS BA 1946; MRCS 1948; MB BChir 1948; MA 1951; FRCS Eng 1954; MChir 1956; MD 1964.

SERVICES National Service RAMC 1949–51; Lieut 1949, Captain 1950; RAMC(V).

CAREER Cons Surgeon Bath Health District 1966–90.

HON APPTS Professional & Linguistic Assessment Board 1976–83, Vice Chairman 1983, Chairman 1984–87.

SOCIETY Proposed for the Society by Guy Blackburn (Master 1980–81). Yeoman 1950; Liveryman 1954; elected to the Court 1974 *vice* PMF Bishop. Chairman Examinations Cttee 1981–85. Junior Warden 1984–85, Senior Warden 1985–86, Master 1986–87. Hon Treasurer 1989–99; Assistant Emeritus 1999; Hon Freeman 2000.

CITY AND CIVIC Gunmakers' Company: Liveryman 1989.

Presented various books for the Library, the photo reproduction of Anne of Denmark, a silver rhinoceros 6¼" x 3", a silver butter dish, his miniature portrait, his stained glass Arms panel and £5,000 for the rhinoceros Court crockery.

Azure, between two Posts raguly palewise each pointed at its lower end a Unicorn rampant Or holding with the forelegs a Salmon Gules; And for the Crest upon a Helm, mantled Azure doubled Or, on a Wreath of the colours, upon a Rock proper arising from Water barry wavy Azure and Argent a Rhinoceros statant also Azure with in the Mouth a Sprig of Oak leaved and fructed of an Acorn pendant Or

Motto: *Manu et Arte*

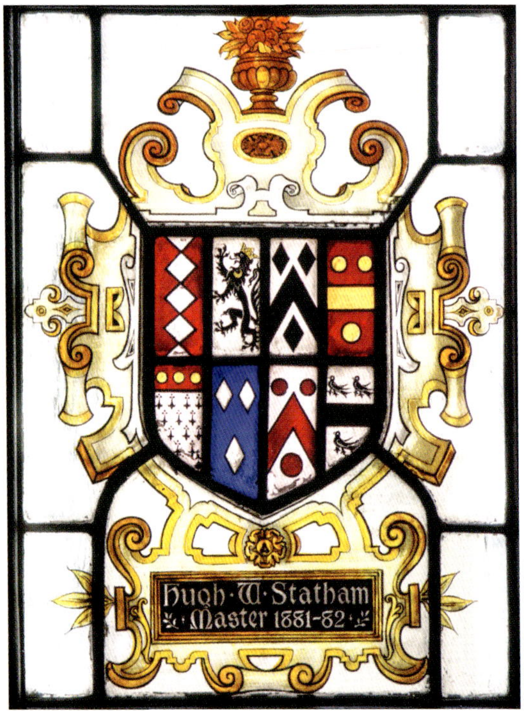

Quarterly of eight: 1. Gules a Pale fussily Argent (Statham); 2. Argent a Lion rampant Sable crowned & charged on the Shoulder with a Crescent Or (Morley); 3. Argent a Chevron between three Lozenges Sable (Mascy); 4. Gules a Fess Or between three Bezants (de la Lande); 5. Ermine on a Chief Gules three Bezants (Okeover); 6. Azure three Lozenges Argent (Freeman); 7. Argent a Chevron between three Roundels Gules (Sherard); 8. Argent a Fess between three Martlets Sable (Briggs)

Crest (not shown): *Upon a Helm on a Wreath of the colours an armoured Arm embowed holding a Sword Argent*

Dr Hugh Worthington STATHAM, LSA, MRCS

This stained glass panel was given by his granddaughter Miss Barbara Gardiner in 1938 but these Arms are not recorded at the College of Arms.

The Arms represent the families of Statham,[17] Morley, Mascy, de la Lande, Okeover, Freeman, Sherard and Briggs. In the fourteenth century, Sir Ralph Statham of Morley married Goditha de Mascy, heiress of her father, and also a co-heiress of Morley, de la Lande & Okeover on her mother's side. In 1744 Samuel Statham married Susannah Freeman whose mother was the Sherard heiress. The relationship to Briggs is not clear.

The stained glass panel was made by James Powell & Sons in 1938 and was installed in window W4-10 or 14 in 1938, showing the shield in Cartouche A. From Sep 1941 to Jan 1946, all stained glass was removed from the Hall during hostilities and on return in 1946 these Arms were placed in window W1-13.

BORN 12 Jan 1809; *s* of Edwyn Statham and Sophia Hall; *m* 1st 1826 Eliza Clarke, one dau; *m* 2nd 1847 Harriet Russell, one dau; *ob.* 16 Jan 1892.

EDUC St Thomas's Hosp Medical Sch.

QUALIFICATIONS LSA 1830; MRCS 1831.

CAREER Partnership with John Keal in Russell Square until 1860; Medical Attendant Foundling Hosp.

SOCIETY Apprenticed to Richard Clewin Griffith 1823; Yeoman 1830; Liveryman 1860; elected to the Court 1874. Junior Warden 1879–80, Senior Warden 1880–81, Master 1881–82.

FAMILY LIVERYMEN (nephew) Reginald Whiteside Statham, Master 1927–28.

In 1872 he donated 10 guineas to the Widows' Fund and in 1882 10 guineas to the Distressed Members' Fund.

Dr Reginald Whiteside STATHAM JP, LSA, MRCS

The stained glass panel was given by his widow but these Arms are not recorded at the College of Arms.

The Arms represent the families of Statham,[18] Morley, Mascy, de la Lande, Okeover, Freeman, Sherard and Briggs. In the fourteenth-century, Sir Ralph Statham of Morley married Goditha de Mascy, heiress of her father, and also a co-heiress of Morley, de la Lande and Okeover on her mother's side. In 1744 Samuel Statham married Susannah Freeman whose mother was the Sherard heiress. The relationship to Briggs is not clear.

The stained glass panel was made by James Powell & Sons in 1938 and was installed in window W4-10 or 14 in 1938, showing the shield in Cartouche A. From Sep 1941 to Jan 1946, all stained glass was removed from the Hall during hostilities and on return in 1946 these Arms were placed in window W1-15.

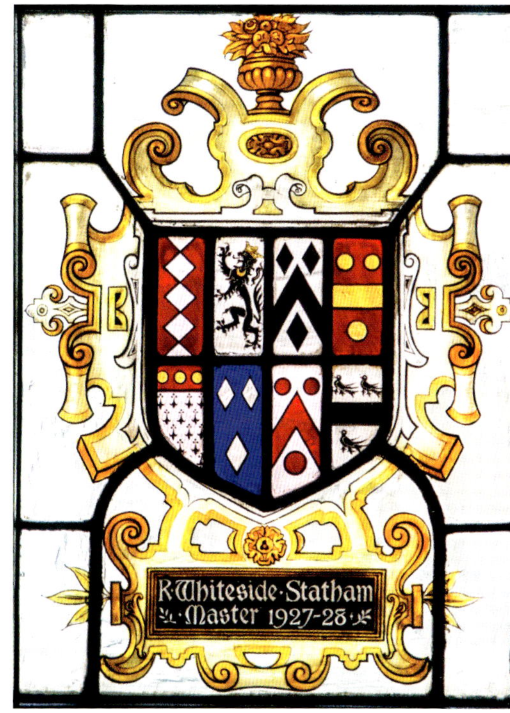

BORN 1861; *s* of Francis Statham and Jane Kingdon; *m* 1887 Nessy Gill, *no children*; *ob.* 30 Jun 1934.
EDUC St Thomas's Hosp Medical Sch.
QUALIFICATIONS LSA 1882; MRCS 1882.
SERVICES Lieut RAMC 1915–?
CAREER GP Cheddar (for 52 years); Medical Offr & Public Vacc No 8 District Axbridge; Medical Offr St Michael's Home for Tuberculosis Axbridge.
SOCIETY Yeoman 1885; Liveryman 1891; elected to the Court 1921 *vice* Dr George Wilks. Examinations Cttee 1924–29. Junior Warden 1925–26, Senior Warden 1926–27, Master 1927–28.
FAMILY LIVERYMEN (uncle) Hugh Worthington Statham, Master 1881–82.
CITY AND CIVIC JP (1922–33); Deputy Coroner for North Somerset (1903–13). Between 1925–27 he donated 10 guineas to the Widows' Fund.

Quarterly of eight: 1. Gules a Pale fussily Argent (Statham); 2. Argent a Lion rampant Sable crowned & charged on the Shoulder with a Crescent Or (Morley); 3. Argent a Chevron between three Lozenges Sable (Mascy); 4. Gules a Fess Or between three Bezants (de la Lande); 5. Ermine on a Chief Gules three Bezants (Okeover); 6. Azure three Lozenges Argent (Freeman); 7. Argent a Chevron between three Roundels Gules (Sherard); 8. Argent a Fess between three Martlets Sable (Briggs)

Crest (not shown): *Upon a Helm on a Wreath of the colours an armoured Arm embowed holding a Sword Argent*

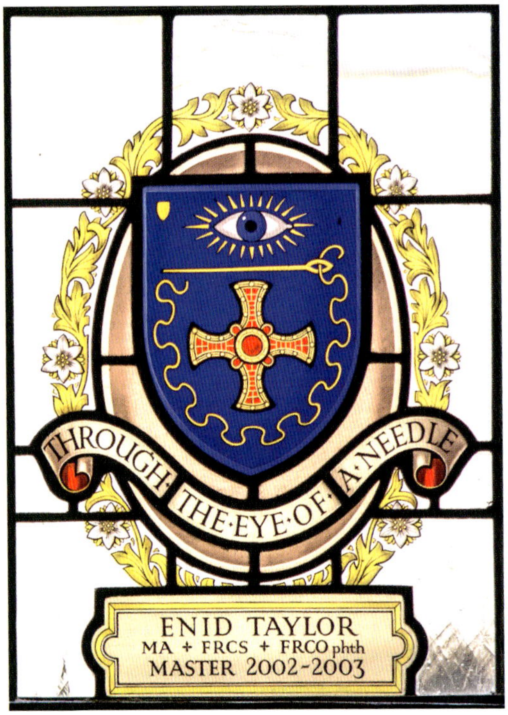

Azure, St Cuthbert's Cross proper within a Thread nebuly enfiling a Needle fesswise in chief point to the dexter Or, the whole ensigned by a Blue Eye proper irradiated Or

Motto: *Through the Eye of a Needle*

Mrs Enid TAYLOR, MA, MB BChir, FRCS, DO, FRCOphth

The Arms were designed by David White, Somerset Herald, in 2004 and are recorded at the College of Arms in Volume Gr 170, Folio 277.

The stained glass panel was made by Messrs Goddard & Gibbs of London and was installed in window W1-9 in 2006, showing a lady's Arms and motto, without a cartouche.

The eye represents ophthalmology and St Cuthbert alludes to origins in County Durham. The needle and thread represents an interest in needlework but also to surgery.

The golden escutcheon indicates the Arms of a married woman. The oval floral surround is not part of the Arms and merely inserted as decoration possibly to give more depth with the lack of helm and mantling.

BORN 8 Jun 1933; *d* of Joseph William and Jane Wheldon; *m* 1959 Thomas Taylor, two sons; *ob.* 9 Apr 2020.

EDUC Girton Coll Cambridge (MA, MB BChir); London Hosp Medical Coll.

QUALIFICATIONS MA; MB BChir 1963; DO 1963; FRCS Eng 1965; FRCOphth 1988.

CAREER Cons Ophthalmic Surgeon Elizabeth Garrett Anderson Hosp 1966–73, Cons Ophthalmic Surgeon North Middx Hosp 1974–98.

HON APPTS Chairman N. E. Thames Ophthalmic Adv Cttee DHSS 1979–86.

SOCIETY Proposed for the Society by Past Master Dr Dinty Moore. Yeoman 1969; Liveryman 1973; elected to the Court 1988 *vice* Prof Norman Ashton. Junior Warden 2000–01, Senior Warden 2001–02, Master 2002–03. Past Master Emeritus 2008.

The first lady to serve on the Court and the first Lady Master.

FAMILY LIVERYMEN (husband) Thomas Henry Taylor, (son) Hugo Wheldon Taylor, (son) Simon Wheldon Taylor.

Embroidered the lectern Arms banner in 1987 and presented the box to keep them in, books for the library, her miniature portrait and her stained glass Arms panel.

Professor Rodney Hemingfield TAYLOR, LRCP MRCS, MB BS, MD, FRCP, MA, DHMSA, DPMSA, FRSPH, MBA

The Arms were designed by Timothy Duke, Chester Herald, in 2012 and are recorded at the College of Arms in Volume Gr 175, Folio 206.

The stained glass panel was made by Richard Scowen of Cornwall in 2013 and was installed in window W1-3 in 2013, showing the full Arms and motto without a cartouche.

The field is divided per fess wavy to represent the surface of the sea, with the sky above. The demi sealions are a marine allusion symbolising dauntless courage at sea. In base are three escallops standing for the church of St James, Hampton Hill, and representing pilgrims.

The crest, a sealion with a naval crown on its head, refers to service in the Royal Navy.

The colours of blue and gold and the unicorn horn are associated with the Society and therefore medicine.

The lyre was originally the attribute of the Greek god Apollo and is a clear symbol representing music.

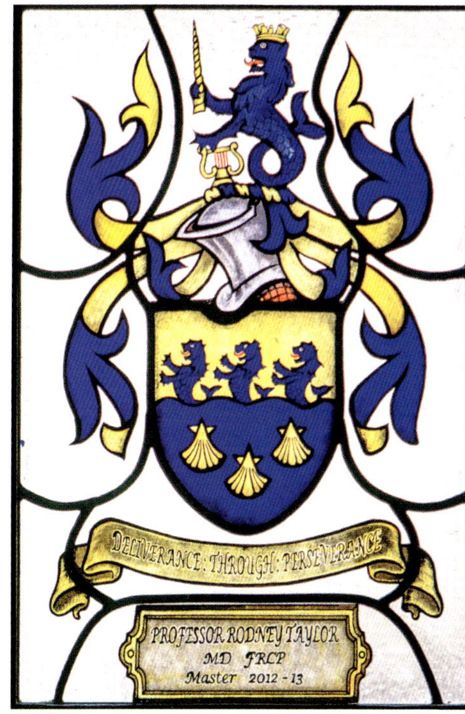

Per fess wavy Or and Azure, three Demi Sealions and in base three Escallops counterchanged. And for the Crest upon a Helm, mantled Azure doubled Or, on a Wreath of the colours, a Sealion Azure crowned with a Naval Crown, holding in the dexter Paw a Unicorn's Horn erect and in the sinister Paw a Lyre Or

Motto: *Deliverance Through Perseverence*

BORN London, 21 Dec 1942; *s* of Dr Alan Taylor and Margaret Paine; *m* 1st 1965 Jean Williams *diss* 1972; *m* 2nd 1972 Janet Baldwin, one son, two daus; *ob.* 3 May 2017.

EDUC U of Bristol (BSc Psychol); University Coll Hosp Medical Sch (MB BS, MD); Open U (MBA); U Surrey (MA Bioethics).

QUALIFICATIONS BSc 1965; LRCP MRCS 1972: MB BS 1972; MRCP UK 1976; MD 1984; FRCP Lond 1987; DHMSA 1992; DPMSA 1994; MBA 1996; FRSPH 2001; MA 2008.

SERVICES Surg Cdr RNR 1977–86; Surg Capt RN 1986–2002.

CAREER Hon Cons Gastroenterologist Central Middx 1980–84; Professor of Naval Medicine 1988–94; Medical Director RNH Haslar 1997–2001; Assoc Postgraduate Medical Dean Royal Defence Med Coll 1997–2001; Cons Physician & Gastroenterologist Ealing Hosp 2001–07; Tutor in Med Ethics & Law ICSM 2007–17; Visiting Prof School of Theology, Philosophy & History St Mary's U Coll, Twickenham 2009–17.

SOCIETY Proposed for the Society by Past Master David Hughes. Osler Lecturer 1994; Yeoman 1997; Liveryman 2001; Gideon de Laune Lecturer 2004; President Faculty of History & Philosophy of Medicine 2004–08; elected to the Court 2006 *vice* Sir John Chalstrey. Junior Warden 2010–11, Senior Warden 2011–12, Master 2012–13.

FAMILY LIVERYMEN (wife) Dr Janet Baldwin (Mrs R. H. Taylor).

CITY AND CIVIC Company of Barbers: Freeman 2006; Liveryman 2008; Wandsman St Paul's Cathedral 2010–17.

Presented cushions for the Courtyard benches, his miniature portrait and his stained glass Arms panel.

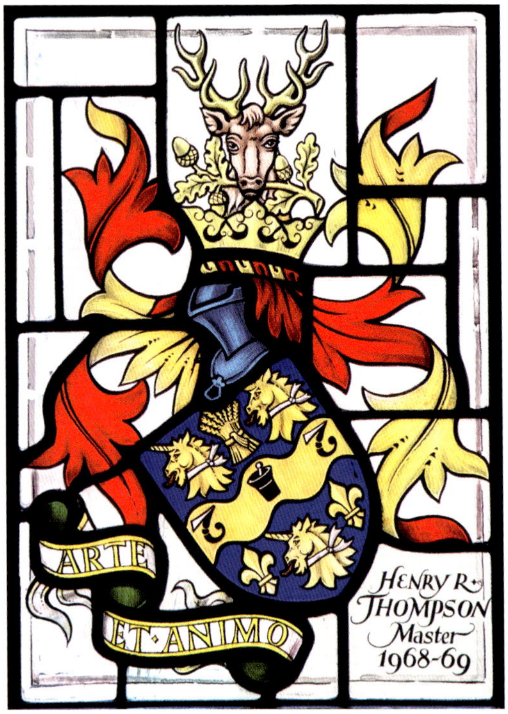

Azure, on a Fess wavy, between in chief a Garb and two Unicorn's Heads erased Or, each gorged with a Ribband Argent, and in base a like Unicorn's Head and two Fleurs-de-Lys Or, a Pestle Argent in a Mortar Sable between two Fleams also Sable their Blades Argent; And for the Crest upon a Helm, mantled Gules doubled Or, on a Wreath of the colours, out of a Crown Or a Stag's Head and Shoulders couped affrontée proper attired also Or holding in its Mouth fess-wise a Branch of Oak leaved and fructed Or

Motto: *Arte et Animo*

Mr Henry Reynolds THOMPSON, MA, LRCP MRCS, MB BChir, FRCS

The Arms were designed by Conrad Swan, York Herald, in 1981 and are recorded at the College of Arms in Volume 144, Folio 103.

The stained glass maker is unknown. The window was installed in window W3-10 in 1983 showing the full Arms and motto without a cartouche.

The three unicorns come from the Paris family (great grandmother) and the wheat-sheaf denotes a connection with Chester. The fleur-de-lys are for Rugby School and the Royal College of Physicians. The fleams denote the connection with surgery and the Barbers' Company and the pestle and mortar is for the Society.

The crest was used as an emblem by his father.

The motto translates as *By skill and courage*.

BORN London 14 Feb 1908; *s* of Harold Theodore Thompson FRCP FRCS and Elinor Waller; *m* 1940 Doreen Holdstock, three sons; *ob.* 9 Dec 1985.

EDUC Christ's Coll Cambridge (BA, MA, MB BChir) and the London Hosp Medical Coll.

QUALIFICATIONS BA 1929; MA 1933; LRCP MRCS 1932; MB BChir 1932; FRCS Eng 1934.

SERVICES Lt Col RAMC 1939–45: 53 Field Surg Unit; CO Surg Div Indian General Hosps.

CAREER Surgeon to the London Hospital; Cons Surgeon St Mark's Hosp for Diseases of the Colon & Rectum 1947–74, Woodford Jubilee Hosp 1947–74 and Forest Hosp 1947–74.

HON APPTS President Hunterian Soc 1977–78; President Medical Soc of London 1966.

SOCIETY Yeoman 1933; Liveryman 1937; elected to the Court 1957 *vice* J. P. Hedley. Junior Warden 1966–67, Senior Warden 1967–68, Master 1968–69.

CITY AND CIVIC Barbers' Company: Freeman 1931, Liveryman 191, Court 1950, Master 1959–60, Barber Emeritus.

Presented *The Apothecary Display'd 1748*, a nineteenth-century physician's mahogany chest, a statuette of Apollo and Daphne, his miniature portrait and his stained glass Arms panel.

Dr John Charles THOROWGOOD, LSA, MRCS, MD, FRCP

These Arms were used by Thorowgood of Thorowgood and Shartfield, Co Herts in 1594 but are not recorded at the College of Arms.[19]

The stained glass panel was made by James Powell & Sons in 1908, the glazier copying the Arms from a bookplate. The panel was installed in window W4-4 in 1908, showing the shield in Cartouche A. It was moved to window W3-9 between 1917 and 1922. From Sep 1941 to Jan 1946, all stained glass was removed from the Hall during hostilities and on return in 1946 these Arms were placed in window W1-5.

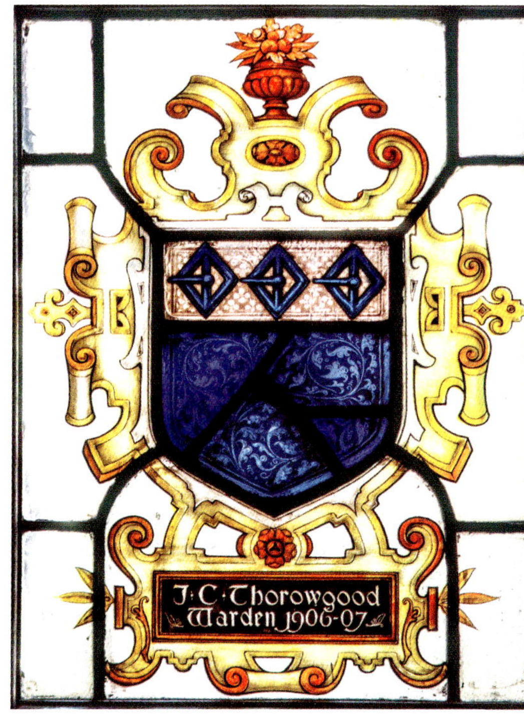

Azure, on a Chief Argent, three lozenge-shaped Buckles, Tongues fesswise, of the field

Crest (not shown): *Either a wolf's head or a fox's head couped Argent charged on the neck with a buckle Azure*

BORN Totteridge 6 Jan 1833; *s* of John Thorowgood and Sarah Napier; *m* 1863 Hester Ashwin, four daus; *ob.* 25 Apr 1913.

EDUC University Coll London (MD).

QUALIFICATIONS LSA 1855; MRCS; MD 1857; FRCP Lond 1874.

CAREER Physician Royal General Dispensary; Cons Physician City of London Chest Hosp 1863–1901; Physician West London Hosp 1873–75.

SOCIETY Yeoman 1860; Liveryman 1879. Elected to the Court 1896 *vice* CA Wakefield; Court of Examiners 1874–1896, Chairman 1892–96; Examinations Cttee 1899–1902. Junior Warden 1905–06 *[not as stated in the window]* but illness prevented his election as Senior Warden and he resigned from the Court in 1908.

Between 1888–1909 he donated 10 guineas in total to the Widows' Fund and he presented his stained glass Arms panel.

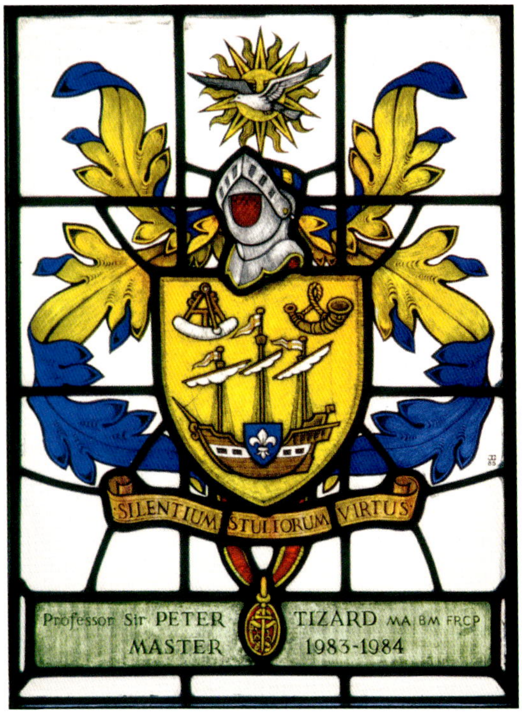

Or, an ancient three-masted Sailing Ship proper, sails furled, pennons flying Argent charged with a Cross Gules, surmounted amidships of an Escutcheon Azure charged with a Fleur-de-Lys of the 2nd, in chief a Quadrant and a Bugle Horn leathered both also proper; And for the Crest upon a Knight's Helm, mantled Azure doubled Or, on a Wreath of the colours in front of a Sun in splendour Or an Albatross Volant proper

Motto: *Silentium Stultorum Virtus*

Professor Sir John Peter Mills TIZARD, BM BCh, DCH, FRCP

The Arms were designed by John Walker, Rouge Croix Pursuivant, and granted to his father, Sir Henry, in 1951. They are recorded at the College of Arms in Volume Gr 113, Folio 281.

The stained glass panel was made by Jane Gray in 1985 and was installed in window W4-12 in 1985 showing the full Arms and motto without a cartouche. Suspended from the shield is the badge of a Knight Bachelor.

The Tizards were Huguenots from France represented by the ship and the fleur-de-lys. The sextant is from his grandfather Captain Thomas Tizard, Hydrographer to the Navy. The crest refers to Sir Henry's service in 1914–18 as a test pilot and aeronautical engineer.

The motto translates as *Silence is the virtue of fools* and is a quotation from the philosopher Francis Bacon (1561–1626).

BORN London 1 Apr 1916; *s* of Sir Henry Thomas Tizard and Kathleen Eleanor Wilson; *m* 1945 Joy Taylor, two sons, one dau; *ob.* 27 Oct 1993.

EDUC Oriel Coll Oxford (MA, BM BCh); Middlesex Hosp Medical Sch.

QUALIFICATIONS BA 1938; MA 1941; BM BCh 1941; MRCP Lond 1944; DCH 1947; FRCP Lond 1958.

SERVICES RAMC 1942–46, Major.

CAREER Cons Paediatrician Paddington Green Children's Hosp 1949–50; Hon Consultant Children's Physician Hammersmith Hosp 1954–72; Reader in Child Health 1954–64; Professor of Paediatrics Royal Postgraduate Medical School 1964–72; Professor of Paediatrics, U Oxford 1972–83; Hon Consultant Children's Physician Oxfordshire Health Authority 1972–83.

HON APPTS President European Paediatric Research Soc 1970–71; President Neonatal Soc 1975–78; President Harveian Soc 1977; President British Paediatric Association 1982–85.

SOCIETY Yeoman 1944; Liveryman 1948; elected to the Court 1971 *vice* WSC Copeman. Junior Warden 1981–82, Senior Warden 1982–83, Master 1983–84. Assistant Emeritus 1991.

FAMILY LIVERYMEN (son) Andrew Henry Tizard; (son) Humphrey Thomas Tizard; (dau) Dr Eleanor Jane Tizard.

HONOURS AND AWARDS Kt Bachelor 1982.

Presented a leather-bound copy of *The Dispensary of the Royal College of Physicians of London* 1754 and his stained glass Arms panel.

Dr Peter John Hocart TOOLEY, LRCP MRCS, MB BS, DObstRCOG, MRCGP, DMJ, DFFP, LLM, MFPM

The Arms were designed by Clive Cheesman, Rouge Dragon Pursuivant, in 2010 and are recorded at the College of Arms in Volume Gr 175, Folio 5.

The stained glass panel was made by Richard Scowen of Cornwall in 2013 and was installed in window W1-1 in 2013, showing the full Arms and motto without a cartouche.

The red and green field represents Wales and Guernsey heritage. The rugby posts depict a passion for rugby and service as Medical Officer for London and Oxfordshire teams. The serpents are for medicine.

On the crest the unicorn horns are for the Society and the ears of wheat for the family association with milling and baking. The donkey is the name given to Guernseymen.

The motto translates as *Stubborn, proud and true* – the characteristics of a donkey – and a Guernseyman.

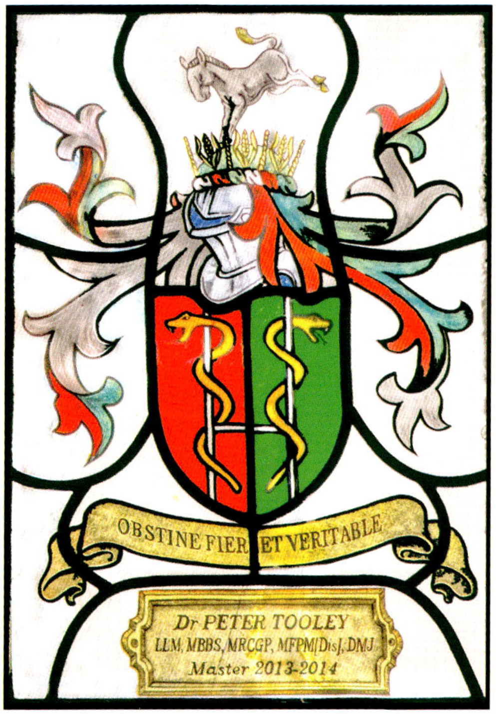

BORN St Helens, Lancs, 28 Feb 1939; *s* of Dr Patrick Tooley and Margaret Williams; *m* 1st 1966 Elizabeth Roche *diss* 1983, one son, two daus; *m* 2nd 1987 Diana Sturdy.
EDUC London Hosp Medical Coll (MB BS); U of Wales Coll, Cardiff (LLM).
QUALIFICATIONS LRCP MRCS 1963; MB BS 1964; DObstRCOG 1965; MRCGP 1971; DMJ (Clin) 1981; DFFP 1993; LLM 1994; MFPM 2012.
CAREER Principal in GP 1966–90; Asst Dep Coroner Reading 1984–89; Medical Director Janssen Pharmaceuticals 1990–98; Consultant Medical Adviser Daiichi Sankyo 1998–2016; Director PT Pharma Consultancy Ltd 1998–2016.
SOCIETY Proposed for the Society by Dr A. Brews, Senior Warden. Yeoman 1965; Liveryman 1970; Chairman of the Livery Cttee 2002–05; elected to the Court 2007 *vice* Dr David Hughes. Junior Warden 2011–12, Senior Warden 2012–13, Master 2013–14.
FAMILY LIVERYMEN (step-dau) Nicola Watley.
Presented the goblet used by the Livery Cttee Chairman, a Courtyard bench, books for the library, his miniature portrait and his stained glass Arms panel.

Per pale Gules and Vert, two Endorses conjoined in base by a Barrulet Argent, each Endorse environed by a Serpent Head outwards Or, langued counterchanged of the field. And for the Crest upon a Helm, mantled per pale Gules and Vert doubled Argent, on a Wreath Argent, Gules and Vert, a Mount of the last within a Palisade of Unicorn Horns Argent alternating with Ears of Wheat Or with an Ass kicking out with its hindlegs Argent unguled and the tail tufted Or

Motto: *Obstine Fier et Veritable*

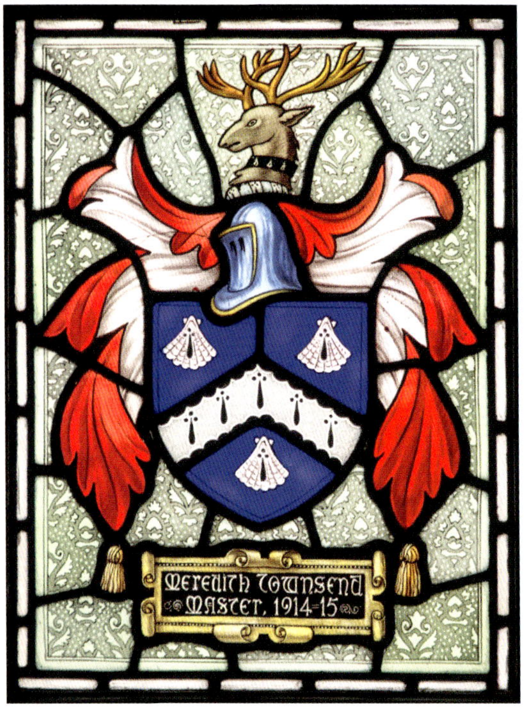

Azure, a Chevron engrailed between three Scallops Ermine; And for the Crest, upon a Helm, mantled Gules doubled Argent, on a wreath Argent, a Buck's head couped proper gorged with a collar Sable charged with three Escallops Argent

Dr Meredith TOWNSEND LSA, MRCS

These Arms with this crest were granted to Townshend of Wincham Hall, Co Cheshire in the seventeenth century. The Townsends/Townshends originated in Denbighshire and quartered the Arms of Leigh on inheriting Wincham at the end of the eighteenth century.

The last male heir of this family died in 1915 and it is not clear how Dr Townsend was related to him so it is likely that these Arms are incorrectly assumed.[20]

It is probable that this panel was commissioned by Dr Meredith's sons. The stained glass panel was made by W. B. Simpson & Sons in 1938 and was installed in window W4-2 in 1938, showing the full Arms without a cartouche. Between Sep 1941 and Jan 1946, all stained glass was removed from the Hall during hostilities and on return in 1946 these Arms were placed in window W2-2.

BORN Newington 1847; *s* of Henry Meredith Townsend LSA and Catherine Morse; *m* 1870 Anne Clara Edith Milton, six sons, six daus; *ob.* 5 Nov 1918.

EDUC St Thomas's Hosp Medical Sch.

QUALIFICATIONS LSA 1868; MRCS 1868.

CAREER Medical Officer & Vaccinator Kensington 1868–1918; Police Surgeon F Division Metropolitan Police for 35 years.

HON APPTS Society Representative on the General Medical Council 1917–1918; Executive Cttee Belgian Doctors & Pharmacists Relief Fund.

SOCIETY Yeoman 1868; Liveryman 1885; elected to the Court 1905 *vice* J. W. Robinson. Examinations Cttee 1911–18. Junior Warden 1912–13, Senior Warden 1913–14, Master 1914–15.

FAMILY LIVERYMEN (father) Dr Henry Meredith Townsend; (son) Dr Meredith Milton Townsend, Assistant 1934–40; (son) Dr Eric Morse Townsend, Assistant 1942–52, Junior Warden 1951–52, Senior Warden 1952.

In 1888 he donated 5 guineas to the Widows' Fund. His family gave, in 1931, a silver two-handled covered cup made in 1789 in his memory.

Sir Cecil Pembrey Grey WAKELEY, Bt of Liss, KBE, CB, DSc, FRCS, LLD, FKC, FRS Ed

The Arms were designed by Alfred Butler, Windsor Herald, in 1942 and are recorded at the College of Arms in Volume Gr 107, Folio 58.

The stained glass panel was made by Carl Edwards *c.*1956 and was installed in window W4-1 *c.*1956, showing the full Arms surrounded by the insignia of the Most Excellent Order of the British Empire and motto without a cartouche.

The Arms have the red hand of an Ulster Baronet in chief.

This is a variant of Wakeley of Charing, viz. *Argent, on a Fess Sable between three Eagles displayed Azure, as many crescents of the field* with the fess changed to a chevron and the third eagle replaced by Asclepius' rod for medicine.[21]

The motto translates as *Nothing without labour.*

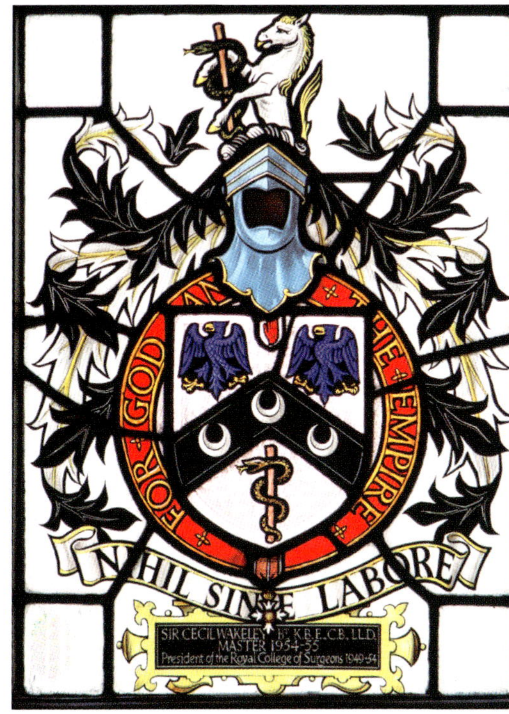

Argent, on a Chevron Sable, between in chief two Eagles displayed Azure and in base a Rod of Asclepius proper, three Crescents of the field; And for the Crest upon a Knight's helm, mantled Sable doubled Argent, on a Wreath of the colours, a demi-Horse Argent supporting between the legs a Rod of Asclepius proper

Motto: *Nihil Sine Labore*

BORN Rainham 5 May 1892; *s* of Percy Wakeley and Mary (May) Sophia Pembrey; *m* 1925 Elizabeth Muriel Nicholson-Smith, three sons; *ob.* 5 Jun 1979.

EDUC King's College Hosp Medical Sch.

QUALIFICATIONS LRCP MRCS 1915; FRCS Eng 1921; DSc 1932.

SERVICES Surg Lieut RN 1915–19; Surg Rear Admiral 1944.

CAREER Surgeon King's College Hosp 1922–, Belgrave Hosp, Maida Vale Hosp for Nervous Diseases and Royal Masonic Hosp; Editor Annals of the RCS, British Journal of Surgery and the Medical & Press Circular; Chairman Imperial Cancer Research.

HON APPTS President Harveian Soc 1932; President Royal College of Surgeons 1949–54; President Hunterian Soc 1961.

SOCIETY Yeoman 1937; Liveryman 1939; elected to the Court 1943 *vice* Vincent Warren Low. Examination Cttee 1944–49. Junior Warden 1952–53, Senior Warden 1953–54, Master 1954–55.

FAMILY LIVERYMEN (son) Sir John Cecil Nicholson Wakeley 2Bt; (son) Dr Richard Michael Wakeley; (nephew) Mr Robin Anthony Wade Wakeley.

CITY AND CIVIC Barbers' Company: Freeman 1930, Liveryman 1930, Court 1948, Master 1954–55.

HONOURS AND AWARDS FRS Edin 1932; FACS 1934; Hon FRACS 1938; Order of the Nile 2nd class 1938; CB 1941; USA Legion of Merit 1944; KBE 1946; France Legion d'Honneur 1948; Hon FRCS Edin 1951; Hon FRCSI 1952; Bart 1953; KStJ; Order of the Southern Cross Brazil.

Presented his portrait by Frank Salisbury which hangs on the Landing in 1962, two brass Navy liquid measures of 1826, eight mortars and five pestles, his miniature portrait and his stained glass Arms panel.

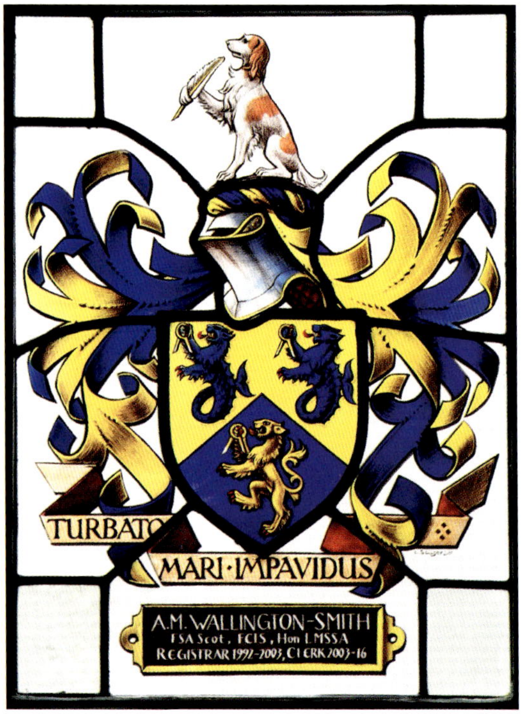

Mr Andrew Marcus WALLINGTON-SMITH, FSA Scot, FCIS, FRGS, Hon LMSSA

The Arms were designed by Thomas Woodcock, Garter King of Arms, in 2016 and are recorded at the College of Arms in Volume Gr 180, Folio 43.

The stained glass panel was made by Leonie Seliger of Canterbury and was installed in window E2-1 in 2017, showing the full Arms and motto without a cartouche.

The colours of the field represent the sea and shore for the family's service in the Navy and are also the Society's colours. The two sealions represent the two current naval members of the family and the lion the land-based son. All have an interest and an ability in navigation represented by the dividers in the dexter paws.

The crest represents a line of springer spaniels and the quill is for a Clerk and also for his father's secretarial specialisation in the Navy.

The motto translates as *Courage in rough waters.*

Per chevron Or and Azure, in chief two Sealions erect and in base a Lion rampant all counterchanged, each grasping in the dexter paw a pair of Naval dividers proper; And for the Crest upon a Helm, mantled Azure doubled Or, on a Wreath of the colours, a liver and white Springer Spaniel sejant its tail docked proper holding in the dexter forepaw a Quill bendwise sinister Argent spined Or

Motto: *Turbato Mari Impavidus*

BORN BMH Singapore 9 Feb 1954; *s* of Captain Anthony Percy Wallington-Smith RN and Moyra Ogilvie Mary Mount-Haes; *m* 1985 Sarah Anne Royle, two sons.

QUALIFICATIONS FSA Scot 1991; ACIS 1993; FCIS 1993; FRGS 2000.

CAREER Royal Navy 1971–92; HM Ships *Scarborough, Cleopatra, Ark Royal, Wakeful, Tartar, Alfriston*, HMY *Britannia*, HM Ships *Alert*, in command, *Coventry, Ajax, Avenger, Active.*

SOCIETY Registrar 1992–2003; Registrar, United Examining Board 1993–2001; Monckton Copeman Lecturer 2003; Clerk 2003–16. Treasurer Faculty of the History and Philosophy of Medicine and Pharmacy 2003–16; Master's Medal 2013; Liveryman by Gift 2016.

CITY & CIVIC Freeman 2013; Chairman Clerks' Assoc 2015–16.

HONOURS AND AWARDS Hon LMSSA 2016.

His stained glass Arms panel was generously donated by the thirteen Masters he served as Clerk.

Mr Michael Phelps WARD, CBE, MA, LRCP MRCS, MB BChir, MD, FRCS, FRGS

The Arms were designed by Robert Noel, Bluemantle Pursuivant, in 1995 and are recorded at the College of Arms in Volume 162, Folio 335.

The stained glass maker is unknown but possibly was Messrs Goddard & Gibbs. The panel was installed in window W2-10 *c.*1995 showing the full Arms and motto without a cartouche.

The field is for Cambridge, the Tibet sky and his operating gown. The snow leopard is native to the Himalayas and the books refer to study and research.

Red signifies blood and white is for snow; the bordure is in the Society colours.

The red knight is a pun for surgery – the warrior steeped in blood with the lance for healing wounds – and the London Pride signifies his long connection with London.

The motto translates as *Advance through knowledge.*

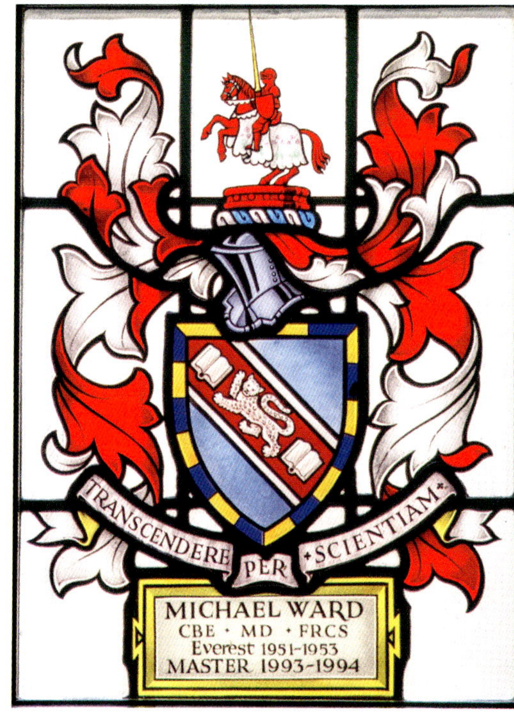

BORN London 26 Mar 1925; *s* of Wilfred Arthur Ward and Norah Anne Phelps; *m* 1957 Jane Ewbank, one son; *ob.* 7 Oct 2005.

EDUC Ironmongers' Company Exhibition to Peterhouse Coll, Cambridge (BA, MA, MB BChir, MD); London Hosp Medical Coll.

SERVICES Captain RAMC 1950–52.

QUALIFICATIONS BA 1945; LRCP MRCS 1949; MB BChir 1949; MA 1961; MD 1968; FRCS Eng 1955; FRGS.

CAREER Medical Officer and Climbing Member of Everest Expedition 1953; Cons Surgeon Poplar Hosp 1964–75; St Andrew's Hosp Bow 1964–93; Newham Hosp 1983–93.

SOCIETY Proposed for the Society by Past Master Dr Dinty Moore. Yeoman 1966; Liveryman 1969; elected to the Court 1985 *vice* Keith Lyle. Junior Warden 1992–93, Master 1993–94. Monckton Copeman Lecturer 1994; Past Master Emeritus 2000. He progressed from Junior Warden straight to Master as Sir John Chalstrey was elected a Sheriff of the City of London that year and spent two years as Senior Warden.

MOUNTAINEERING In early 1951, examining forgotten photographs and maps in the Royal Geographical Society archives, he identified a possible route up the Nepalese side of Everest. Together with Murray, he initiated and took part in Shipton's 1951 reconnaissance. In 1951–52, he worked with Pugh on the high-altitude medical problem; Chairman Mt Everest Foundation 1978–80.

HONOURS AND AWARDS Founder's Gold Medal of the Royal Geographical Society 1982, CBE 1983.

Presented his miniature portrait and his stained glass Arms panel.

Bleu celeste, on a Bend Argent a Bend Gules thereon a Snow Leopard passant guardant between two open Books proper bound Sable, a Bordure compony Or and Azure; And for the Crest upon a Helm mantled Gules doubled Argent, on a wreath Argent and Bleu Celeste, a Chess Piece of a base thereon a Knight in Plate Armour Gules holding in the dexter Hand a Lance point upwards Or and bearing on the sinister Arm a Shield and seated upon a Horse forcene Gules caparisoned Argent semy of blooms of London Pride proper

Motto: *Transcendere Per Scientiam*

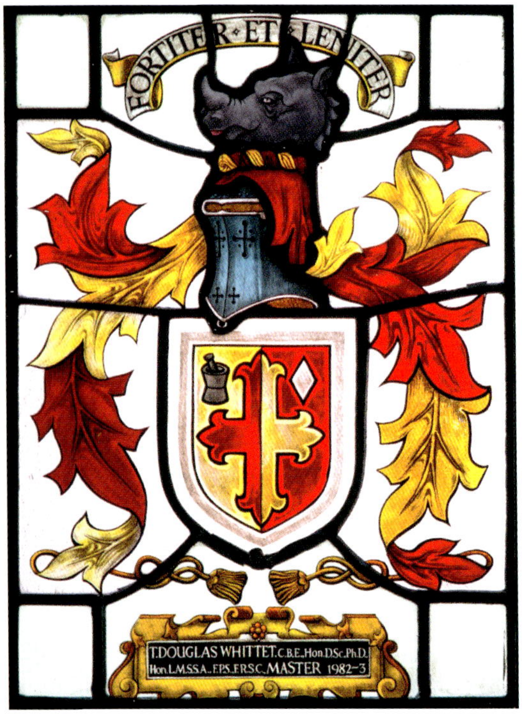

Per pale Or and Gules, a Cross flory counterchanged between, in dexter chief a Mortar and Pestle Sable and in sinister chief a Fusil paleways Argent; a Bordure of the last for difference; And for the Crest upon a Helm mantled Gules doubled Or, on a Wreath of the colours, the Head of a Rhinoceros erased proper

Motto: *Fortiter et Leniter*

Dr Thomas Douglas WHITTET, CBE, BSc, PhD, FPS, MCPP, CChem, FRSC, DBA, Hon LMSSA

The Arms were granted by Lord Lyon King of Arms on 1 May 1979 and the panel was donated by Mr John Evans, MPS.

The maker of the stained glass panel is unknown but it was installed in window W4-10 in 1984, showing the full Arms with motto without a cartouche.

The Arms are based on those of the family of his maternal grandmother, the Carlyles of Torthorwald (*Or a cross flory Gules*) with the pestle and mortar for his work as Chief Pharmacist, the fusil representing a shuttle of his weaving ancestors in Scone and the rhino crest for his connection with the Society.

The motto is adapted from his school, Rosebank in Hartlepool and translates as *Bravely and gently.*

BORN Hartlepool 4 Jan 1915; *s* of Thomas Douglas Whittet and Ellen Sloan Scott; *m* 1942 Doreen Mary Bowes, two sons; *ob.* 15 Apr 1987.

EDUC Sunderland (DBA); University Coll London (BSc, PhD).

QUALIFICATIONS BSc 1953; PhD 1958; FPS 1938; MCPP 1980; CChem 1975; FRSC 1955; Dip Biochemical Analysis 1942; FRIC 1955.

CAREER Chief Chemist Nuol Ltd 1939–41; Chief Pharmacist Baguley Sanatorium Manchester 1943; Chief Pharmacist & Lecturer in Pharmacy Charing Cross Hosp 1943–47; Chief Pharmacist and Cons Pharmacist to Faculty Medical Sciences University Coll Hosp 1947–65; WHO on Cttee International Pharmacopoeia 1948; Recognised Teacher Faculty Medicine U London 1953; Ministry of Health: Deputy Chief Pharmacist 1965–67, Chief Pharmacist 1967–78.

HON APPTS European Pharmacopoeia Commission 1967–71; Council of Europe Pharmaceutical Cttee 1967–77; British Pharmaceutical Codex Revision Cttee 1967–75; Joint Formulary Cttee 1967–78; Chairman British Society for the History of Pharmacy 1972–74.

SOCIETY Yeoman 1955; Liveryman 1958; Sydenham Lecturer 1965; Chairman Faculty of the History & Philosophy of Medicine and Pharmacy 1975–78; elected to the Court 1972 *vice* Sir Cecil Wakeley. Gideon de Laune Lecturer 1977. Junior Warden 1980–81, Senior Warden 1981–82, Master 1982–83.

FAMILY LIVERYMEN (son) Dr David Brian Bowes Whittet; (son) Douglas Carlyle Bowes Whittet.

HONOURS AND AWARDS Hon DSc U Bath 1968; Hon DSc U Aston 1974; CBE 1977; Hon LMSSA 1984.

Presented many books for the Library including a complete set of pharmacopoeia and several specie jars, a specially cast mortar and pestle bearing the Society's Arms, the burnished and restored old pestle and mortar shop sign from St Albans in the Courtyard, an Apothecary token.

Dr George WILKS
BA, MB MC, LSA, MRCS

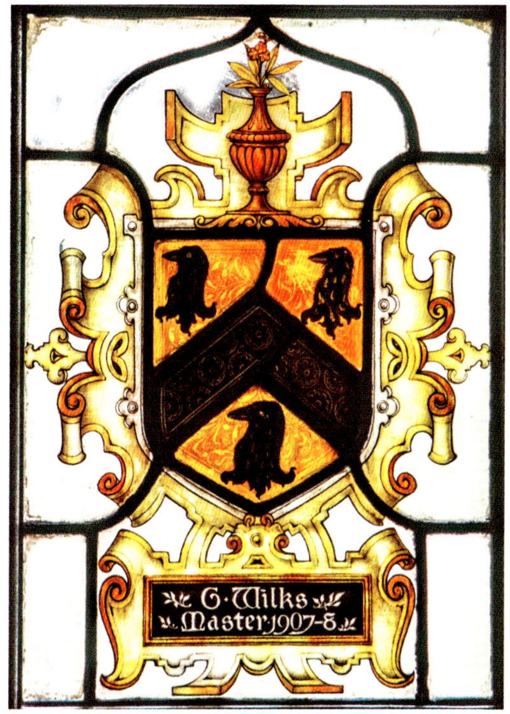

Or, a Chevron Sable between three Raven's heads erased of the last gutté d'or

There are examples of similar Arms being used by families of Wilkes,[22] but no connection with these armigers has been established. A grant of Arms to Sir Samuel Wilks Bt PRCP, using these colours and a variant of the chevron and ravens was made in 1897,[23] but he is also apparently unrelated to Dr Wilks.

The stained glass panel was made by James Powell & Sons in 1908 and was installed in window W4-5 in 1908, showing the shield in Cartouche B. It was moved to window W3-8 between 1917 and 1922 and probably moved again to window W4-13 in 1938. From Sep 1941 to Jan 1946, all stained glass was removed from the Hall during hostilities and on return in 1946 these Arms were placed in window W1-11.

It would appear that these unrecorded Arms have been assumed by Dr Wilks without the sanction of the College of Arms.

BORN Ashford 1840; *s* of Dr George Frederick Wilks and Elizabeth Philpott; *unmarried*; *ob.* 11 Jun 1919.
EDUC Trinity Coll Cambridge (BA, MB MC); St Bartholomew's Hosp Medical Coll.
QUALIFICATIONS BA 1863; MB MC 1867; LSA 1867; MRCS 1867.
CAREER In practice in Ashford with his father 1867–86; Medical Officer to the General Post Office; Physician in Ordinary to HRH Prince Alfred, Duke of Edinburgh; Medical Officer to HIH the Duchess of Edinburgh.
HON APPTS Society representative on the General Medical Council 1912–17.
SOCIETY Yeoman 1863; Liveryman 1880; elected to the Court 1897 *vice* William Smith. Examinations Cttee 1905–10. Proceeded straight to Senior Warden 1906–07 (in place of Dr John Thorowgood who was too ill to proceed), Master 1907–08. Retired from the Court 1917.
FAMILY LIVERYMEN (father) Dr George Frederick Wilks; (uncle) Dr Charles Wilks.
CITY AND CIVIC Conductor of the Ashford Choral Society 1891–1905; Ashford philanthropist.
Between 1876–1908 donated 20 guineas to the Widows' Fund and £10 to the Distressed Members' Fund and his stained glass Arms panel.

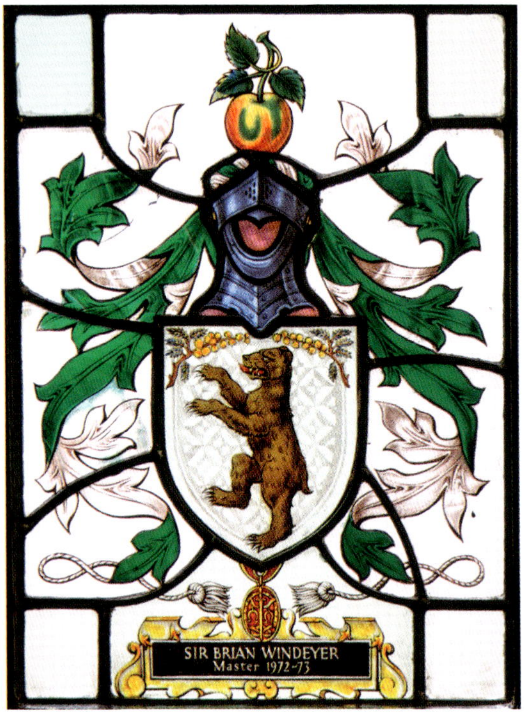

Professor Sir Brian Wellingham WINDEYER, MB BS, FRCS Ed, FRCP, FRCR, DMRE

The Arms were designed by John Walker, Lancaster Herald, in 1956 and granted to Sir Brian's first cousin Maj Gen Sir Victor Windeyer of Turramurra and are recorded at the College of Arms in Volume Gr 118, Folio 261. The grant was made to the descendants of his late grandfather Sir William Charles Windeyer.

The stained glass panel was made by Carl Edwards in 1975 and was installed in window E1-14 in 1975, showing the full Arms without a cartouche. Suspended from the shield is the badge of a Knight Bachelor.

The family has Swiss origins and the bear is from the Arms of the City of Bern with the wattle blossom referring to the Australian settlement of the family by their great grandfather. The apple also has Swiss origins.

Sir Victor was a very successful Australian general in the Second World War and it seems that Sir Brian has adapted the Arms by omitting the Brigade patch on the bear's shoulder.

Argent, a Bear rampant, charged on the shoulder for distinction with a representation of the Colour Patch of the Headquarters of the 20th Australian Infantry Brigade Imperial Force, in chief two Sprigs of Wattle all proper; And for the Crest upon a Knight's Helm, mantled Vert doubled Argent, on a Wreath of the colours, an apple slipped and leaved proper

BORN Sydney 7 Feb 1904; *s* of Richard Windeyer QC and Mabel Robinson; *m* 1st 1928 Joyce Russell, one son, one dau; *m* 2nd 1948 Anne Bowry, one son, two daus; *ob.* 26 Oct 1994.

EDUC U Sydney Medical Sch (MB BS); U Cambridge (DMRE).

QUALIFICATIONS MB BS 1927; FRCS Edin 1930; DMRE 1932; FFR 1940; MRCP Lond 1957; FRCP Lond 1962; FRCR 1975.

SERVICES Consultant in Radiotherapy to RN 1968–70.

CAREER Director Meyerstein Inst Radiography 1936–54; Director of Radiotherapy, Emergency Medical Service Mount Vernon 1939–45; Professor of Therapeutic Radiology U London 1942; Dean Middlesex Hosp Med Sch 1954–67; Dean of the Faculty of Medicine U London 1964–68; Vice Chancellor U London 1969–72.

HON APPTS Royal Coll Surgeons Council 1948–53; President Faculty of Radiologists 1949–52; Chairman Radioactive Substances Advisory Cttee 1961–70; Royal Commission on Medical Education 1965–68; Chairman National Radiological Protection Bd 1970–78; Chairman Academic Council U London 1967.

SOCIETY Yeoman 1951; Liveryman 1954; elected to the Court 1963 *vice* Dr Reginald Fisher. Junior Warden 1970–71, Senior Warden 1971–72, Master 1972–73. Assistant Emeritus 1979.

HONOURS AND AWARDS FRCS Eng *ad eundum* 1948; Hon FRACS 1951; Hon DSc U British Columbia 1952; Hon FCRA 1955; Kt Bachelor 1961; Hon DSc U Wales 1965; Hon FACR 1966; Hon LLD U Glasgow 1968; Hon ScD U Cambridge 1971; Hon Fellow BIR 1972; Hon MD U Sydney 1979.

Presented various books for the Library, a silver cigar box, his miniature portrait and his stained glass Arms panel.

Sir Gordon Ethelbert Ward WOLSTENHOLME, OBE, MA, MB BChir, FRCP, FIBiol, FRSA

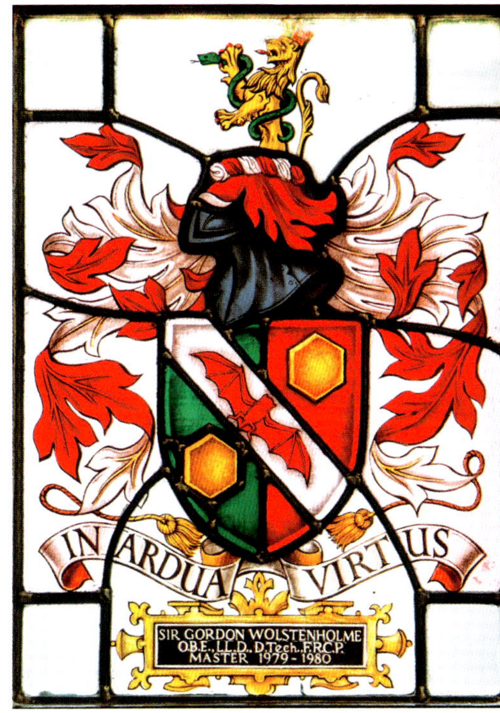

The Arms were designed by Walter Verco, Norroy and Ulster King of Arms, in 1979 and are recorded at the College of Arms in Volume Gr 141, Folio 241.

The stained glass panel was made by Carl Edwards and was installed in window E1-12 *c.*1981, showing the full Arms and motto without a cartouche.

The benzene hexagons refer to chemistry and the bat to his work in blood transfusion.

The helm is incorrect as the visor should be open for a knight.

The motto translates as *Virtue amid difficulties* and is adapted from Ovid's *Epistulae ex Ponto.*

Per pale Vert and Gules, on a bend Argent, between two regular Hexagons Or, a Bat volant affrontée bendwise Gules; And for the Crest upon a Knight's Helm, mantled Gules doubled Argent, on a Wreath of the colours, a demi-Lion rampant Or crowned with a Crown per pale Vert and Gules, the dexter Leg and Body entwined of a Serpent Vert

Motto: *In Ardua Virtus*

BORN Sheffield 28 May 1913; *s* of George Ethelbert Wolstenholme and Clementina Ward; *m* 1st 1939 Mary Elizabeth Spackman, one son, two daus; *m* 2nd 1948 Edita (Dushanka) Messinger, one dau; *ob.* 29 May 2004.

EDUC Corpus Christi Coll Cambridge (BA, MA, MB BChir); Middlesex Hosp Medical Sch.

QUALIFICATIONS BA 1936; MA 1940; MB BChir 1948; MRCP 1959; FRCP Lond 1964; FIBiol; FRSA 1979.

SERVICES RAMC Lt Col 1940–47.

CAREER founding Director of the Ciba Foundation 1949–78; Founder Action in International Medicine 1988, Chairman 1988–95.

HON APPTS Genetic Manipulation Adv Gp – Member 1954, Treas 1955–61, Board 1961–70, Chairman 1976–78; Society Rep General Medical Council 1973–83; Royal Soc Medicine – Hon Secy 1964–70, President 1975–77 & 1978; Vice President Zoological Society; Harveian Librarian 1979–89.

SOCIETY Yeoman 1950; Liveryman 1954; elected to the Court 1969 *vice* Richard Traill. Chairman Faculty of History & Philosophy of Medicine & Pharmacy 1973–75. Junior Warden 1977–78, Senior Warden 1978–79, Master 1979–80. Locke Lecturer 1979; Assistant Emeritus 1988.

HONOURS AND AWARDS OBE 1944; Yugoslav Lik decoration 1945; France Chevalier of the Legion d'Honneur 1959; Star of Ethiopia 1966; Hon LLD U Cambridge 1968; Hon FACP 1975; Kt Bachelor 1976; Hon DTech Brunel U 1981; Hon MD St George's Med Sch Grenada 1982; Fellow Green Coll Oxford 1986; Hon FDS RCS 1991.

Presented various books for the Library, his miniature portrait and his stained glass Arms panel.

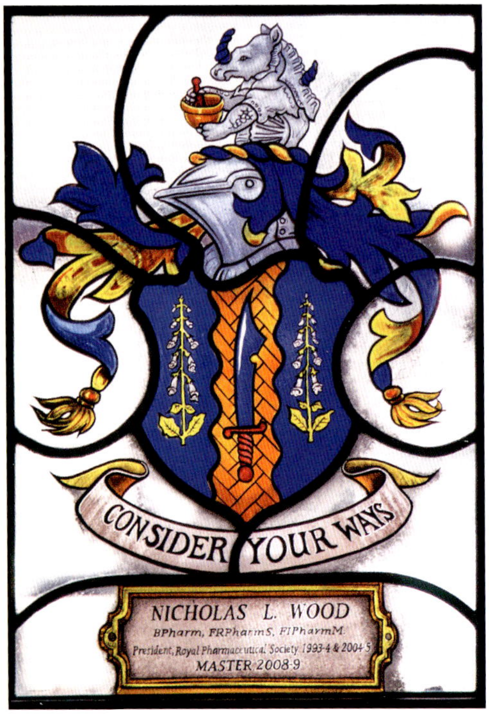

Azure, on a Pale wavy Or parqueted Sable between two Foxgloves Argent slipped and leaved Or, a Seax Blade upwards Azure Hilt Pommel and Quillons Gules. And for the Crest upon a Helm, mantled Azure doubled Or, on a Wreath of the colours, a demi Rhinoceros Argent armed with one Horn on the Nose and another on the Back Azure holding with the Feet a Mortar Or and a Pestle Gules

Motto: *Consider Your Ways*

Mr Nicholas Leslie WOOD, BPharm, FRPharmS, FIPharmM

The Arms were designed by William Hunt, Windsor Herald, in 2009 and are recorded at the College of Arms in Volume Gr 172, Folio 288.

The stained glass panel was made by Richard Scowen of Cornwall in 2010 and installed in window W1-4 in 2010, showing the full Arms and motto without a cartouche.

The seax is from the Arms of Essex and of Epping Forest, where the Woods came from. The hatched gold centre is a pun on the name as it looks like wood block flooring.

The Arms allude to the three bodies with which he has been involved: the Apothecaries, the Royal Pharmaceutical Society of Great Britain (RPSGB), and the London School of Pharmacy. The rhinoceros is from the Apothecaries Arms, the mortar and pestle is from the RPSGB Arms and additionally represents the family's pharmacy businesses. The foxglove, the source of the cardiac drug digitalis, from the School's Arms, represents medicine in general.

The wavy lines allude to the sea and power boating, and the overall gold and blue colours are those of the Apothecaries. The motto is taken from an annotation in the Ketteridge family Bible and refers to the book of Haggai 1:7, which reads 'Thus said the Lord of hosts; Consider your ways.'

BORN 25 Sep 1948; *s* of Harold Edward Wood and Joyce Winifred Clark; *m* 1974 Elizabeth Ketteridge, two sons.

EDUC Sch of Pharmacy U London (BPharm).

QUALIFICATIONS BPharm 1972; MRPharmS 1973; FRPharmS 1993; FIPharmM 2006.

CAREER Man Dir NL Wade Ltd 1982–2000; Exec Chairman Leach & Burton Ltd 1988–2012; Inst of Pharmacy – Gen Sec 1999–2003, Pres 2007–15.

HON APPTS Standing Pharmaceutical Advice Cttee DoH 1987–96; Joint Formulary Ctte BNF 1987–2007; Pet Health Council 1990–97; Fedn International Pharmaceutique Council 1992–94; Royal Pharmaceutical Society – Vice Pres 1992–93, Pres 1993–94 & 2004–05; Nurse Prescribers Formulary Cttee 1998–2007; Council for Healthcare Regulatory Excellence 2004–05; Vice Chairman Sch of Pharmacy 2006–09.

SOCIETY Proposed for the Society by Past Master Douglas Whittet. Yeoman 1986; Liveryman 1990; elected to the Court 1995 *vice* Dr Malcolm Godfrey. Junior Warden 2006–07, Senior Warden 2007–08, Master 2008–09. Gideon de Laune Lecturer 2009; Hon Curator 2013–d.

FAMILY LIVERYMEN (wife) Elizabeth Wood.

Presented several books for the library, his miniature portrait and his stained glass Arms panel.

APPENDIX II

Important Windows made at Apothecaries' Hall by Carl Edwards

This appendix contains a list of the major commissions made by Carl Edwards in his studio at Apothecaries' Hall between 1952 and 1972. In addition, he completed more than sixty-four parish church commissions in the United Kingdom and at least fourteen overseas.

In the table a commission consisting, for example, of four windows, each of two lights would be shown as '4 × 2 lights'.

YEAR	ESTABLISHMENT	LOCATION	POSITION	COMMISSION
1953	St John's Church	Kingston	North Transept	1 × 5 lights
1954	Temple Church	City of London	East Windows	3 × 3 lights
1954	Cathedral Church of Christ	Liverpool	Library Windows	
1955	Lambeth Palace Chapel	London	East Window	1 × 5 lights
1956	Tabley House	Knutsford, Cheshire	Tea Room	1 × 3 lights
1956	Lambeth Palace Chapel	London	North Windows South Windows	3 × 3 lights 3 × 3 lights
1956	Cathedral Church of St Thomas of Canterbury	Portsmouth	South Transept D-Day window	single light
1956	House of Lords	Westminster Palace	Prince's Chamber Debating Chamber	6 × 3 lights + tracery 12 × 4 tiered lights + tracery
1957	Guildhall	City of London		panel for screen
1958	Temple Church	City of London		repairs to works by Willement & Powell
1958	St Clement Danes Church	London	East Windows	3 × 1 lights
1958	Tabley House	Knutsford, Cheshire	Transom Window	1 × 3 lights
1958	Garrison Church	Portsmouth	East Window	1 × 3 lights
1958	St David's Cathedral	Wales	East Chancel	1 × 3 lights + tracery

1959	Elizabeth Garrett Anderson Hospital	London		single light
1959	Westminster School	London	Heraldic window	1 × 3 lights
1960s	St Patrick's Cathedral	Bunbury, Australia		various
1960	Cathedral Church of Christ	Liverpool	Nave Window	1 × 2 lights + tracery
1960	King Edward's School	Whitley, Surrey		4 × 2 lights
1962	Temple Church	City of London		repairs to works by Willement
1962	St Francis Xavier's Cathedral	Geraldton, Western Australia	North Nave East Window	1 × 3 lights
1963	Cathedral Church of Christ	Liverpool	North Aisle	1 × 2 lights + tracery
1963	Blue Coat School	Wavertree, Lancs	South Aisle	single light
1965	Holy Trinity Cathedral	Auckland, New Zealand		Rose Window
1965	Cathedral Church of Christ	Liverpool	South Aisle North Aisle	1 × 2 lights 1 × 2 lights
1965	Worcester College	University of Oxford	Library	single light
1966	Cathedral Church of Christ	Liverpool	Nave – Layman's Window	1 × 2 lights
1970	Tallow Chandlers' Hall	City of London	Great Hall – Oriel Window	2 × 2 lights 1 × 3 lights

APPENDIX III

Stained glass Companies and Artists

The makers of all but sixteen of the seventy-seven panels to date in the Great Hall are known. Ten of the unknown panels simply show arms on a shield within a cartouche, and this often makes identification of the maker difficult. However, for thirteen of these unknowns the makers can be reasonably deduced.

The firm of W. B. Simpson, for example, is very likely to have made more than the one panel listed but with the loss of the company's records in the Blitz this cannot be proven. It is also a shame that only three of the panels bear a maker's mark or signature. Some stained glass artists 'sign' their work (see Figures 4.23 and 4.24), but unfortunately most do not.

Caroline Benyon

The daughter of Carl Edwards, Caroline Benyon started working at the Glass-House in Fulham in 1972 when the Carl Edwards Studio moved there from Apothecaries' Hall. She continued there after his death in 1985, until 1993 when she moved to Hampton and formed her own studio, Benyon Stained Glass.

Benyon is a Court Assistant of the Company of Glaziers and Painters of Glass and currently Chairman of the British Society of Master Glass Painters.

Active for the Society with her father and again in 2017 (one stained glass panel: Moore-Gillon 2017).

Chapel Studio 1973: Chapel Studio Stained Glass Ltd 2005

Chapel Studio was established in King's Langley in 1973 by Alfred Fisher and Peter Archer, who brought extensive knowledge of traditional craftsmanship acquired at the Whitefriars Studios.

In 1975 Robert Holloway, a second-generation stained glass craftsman also from the Whitefriars glassworks, joined the studio. Over the following decades, the studio grew in both size and reputation. In 1999, following the retirement of Fisher and Archer, Holloway became sole owner of Chapel Studio. In 2005 it became Chapel Studio Stained Glass Limited and continues to be recognised as a leading authority for new designs, conservation of medieval and restoration of Victorian stained glass, as well as for repair and protective work countrywide of vandalised or deteriorating windows, many of historical importance.

Alfred Fisher was Master of the Company of Glaziers and Painters of Glass in 1991–92.

Peter Archer is a Liveryman of the Company of Glaziers and Painters of Glass.

Alfred Fisher was active for the Society 1990–97 (two stained glass panels: Fisher 1990, Jay 1997).

Clayton & Bell

The Company of Clayton & Bell, based in Regent Street in London, was founded in 1855 by John Richard Clayton (1827–1913) and Alfred Bell (1832–1895) and became one of the largest stained glass firms of the nineteenth and twentieth centuries in this country. The panel in the Hall by this Company was made by Bell's great-grandson Michael Charles Farrar Bell (1911–1993). The firm closed down in 1993 on the death of Michael.

Michael Charles Farrar Bell was Master of the Company of Glaziers and Painters of Glass in 1974.

Active for the Society 1992 (one stained glass panel: Eadie 1992 – this panel bears the maker's monogram).

Carl Edwards Studio

See Chapter 7 for a biography of Carl Edwards (1914–1985).

Active for the Society *c.*1955–85 (thirteen confirmed stained glass panels: Morley *c.*1955, Wakeley *c.*1956, Copeman *c.*1960, Ironside *c.*1965, Dodds *c.*1965, Porritt *c.*1967, Lyle *c.*1972, Sinclair *c.*1972, Cohen 1975, Richardson 1975, Windeyer 1975, Grey-Turner 1978, Wolstenholme *c.*1981; and two probables: Moore *c.*1967, Jackson 1979).

Goddard & Gibbs

This firm was first established in 1868 as Walter Gibbs & Sons of Blackfriars Road, London. As with other decorative glass firms, it went through some major changes, first of all becoming part of the firm James Clark & Eaton Ltd, also based in the Blackfriars Road area. In 1938 the firm acquired Goddard's Glass House in Kingsland Road, Shoreditch, thus establishing the name Goddard & Gibbs. In 1978 the firm was taken over by another Clark, Charles Clark, but retained its name.

Then in 2006 Goddard and Gibbs was again taken over, this time by the stained glass company John Hardman of Birmingham (established 1838). This company went bankrupt two years later and unfortunately all the old Goddard & Gibbs archives had been removed to that company. It is not certain what happened to the archives when Hardman's was liquidated.

Goddard & Gibbs was re-established by a group of former workers under its long-time chief designer John Lawson (1932–2009), who had joined the firm in 1970. There have been other excellent designers as well, such as Arthur Edward Buss (1905–1999), whom Lawson succeeded, and Caroline Swash. The firm is now based in Corsham, Wiltshire, and has an international reputation for its contemporary stained glass and for the restoration of older stained glass.

Active for the Society in the 1990s (five confirmed stained glass panels: Hughes 1994, Chalstrey 1998, Gibberd 1998, Field 2000, E. Taylor 2004; and possibly four others: Southwood 1991, Neild 1991, Glenister 1993, Ward *c.*1995).

Jane Gray

Jane Gray trained at the Kingston School of Arts and then the Royal College of Art. On graduation, she became assistant to Lawrence Lee and assisted him in his seminal work on the new Coventry Cathedral.

Gray is a Liveryman of the Company of Glaziers and Painters of Glass.

Active for the Society 1985–88 (two stained glass panels: Tizard 1985, Dudgeon 1988 – both panels bear her monogram).

Melanie Howse

Melanie Howse studied at the Portsmouth College of Art and the Swansea Institute before opening her studio in Chichester in 1996. She was recently commissioned to design in stained glass the Arms of Alderman Sir Andrew Parmley, Lord Mayor of the City of London 2016–17.

Active for the Society only in 2007 (one stained glass panel: Livesley 2007).

Lawrence Lee

Lawrence Stanley Lee (1909–2011) graduated from the Royal College of Art in 1930 and worked for his tutor, Martin Travers (1886–1948), returning to Travers' studio after war service. The studio was much involved in restoring war damage and Lee established his own studio on Travers' death in 1948, when he also succeeded Travers as Head of Stained Glass at the Royal College of Art. His most famous work is the ten large windows in the new Coventry Cathedral in collaboration with Keith New and Geoffrey Clarke.

Lee was Master of the Company of Glaziers and Painters of Glass in 1973.

Active for the Society only in 1975 (one stained glass panel: Mitchell-Heggs 1975).

Lowndes & Drury and the Glass-House

Mary Lowndes (1856–1929) and Alfred John Drury (1868–1940) went into partnership in 1896 and built the Glass-House in Fulham in 1906 for use by independent stained glass artists. In 1953 Drury's son Victor (1899–1988) established Lowndes & Drury Ltd. The company closed down on Victor's retirement in 1973. In 1972 the Glass-House was taken over by an independent trust until its closure in 1993.

Active for the Society with the work of Francis Spear.

James Powell & Sons

The Whitefriars Glass Company, based in Fleet Street and which had its origins in around 1680, was purchased in 1834 by James Powell (1774–1840) and renamed James Powell & Sons (Whitefriars Glass). They were all newcomers to glass-making but developed a specialty in church stained glass, particularly decorative quarry glass which was mass produced by moulding and printing rather than hand-cutting and painting.

The name was changed to James Powell & Sons (Whitefriars) Ltd in 1919 and a new factory opened in Wealdstone in 1923. The firm enjoyed great prosperity under its designer and chairman James Humphries Hogan (1883–1948) until the Second World War. Hogan was succeeded as head designer by Carl Edwards (1914–1985) until 1952. In 1962 the firm changed its name back to Whitefriars Glass Ltd until its purchase in 1981 by Caithness Glass. It is now part of Dartington Glass.

Note: Christopher Charles Powell (1876–1955), his brother Albert Frederick Powell and their father Charles Powell (d.1934) do not appear to be related to these Powells and operated independently from workshops in Lincoln and Highgate. Although Christopher tendered for work in 1937, it does not appear that he made any of the Hall panels.

Active for the Society 1906–48 (fifteen confirmed stained glass panels: Cooper 1906, Day 1906, Jeffcoat 1906, Griffith 1906, Wilks 1908, Thorowgood 1908, H. W. Statham 1938, R. W. Statham 1938, Nuffield 1938, MacNalty 1938, Dawson 1938, Browne 1939, Hayes 1941, Lett 1943, Cargill 1948 – and possibly also Haydon 1938).

Richard Scowen

Richard Scowen was the chief designer at Lead and Light, a studio and stained glass establishment in Camden Lock in London. He subsequently set up his own private stained glass business in Cornwall.

Active for the Society 2007–present (eight stained glass panels, Shand 2007, Knapman 2009, Paris 2010, Wood 2010, Chambers *c.*2013, R. H. Taylor 2013, Tooley 2015, Adams 2017).

Leonie Seliger

Leonie Seliger studied glass and painting at Hadamar College in Germany and qualified from the University of York. She joined the Cathedral Studios Glass Workshop at Canterbury Cathedral in 1972 and became its Director and head of the stained glass conservation department in 2005. The Workshop was established in 1972 and is used for conservation work by all the major keepers of stained glass in the country.

Seliger is a Liveryman of the Company of Glaziers and Painters of Glass.

Active for the Society 2001–present (eight stained glass panels: Briscoe 2001, Jourdan 2004, Berry 2005, Beedham 2014, Bethel 2015, Palmer 2016, Wallington-Smith 2017, Mackworth-Young 2019).

W. B. Simpson

The firm of W. B. Simpson was established in 1833 by William Butler Simpson (1798–1882), mainly making painted tiles but with a sideline in ecclesiastical stained glass. His two sons, William Frederick Simpson and Edward Henry Simpson, were made partners in 1860 when the name was changed to W. B. Simpson & Sons, moving to St Martin's Lane in 1868. The founder's great-grandsons, Graham Colin Simpson and Lionel Simpson, changed the name of the firm to W. B. Simpson & Sons Ltd in 1925 on becoming directors. The Second World War provided a check to Simpsons' activities and their premises were damaged in the Blitz. However, the firm's fortunes revived after the war with rebuilding and repair work and it continues to this day in Redhill in Surrey.

Active for the Society *c.*1920–1938 (thirty-seven cartouches *c.*1920 and one confirmed stained glass panel: Townsend 1938; possibly also F. G. Brown *c.*1920, T. E. B. Brown *c.*1920, Crosby *c.*1920, Connolly *c.*1920, Osborn *c.*1920).

Francis Spear

Francis Howard Spear (1902–1979) graduated from the London County Council Central School of Arts & Crafts in 1923, to which he returned as a part-time instructor in stained glass from 1929 to 1953. He set up his own studio in Chelsea in 1946. See also Chapter 6.

Active for the Society in the 1930s (the Apothecary round window and one confirmed stained glass panel: Hepburn 1931, and probably a second, Brenchley *c.*1931).

Stella Timmins

Stella Timmins set up the Stained Glass Design studio in London NW1. Her work for six other livery companies is installed in the Guildhall Art Gallery.

Active for the Society only in 1997 (one stained glass panel: Pugh 1997).

Panels whose makers are unknown or not confirmed

F. G. Brown *c.*1920[**], T. E. B. Brown *c.*1920[**], Crosby *c.*1920[**], Connolly *c.*1920[**], Osborn *c.*1920[**],

Brenchley *c.*1931[††],

Haydon *c.*1938[@@],

Moore *c.*1967[##], Jackson 1979[##],

Cashell 1972, Thompson 1983, Whittet 1984,

Southwood 1991[ϕϕ], Neild 1991[ϕϕ], Glenister 1993[ϕϕ], Ward *c.*1995[ϕϕ].

** *possibly W. B. Simpson;* †† *probably Spear;* @@ *probably James Powell;* ## *probably Edwards;* ϕϕ *probably Goddard & Gibbs – these assumptions are based on the fact that particular stained glass makers were popular at specific times and that the Society seemed to encourage uniformity where possible: see the Clerk's letter of December 1937 quoted in Chapter 4*

APPENDIX IV

The Great Hall West Windows 1908–2020

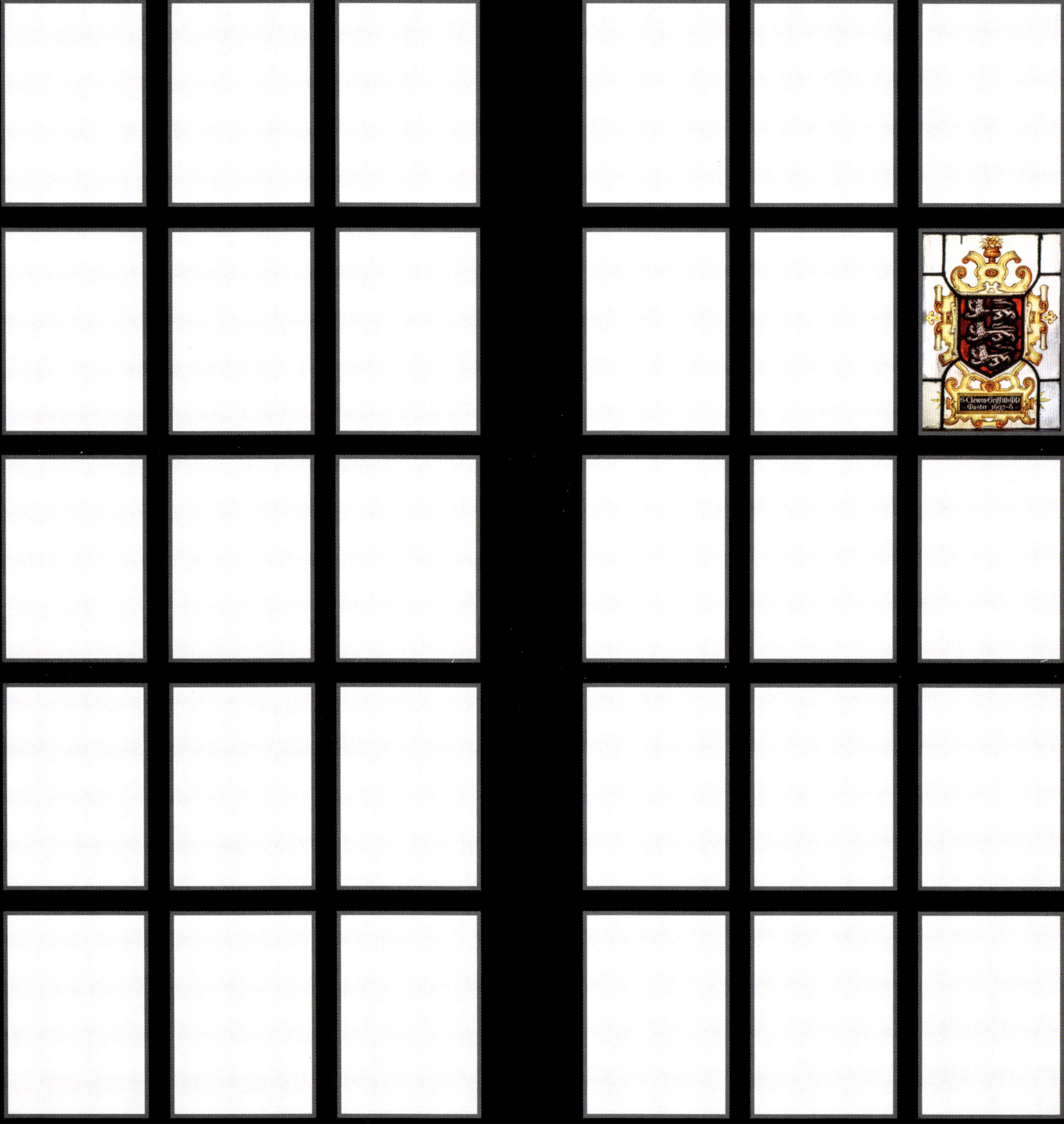

West 1

West 2

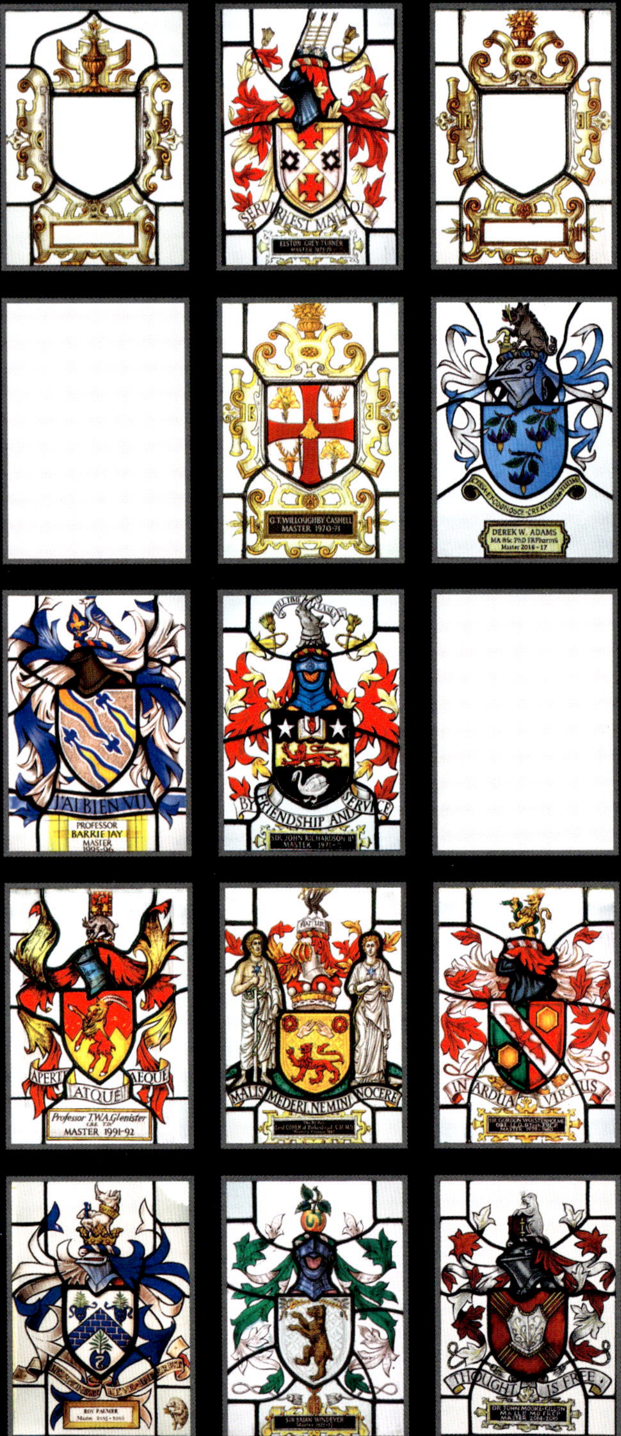

G.T. WILLOUGHBY CASHELL
MASTER 1970–71
DEREK W. ADAMS
PROFESSOR
BARRIE JAY
MASTER
J'ALBIEN VU
BY FRIENDSHIP AND SERVICE
APERTE ATQUE AEQUE
Professor T.W.A. Glenister
MASTER 1991–92
MALIS MEDERI NEMINI NOCERE
IN ARDUA VIRTUS
THOUGHT IS FREE

East 1

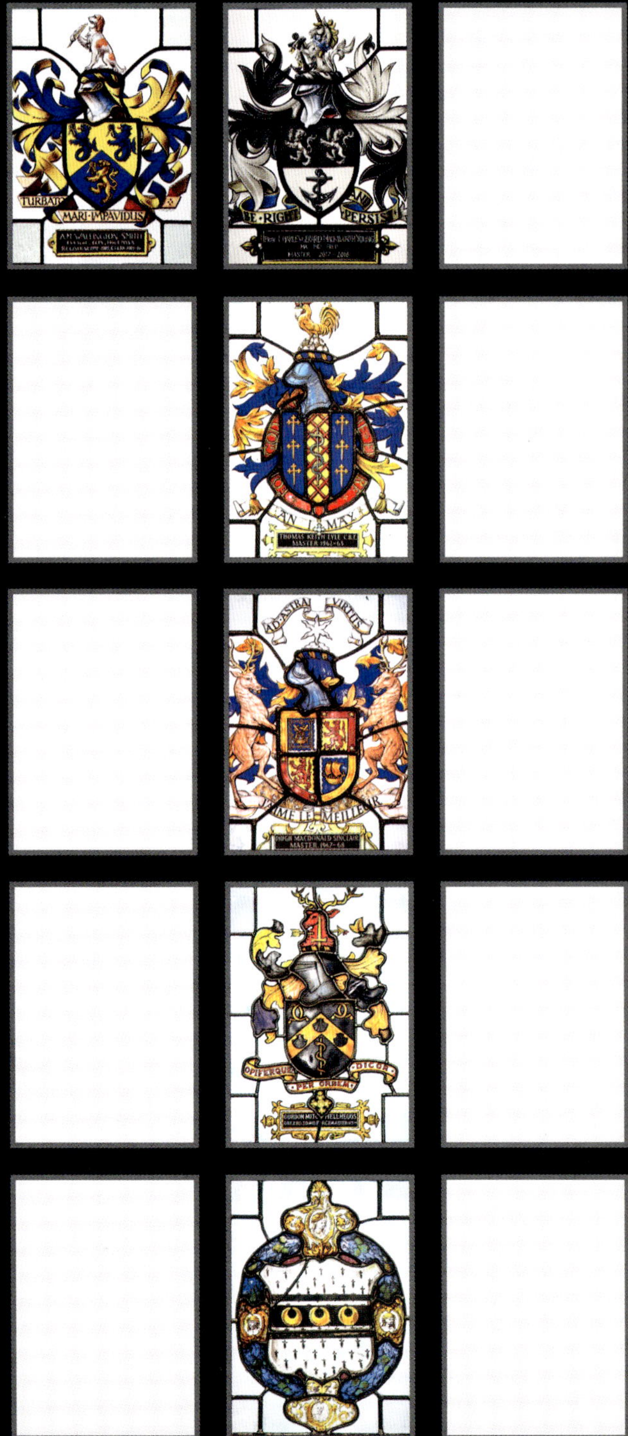

MARI IMPAVIDUS
BE RIGHT PERSIST
THOMAS KEITH LYLE C.B.E.
HUGH MACDONALD SINCLAIR

East 2

Bibliography

Primary Sources

Worshipful Society of Apothecaries Archive at Apothecaries' Hall

WSA CM	Society of Apothecaries Court Minutes
WSA PCM	Society of Apothecaries Private Court Minutes
WSA L	Society of Apothecaries Ledger
WSA CB	Society of Apothecaries Cash Book
WSA WA	Society of Apothecaries Wardens' Accounts
WSA CPGC	Society of Apothecaries Court of Proprietors and General Committee Book
WSA CCB	Society of Apothecaries Corporation Cash Book
WSA Year Book	Society of Apothecaries Year Books

James Powell and Sons Archive at the Victoria and Albert Museum Archive of Art and Design

JP&S WGOB	James Powell and Sons Window Glass Order Books
JP&S WD	James Powell and Sons Journal Window Department Books
JP&S EB	James Powell and Sons Estimate Book

Lowndes and Drury Archive at the Victoria and Albert Museum Archive of Art and Design

LS&D ADB	Lowndes and Drury Archive Day Book
LS&D AI	Lowndes and Drury Archive Invoices
LS&D AL	Lowndes and Drury Archive Ledger

Secondary Sources

Anton, C. *Sallust's Jugurthian War and Conspiracy of Cataline* (New York, 1846)

Balfour-Paul, Sir J. *Heraldry in Relation to Scottish History and Art* (Edinburgh, 1900)

Barrett, C. R. B. *The History of the Society of Apothecaries of London* (London, 1905)

Beavan, A. *The Aldermen of the City of London temp Henry III–1912* (London, 1908)

Bedini, S. A. *The Pope's Elephant* (Manchester, 1997)

Brooke-Little, J. P. *Boutell's Heraldry* (London: Frederick Warne, revised 1970)

Brooke-Little, J. P. *Boutell's Heraldry*, 9th edn (London: Frederick Warne, 1983)

Brookes, A. *The Stained Glass of Francis Spear* (Chippenham, 2012)

Burke, J. B. *A Genealogical and Heraldic History of the Extinct and Dormant Baronetcies of England* (London, 1838)

Burke, Sir B. *The General Armory of England, Scotland and Wales* (London, 1842)

Burke, Sir B. *The General Armory of England, Scotland and Wales* (London, 1884)

Burke, Sir B. *The General Armory of England, Scotland and Wales* (London, 1888)

Chauncy, Sir H. *The Historical Antiquities of Hertfordshire* (London, 1700)

Clarke, T. H. *The Rhinoceros from Dürer to Stubbs: 1515–1799* (London, 1986)

Cobbett, W. *Parliamentary History of England: Vol. 1 1066–1625* (London, 1806)

Corfe, G. *The Apothecary Ancient and Modern of the City of London* (London, 1885)

Dennis, M. *Emblems of Scotland: the Unicorn* (Heraldry Society of Scotland, 1997)

Edmondson, J. *A Complete Body of Heraldry Vol. II* (London, 1780)

Fairburn, J. *Book of Crests of the Families of Great Britain and Ireland Vol. I* (London, 1905)

Fox-Davies, A. C. *Armorial Families* (Edinburgh, 1895)

Fox-Davies, A. C. *Armorial Families* (Edinburgh: TC & EC Jack, 1905)

Fox-Davies, A. C. *The Book of Public Arms* (London: TC & EC Jack, 1915)

Fox-Davies, A. C. *Armorial Families* (London, 1929)

Hobbes, T. *Behemoth or the Long Parliament* (London, 1889)

Hunting, P. *A History of the Society of Apothecaries* (London: Society of Apothecaries, 1998)

James, R. *Pharmacopoeia Universalis or a New Universal English Dispensatory* (London, 1747)

Lavers, C. *The Natural History of Unicorns* (London, 2010)

Metcalf, W. C. (ed.) *The Visitations of Hertfordshire made by Robert Cooke 1572 & Sir Richard St George 1634: Harleian Society Vol. XXII* (London, 1886)

Nisbet, A. *A System of Heraldry Vol. I* (Edinburgh, 1816)

Oman, C. *Ayot Rectory* (London: Hodder & Stoughton, 1965)

Page, W. (ed.) *A History of the County of Hertford: Vol. 3* (London, 1912)

Ranger, T. and Slack, P. (eds) *Epidemics and Ideas: Essays on the Historical Perception of Pestilence* (Cambridge: Cambridge University Press, 1999)

Rylands, W. H. *Grantees of Arms Named in Docquets and Patents 1687–1898: Harleian Society Publications Vol. 67* (London, 1916)

Ridley, G. *Clara's Grand Tour: Travels with a Rhinoceros in Eighteenth-Century Europe* (Atlantic Books, 2004)

Robson, T. *The Cabinet of Armorial Bearings Vol. I* (Sunderland, 1830)

Rookmaaker, L. C. *Bibliography of the Rhinoceros* (Rotterdam, 1983)

Royal Commission on Historical Monuments of England survey *An Inventory of the Historical Monuments in Hertfordshire* (London: HMSO, 1910)

Salmon, N. *The History of Hertfordshire Vol. I* (London, 1728)

Salmon, W. (trans) *Pharmacopoeia Londinensis or the New London Dispensatory* (London, 1691)

Smith, P. C. *Royal Navy Ships' Badges* (Balfour, 1974)

Statham, Rev. S. P. H. *The Descent of the Family of Statham* (London: Times Book Company, 1925)

Thomas Parker, J. *The Mythic Chinese Unicorn* (Friesen Press, 2013)

Thomson, J and Hacker, L. *The Windows of Lambeth Palace Chapel: the Story of Salvation* (Blurb Inc, 2014)

Wall, C., edited by Cameron, H. C. and Underwood, E. A. *A History of the Worshipful Society of Apothecaries of London Vol. I, 1617–1815* (Oxford: Oxford University Press, 1963)

Wall, C. *The London Apothecaries, their Society and their Hall* (Harrison, 1932)

Wegeler, J. *Philosophia patrum versibus praesertim leoninis, rhythmis Germanicis adiectis* (1869)

Whittet, T. D. *Clerks, Bedels and Chemical Operators of the Society of Apothecaries* (London, 1977)

Willement, T. *The Armorial Insignia of the Kings and Queens of England from Coeval Authorities* (London, 1821)

Journals and Articles etc.

Anon 'Scientific tests fail to show rhino horn effective as medicine' *Environmentalist* 3.2 (1983): 153

Anon 'Pharmacopoeia Londinensis 1618 (the London pharmacopoeia)' *Pharmaceutical Journal* 273 (28 August 2004)

Anon 'The City Arms' *London Metropolitan Archive Research Guide 11* (2010)

Anon 'Hennell's Obituary': *Gentleman's Magazine* Vol. 18 (London, 1842)

Anon 'Questions and Answers', *Notes and Queries* 11 (London, 1855)

Amin, R. Zoological Society of London Report 2008

Chessyre, H. 'The Worshipful Society of Apothecaries' in *British Heritage* (Dec/Jan 1981/82)

Cole, F. J 'The History of Albrecht Durer's Rhinoceros in Zoological Literature', in Underwood, E. A. (ed.), *Science, Medicine and History: Essays on the Evolution of Scientific Thought and Medical Practice, Written in Honour of Charles Singer, Volume 1* (Oxford: Oxford University Press, 1953)

Dickinson, T. V. 'The Armorial Bearings of the Worshipful Society of Apothecaries', *Proceedings of the Royal Society of Medicine XXIII Part I 1929–30*

Ford, J. M. T. 'Thomas Basden, Apothecary of London', January 2017

Jackson, W. 'The Use of Unicorn Horn in Medicine', *The Pharmaceutical Journal* 273, 18/25 December 2004

Oswald, A. 'The Hall of the Worshipful Society of Apothecaries', *Country Life*, 10 October 1947

Reczek, K. 'Polychrome Gilded Coat of Arms', DBR Conservation Report, December 2016

Reczek, K. DBR Conservation Report, January 2017

Shand, W. S. 'The Pill Tile', Lecture given at Barber-Surgeons' Hall, March 2000

Tindall, I. W. L. 'Notes on 217 (London) General Hospital RAMC(V)', Paper dated 1998

Whittet, T. D. 'The 1671 Windows at Apothecaries' Hall', *Chemist & Druggist* (30 July/6 August 1983)

Sources for Appendix 1

Royal College of Physicians of London: Munk's Roll (Biographies of the Fellows of the College in twelve volumes, 1518–present; volumes 6–7 were edited by Past Master Sir Gordon Wolstenholme)

Royal College of Surgeons of England: Plarr's Lives of the Fellows (Biographies of the Fellows of the College in nine volumes, 1843–present)

Who's Who 1946–2014 (London: A & C Black)

Medical Directories 1911–98 (London: 1871–1971 J & A Churchill; 1972–94 Churchill Livingstone; 1997–8 Cartermill International)

Wall's Index Unbound directory of members of the Society of Apothecaries compiled from 1929 onwards by Past Master Cecil Wall (1869–1947)

Past Master G. T. W. Cashell's 1984 catalogue of the windows in the Great Hall

Research at the College of Arms by Court Assistant Dr Peadar O'Mordha

Notes

Introduction

1. William Cobbett, *Parliamentary History of England*, vol. 1 1066–1625 (London, 1806), p. 1503.

Chapter 1

1. C. R. B. Barrett, *The History of the Society of Apothecaries of London* (London: Elliot Stock, 1905), p. 276.
2. The Oath of Hippocrates of Kos.
3. T. Ranger and P. Slack (eds), *Epidemics and Ideas: Essays on the Historical Perception of Pestilence* (Cambridge University Press, 1999), p. 61.
4. Ibid., p. 46.
5. Ibid., p. 58.
6. Ibid., p. 61.
7. Ibid., p. 71.
8. Personal communication, Bryony Hudson, August 2017.
9. J. Thomas Parker, *The Mythic Chinese Unicorn* (Fort St, Victoria, BC: Friesen Press, 2013), p. 93.
10. Ibid., p. 185.
11. M. Dennis, *Emblems of Scotland: The Unicorn* (The Heraldry Society of Scotland, 1997), p. 27.
12. C. Lavers, *The Natural History of Unicorns* (London, 2010), p. 50.
13. Dennis, *Emblems of Scotland: The Unicorn*, p. 27.
14. Sir James Balfour-Paul, *Heraldry in Relation to Scottish History and Art* (Edinburgh: David Douglas, 1900), p. 95.
15. J. P. Brooke-Little, *Boutell's Heraldry* (London: Frederick Warne, 1970), p. 154.
16. Ibid., p. 157.
17. *Pharmacopoeia Londinensis* 1618 (the London pharmacopoeia), Pharmaceutical Journal, Vol. 273, 28 August 2004, p. 229.
18. W. Salmon (trans), *Pharmacopoeia Londinensis or the New London Dispensatory* (London, 1691).
19. R. James, *Pharmacopoeia Universalis or a New Universal English Dispensatory* (London, 1747).
20. I am grateful to Past Master Nicholas Wood for making available to me his paper on uses of the rhinoceros horn and on which this paragraph is based.
21. W. Jackson, 'The Use of Unicorn Horn in Medicine', *The Pharmaceutical Journal*, Vol. 273, 18 December 2004, pp. 925–27.
22. 'Scientific tests fail to show rhino horn effective as medicine', *Environmentalist*, Vol. 3(2), 1983, p. 153 (Hoffman-LaRoche 1980 tests on behalf of World Wildlife Fund).
23. R. Amin, Zoological Society of London report, 2008.
24. http://voices.nationalgeographic.com/2010/07/07/rhino_horn_and_traditional_chinese_medicine_facts/ accessed 28 June 2017.
25. G. Ridley, *Clara's Grand Tour: Travels with a Rhinoceros in Eighteenth-Century Europe* (Atlantic Books, 2004).
26. S. A. Bedini, *The Pope's Elephant* (Manchester: *Carcanet Press*, 1997), p. 128.
27. L. C. Rookmaaker, *Bibliography of the Rhinoceros* (Rotterdam, 1983), p. 247.
28. Bedini, *The Pope's Elephant*, p. 121.
29. F. J. Cole, 'The History of Albrecht Dürer's Rhinoceros in Zoological Literature' in *Science, Medicine and History*, Vol. I (Oxford University Press, 1953), pp. 339–40.
30. Ridley, *Clara's Grand Tour*.
31. T. H. Clarke, *The Rhinoceros from Dürer to Stubbs 1515–1799* (London, 1986), p. 20.
32. Cole, 'The History of Albrecht Dürer's Rhinoceros in Zoological Literature', pp. 339–40.
33. Bedini, *The Pope's Elephant*, p. 121.
34. Cole, 'The History of Albrecht Dürer's Rhinoceros in Zoological Literature', pp. 339–40.

Chapter 2

1. Vexillology is the study of flags, their history, symbolism and usage.
2. C. R. B. Barrett, *The History of the Society of Apothecaries of London* (London: Elliot Stock, 1905), p. 139.
3. Ibid., p. 144.
4. WSA Private Court Minute 282, 1 July 1988.
5. WSA Private Court Minute 110, 12 January 2005.
6. Barrett, *History of the Society of Apothecaries of London*, pp. 82 and 269.
7. Ibid., p. 272.
8. Ibid., p. 156.
9. DBR Conservation Report, January 2017.
10. Barrett, *History of the Society of Apothecaries of London*, p. 184.
11. WSA Year Books 1958–59 and 1959–60.
12. http://www.farebrother.com/about/history accessed 29 September 2018.
13. C. Wall, *The London Apothecaries, their Society and their Hall* (Harrison, 1932), p. 25.
14. 'Herbarising expeditions also known as simpling days were botanical excursions by barge for apprentices and others to collect and study medicinal plants at the Hall. Up to six expeditions were held annually between 1620–1813 and in those days uncatalogued and rare plants were to be found growing in open spaces within reach of the City.' See P. Hunting, *A History of the Society of Apothecaries*, (London, 1998), p. 41.
15. Personal communication, Archivist Company of Joiners & Ceilers, 27 March 2019.
16. Personal communication, Asst Archivist Company of Mercers, 29 March 2019.
17. WSA Archive File 71.
18. C. Wall, *'The Barges and the Banners of the Society of Apothecaries of London'* WSA Year Book 1937–38 p viii.
19. WSA Private Court Minute 246, June 1989.
20. WSA Archive File 71.
21. Barrett, *History of the Society of Apothecaries of London*, p. 161.
22. WSA Archive File 71.
23. C. Wall, 'The Barges and the Banners of the Society of Apothecaries of London', p. iii.
24. C. Wall, *History of the Worshipful Society of Apothecaries of London, Vol. I 1617–1815*, edited by H. C. Cameron and E. A. Underwood (Oxford: Oxford University Press, 1963), p. 141.
25. Wall, 'The Barges and the Banners of the Society of Apothecaries of London', p. ix.
26. Court Minute, 18 August 1797.
27. Barrett, *History of the Society of Apothecaries of London*, p. 145.
28. WSA Private Court Minutes, December 2012 and Sustentation Committee Minutes, January 1988.
29. WSA Court Minute 68, 19 March 2012.

Chapter 3

1. C. R. B. Barrett, *The History of the Society of Apothecaries of London* (London: Elliot Stock, 1905), p. 142.
2. P. Hunting, *A History of the Society of Apothecaries* (London, 1998), p. 102.
3. Barrett, *The History of the Society of Apothecaries of London*, pp. 140–41.
4. WSA 1947 inventory of furniture and silver.
5. WSA Court Minute, June 1941, p. 204.
6. WSA Year Book 1962–63.
7. Hunting, *A History of the Society of Apothecaries*, p. 122.
8. WSA Private Court Minute 2, September 1947.
9. WSA Court Minute 62, March 1987.
10. WSA Private Court Minute 240; May 1988.
11. WSA Private Court Minute 290, July 1988; and Minute 43, October 1988.
12. WSA Court Minute 13, October 1997.
13. WSA Private Court Minute 225, May 2007.
14. WSA Court Minute 4, October 2015.
15. WSA Year Book 1968–69.
16. WSA Court Minute 7, October 2003.
17. WSA Court Minute 6, October 1989.
18. I. W. L. Tindall, *Notes on 217 (London) General Hospital RAMC(V)*, 1998.
19. WSA Private Court Minute 100, January 2012.
20. WSA Private Court Minute 18, September 1994.
21. A pill masser is a machine that mixes the ingredients for pills.

22. W. S. Shand, 'The Pill Tile', lecture given at Barber-Surgeons' Hall, March 2000.
23. WSA Private Court Minute 226, 1 April 1987.
24. WSA Court Minute 4, 29 October 2007.
25. Barrett, *The History of the Society of Apothecaries of London*, p. 157.

Chapter 4

1. C. R. B. Barrett, *The History of the Society of Apothecaries of London* (London: Elliot Stock, 1905), frontispiece and p. 287.
2. James Powell & Sons (JP&S) *Window Glass Order Book* (1904–1906), AAD 1/17 – 1977, p. 313.
3. JP&S *Journal Window Department (1905–1910)* AAD 1/65 – 1977, p. 49.
4. JP&S *Window Glass Order Book (1904–1906)* AAD 1/17 – 1977, p. 392.
5. JP&S *Journal Window Department (1905–1910)* AAD 1/65 – 1977, p. 97.
6. JP&S *Window Glass Order Book (1906–1909)* AAD 1/18 – 1977, p. 259.
7. WSA File 44, *The Builder*, 7 Dec 1917.
8. JP&S *Window Glass Order Book (1906–1909)* AAD 1/18 – 1977, p. 259.
9. JP&S *Journal Window Department (1905–1910)* AAD 1/65 – 1977, p. 215.
10. WSA File 44.
11. WSA C&PCM (1897–1913) pp. 359, 408, 410, 447 and 500.
12. WSA *Ledger (1918–1925)* p. 220.
13. WSA File 209.
14. WSA File 209.
15. WSA File 209.
16. WSA File 209.
17. WSA File 209.
18. JP&S *Journal Window Department (1939–1951)* AAD 1/73 – 1977, pp. 87, 107 and 252.
19. JP&S *Journal Window department (1934–1939)* AAD 1/73 – 1977, p. 347.
20. WSA *Ledger (1936–1943)*, p. 156.
21. WSA File 209.
22. WSA File 209, Carl Edwards folder.
23. WSA File 209, Carl Edwards folder.
24. WSA File 209, Carl Edwards folder.
25. WSA C&CPM (1938–1948), p. 184.
26. JP&S *Journal Window Department (1939–1951)* AAD 1/73 1977, p. 82.
27. WSA *Ledger (1936–1943)*, p. 185.
28. WSA C&PCM (1938–1948); p. 326.
29. WSA File 71.
30. WSA C&PCM (1938–1948); p. 328.
31. WSA File 71.
32. WSA C&PCM (1938–1948); p. 458.
33. JP&S *Estimate Book (1937–1948)* AAD 1/46 – 1977, pp. 175 and 176.
34. JP&S *Journal Window Department (1939–1951)* AAD 1/73 – 1977, p. 153.
35. WSA *Ledger (1943–1947)*, p. 75.
36. WSA C&PCM (Current volume), 10 March 2009, item 178.

Chapter 5

1. WSA *Accounts (1669–1694)*, 5 September 1670, pages unnumbered.
2. WSA *Wardens Accounts (1668–1691)*, 5 September 1670; 1671, exact date not recorded, pages unnumbered.
3. C. R. B. Barrett, *The History of the Society of Apothecaries of London* (London: Elliot Stock, 1905), pp. 273 and 285.
4. WSA C&PCM (1926–38) 1928: 14 February, p. 130; 6 March, p. 136; 8 May, p. 145.
5. WSA File 303, Reginald Cecil Wall papers.
6. WSA File 44, *The Builder.*
7. JP&S *Journal Window Department (1939–1951)* AAD 1/73.1977, p. 153.
8. *The Civil Engineer & Architect's Journal* Vol 1 (1838), p. 156. Description of how the panel 'Tournament of the Field of Cloth of Gold' was painted with enamels by Thomas Wilmshurst in 1830: 'Painted on Newcastle crown glass (not too thick or it will fly in firing) first covered in a light neutral tint for ground outline drawn on reverse side with Indian ink fired lightly not to melt. Glass removed and placed on a large sheet of plate glass supported by a frame easel against strong light "the stains are then put in" with the lights and shadows in enamels strengthened several times, fired each time "until a proper depth is obtained".'
9. WSA *Wardens Accounts (1668–1691)* 1670/71, Edward Pilkington, Renter Warden; 1671/72 William Butler, Renter Warden. Pages unnumbered.
10. Ibid.
11. T. Willement, *The Armorial Insignia of the Kings and Queens of England from Coeval Authorities* (London, 1821), plate xxiv.
12. Personal communication, Mr Geoffrey Lane, Librarian of the British Society of Master Glass Painters.
13. WSA Job Weale's Treasurer's accounts, 9 August 1633. Pages unnumbered.
14. London Metropolitan Archives Research Guide 11, *The City Arms*, 2010.
15. Barrett, *The History of the Society of Apothecaries*, p. 67.
16. According to Alfred Beavan in *The Aldermen of the City of London temp Henry III–1912* (London, 1908), pp. 75–119, Lorymer's will is dated 8 November 1666 and proved 16 January 1667, but most authorities date his death to 1663.
17. WSA C&PCM (1651–80), p. 192.
18. Sir Bernard Burke, *The General Armory of England, Scotland and Wales* (London, 1884), p. 626.
19. Ibid., p. 622.
20. J. Edmondson, *Complete Body of Heraldry Vol II* (London, 1780), pages unnumbered.
21. Sir Bernard Burke, *The General Armory of England, Scotland and Wales* (London, 1842), pages unnumbered.
22. W. H. Rylands, *Grantees of Arms Named in Docquets and Patents 1687–1898*, Harleian Society Publications Vol. 67 (London, 1916), p. 291.
23. Coll. Arms Gr 32.225, granted on 15 February 1821 to James-Rivington Wheeler Esq. of Gloucester Place, Marylebone, Middlesex and of Piggotts, Hertfordshire; to him and his descendants and to the descendants of his father, Thomas Wheeler gent. deceased, late of the City of London.
24. *The Chemist and Druggist*, 30 Jul 1983 pp. 196–97 and 6 August 1983, pp. 224, 226, 229.
25. Personal communication, Caroline and Tony Benyon, January 2020.
26. *Hennell's Obituary: Gentleman's Magazine* Vol. 18 (London, 1842), pages unnumbered.
27. T. D. Whittet, *Clerks, Bedels and Chemical Operators of the Society of Apothecaries* (London, 1977), p. 69.
28. G. Corfe, *The Apothecary Ancient and Modern of the City of London* (London, 1885).
29. Personal communication, Dr Henry Oakeley, Garden Fellow of the Royal College of Physicians of London.
30. Ibid.
31. A. Oswald, 'The Hall of the Worshipful Society of Apothecaries', *Country Life*, 10 October 1947: pp. 726–29.
32. WSA *Court of Proprietors and General Committee Book 1822–1838*, 10 June 1823. Pages unnumbered.
33. WSA Year Book 1960–61.
34. JP&S *Journal Window Department 1939–1951* AAD 1/73.1977, p. 82.
35. WSA *Ledger (1936–43)* 15 October 1941, p. 185.
36. WSA C&PCM (1938–48) pp. 326, 328 and 458.
37. JP&S *Journal Window Department (1939–1951)* AAD 1/73.1977, p. 153.
38. JP&S *Estimate Book (1937–48)* AAD 1/46.1977 pp. 175–76.
39. WSA *Ledger (1943–47)*, p. 75.
40. JP&S *Window Glass Order Book (1948–55)* AAD 1/3.1977, p. 158.
41. JP&S *Journal Window Department (1939–51)* AAD 1/73.1977, p. 328.
42. WSA *Corporation Cash Book (1932–53)*, p. 181.

Chapter 6

1. Francis Spear archive in the Lowndes & Drury archive.
2. WSA C&PCM (1926–38), p. 327.
3. Lowndes & Drury (LS&D) *ADB Day Book (1931–1938)*, AAD/2008/1/61, p. 10.
4. LS&D *AI Invoices (1930–1935)*, AAD/2008/1/48, p. 253.
5. LS&D *AL Ledger (1926–1933)*, AAD/2008/1/15, p. 140.
6. LS&D *AI Invoices (1930–1935)*, AAD/2008/1/48, p. 253.
7. WSA *Ledger (1928–1935)*, File 42, p. 233.
8. WSA *Cash Book (1914–1931)*, File 121, p. 194.
9. A. Malik, F. Afaq, S. Sarfaraz, D.N. Syed, H. Mukhtar, 'Pomegranate Fruit Juice for Chemoprevention and Chemotherapy of Prostate Cancer', *Proceedings of the National Academy of Sciences of the United States of America*, 11 October 2005, 102 (41), pp. 14813-8.

Chapter 7

1. From the lecture *'The Beauty of Stained Glass'* given by Carl Edwards to the Royal Society of Arts in March 1955. Reproduced from the *Journal of the British Society of Master Glass-Painters*, Vol XX No 1 1955-56, p. 50. Reproduced by kind permission of the Chairman,

Caroline Benyon, daughter of Carl Edwards.
2. J. Thomson and L. Hacker, *The Windows of Lambeth Palace Chapel: the Story of Salvation* (Blurb Inc, 2014).
3. WSA 350th Anniversary papers, File 45, Folder 4
4. Ibid.
5. J. P. Brooke-Little, *Boutell's Heraldry* (London: F. Warne, revised 1983).
6. A. C. Fox-Davies, *The Book of Public Arms* (London: TC & EC Jack, 1915).
7. *Questions and Answers, Notes and Queries*, Vol XI (London: G. Bell, 1855), p. 350.

Chapter 8

1. T. Hobbes, *Behemoth or the Long Parliament* (London, 1889), p. 202.
2. C. Wall, *A History of the Worshipful Society of Apothecaries of London Vol I 1617–1815*, edited by H. C. Cameron and E. A. Underwood (Oxford: Oxford University Press, 1963), ch. 7.
3. C. Wall, *Notes on Contemporary Events 1610–1670* (pamphlet), edited by J. M. T. Ford, 2018.
4. The three lions passant of the English Arms are often confusingly called leopards. 'Leopard' was a technical heraldic distinction as the heraldic lion was originally found in only one attitude – rampant. As heraldry spread, new attitudes were needed and the early heralds considered walking lions to behave like a leopard, hence the lion-leopardé or leopard for a lion passant. As with all heraldic animals, the leopard carried some symbolic meaning; it was thought to be the result of an adulterous union between a lion and a mythical beast called a 'pard' (thus, leo-pard). Believed to be incapable of reproducing, leopards were sometimes used for someone born of adultery, or unable to have children – a senior clergyman for example. The English Royal Arms included the three lions from the time of Richard I (r.1189–99) onwards. See J. P. Brooke-Little, *Boutel's Heraldry* (London, 1983), p. 65.
5. C. R. B. Barrett, *The History of the Society of Apothecaries of London* (London: Elliot Stock, 1905), p. 96.
6. WSA Court Minute, 24 October 1990; Private Court Minute 80, November 1990; Sustentation Committee Minute, 7 June 1991.
7. WSA Sustentation Committee Minutes, December 1987, paragraph 13.
8. Barrett, *The History of the Society of Apothecaries of London*, p. 280.
9. WSA Court Minute 3, October 2001.
10. WSA Private Court Minute 66, August 2002.
11. WSA Private Court Minute 13, October 2002.
12. Barrett, *The History of the Society of Apothecaries of London*, p. 149.
13. J. M. T. Ford, 'Thomas Basden, Apothecary of London', Apothecaries' Hall paper, January 2017.

Chapter 9

1. W. Page (ed.), Parishes: Ayot St. Lawrence or Great Ayot, in A History of the County of Hertford: Volume 3 (London, 1912), pp. 59–63. British History Online. http://www.british-history.ac.uk/vch/herts/vol3/pp59–63 accessed 30 January 2019.
2. Sir Henry Chauncy, The Historical Antiquities of Hertfordshire (London, 1700), pp. 322–25.
3. http://www.bodley.ox.ac.uk/dept/scwmss/wmss/online/1500-1900/steele/steele.html accessed 27 February 2018.
4. N. Salmon, The History of Hertfordshire Vol. I (London, 1728), p. 206.
5. W. C. Metcalf (ed.), The Visitations of Hertfordshire made by Robert Cooke 1572, Harliean Society Vol. XXII (London, 1886), p. 130.
6. Sir J. B. Burke, A Genealogical and Heraldic History of the Extinct and Dormant Baronetcies of England (London, 1838), p. 331.
7. Page, *Parishes*, pp. 59–63.
8. Carola Oman, *Ayot Rectory* (London: Hodder and Stoughton Ltd, 1965), pp. 140–41.
9. Royal Commission on Historical Monuments (England), *An Inventory of the Historical Monuments in Hertfordshire* (London, 1910), pp. 42–43. *British History Online* http://www.british-history.ac.uk/rchme/herts/pp42–43 accessed 30 January 2019.
10. Personal communication, Tony Benyon.
11. Personal account of Liveryman Dr Peter Francis White.
12. WSA Archive File 41, Folder 1.
13. Page, *Parishes*, pp. 59-63.
14. Sir J. B. Burke, *The General Armory of England, Scotland, Ireland and Wales* (London, 1884), p. 80.
15. Ibid., p. 49.
16. Burke, *A Genealogical and Heraldic History*, p. 486.
17. J.P. Brooke-Little, *Boutell's Heraldry*, 9th edn (London, 1983), pp. 57, 114 and 118.
18. Ibid., pp. 183–86.
19. WSA Archive File 41, Folder 1.
20. WSA Archive File 41, Folder 1.

Chapter 10

1. C. R. B. Barrett, *The History of the Society of Apothecaries* (London: Elliot Stock, 1905), p. 276.
2. WSA File 44, 'The Society of the Art and Mistery of Apothecaries of London', *The Builder*, 7 December 1917.
3. James Powell & Sons, *Journal Window Department (1939–1951)*, AAD/1/73 1977, p. 82.
4. Personal communication, Dr Jasmine Allen.
5. C. Anthon, *Sallust's Jugurthian War and Conspiracy of Cataline* (New York, 1846), ch. 10.
6. J. Wegeler, *Philosophia patrum versibus praesertim leoninis, rhythmis Germanicis adiectis* (1869), p. 61.
7. WSA Private Court Minute 181, March 1985.
8. Barrett, *History of the Society of Apothecaries*, p. 274.
9. G. Corfe, *The Apothecary Ancient and Modern of the City of London* (London, 1885), p. 35.

Chapter 11

1. WSA Year Book 1960–61.
2. P.C. Smith, *Royal Navy Ships' Badges* (Balfour, 1974), p. 10.
3. https://history.rcplondon.ac.uk/blog/status-symbols-rcp-coat-arms accessed 25 September 2018.
4. WSA Year Book 1959–60.
5. Private Court Minute 193, March 1988.
6. P. Hunting, *A History of the Society of Apothecaries* (London, 1998), p. 135.
7. C. R. B. Barrett, *The History of the Society of Apothecaries of London* (London: Elliot Stock, 1905), p. 246.
8. Hunting, *A History of the Society of Apothecaries*, p. 136.
9. WSA Year Book 1958–59.
10. Dictionary of National Biography, 1885–1900, Volume 23.
11. WSA File 209, letter 30 June 1977.
12. Barrett, *The History of the Society of Apothecaries of London*, p. 166.
13. Ibid., p. 204.
14. http://munksroll.rcplondon.ac.uk/Biography/Details/4888 accessed 25 September 2018.
15. WSA Year Book 1948–49.

Appendix I

1. Burke Sir Bernard, *General Armory of England, Scotland and Wales* (London, 1884), p. 119.
2. A. C. Fox-Davies, *Armorial Families* (London, 1929), p. 139.
3. Robson T, *The Cabinet of Armorial Bearings Vol I* (Sunderland, 1830), p. 376; J. Fairburn, *Book of Crests of the Families of Great Britain and Ireland Vol I* (London, 1905), p. 99.
4. WSA, *Minutes of the Future Activities Cttee*, 7 Mar 1980 para 13.
5. Burke, *General Armory*, p. 221; Fox-Davies, *Armorial Families*, p. 416.
6. Burke, *General Armory*, p. 270.
7. http://www.glenister.org/items/glenArms3grant.asp accessed January 2020.
8. Burke, *General Armory*, p. 472.
9. A. C. Fox-Davies, *Armorial Families* (Ulster Office, 1905), p. 644.
10. Fox-Davies, *Armorial Families* (London, 1929) p. 921.
11. Fox-Davies, *Armorial Families* (Edinburgh, 1905), p. 736; Fox-Davies, *Armorial Families*, Vol. II: p. 1046; W. H. Rylands, *Grantees of Arms Named in Docquets and Patents 1687–1898*, Harleian Society Publications Vol. 67 (London, 1916), p. 202.
12. Burke, *General Armory*, de Lyle (Lord Lyle), p. 632; A. Nisbet, *A System of Heraldry Vol I* (Edinburgh, 1816), p. 215.
13. Burke, *General Armory*, p. 1152.
14. Ibid., p. 691.
15. Ibid., p. 707.
16. Ibid., p. 764.
17. Rev S. P. H. Statham, *The Descent of the Family of Statham* (London: Times Book Company, 1925).
18. Statham, *The Descent of the Family of Statham*.
19. Burke, *General Armory*, p. 1011.
20. Burke, *General Armory* (London, 1888), p. 1023; Burke, *Landed Gentry* (London, 1939), p. 2267.
21. Burke, *General Armory*, p. 1062.
22. https://www.americanheraldry.org/heraldry-in-the-usa/roll-of-early-american-Arms/P80 accessed January 2020: Burke, *General Armory*, p. 1111.
23. J. Foster, *Grantees of Arms named in Docquets and Packets between the Years 1687–1898 Vol K–Z* (London, 1917), p. 396.

Picture Credits

The Heraldry of the Society

1.1 Brian Ellis
1.2 Ian Lomas
1.3 The Elisha Whittelsey Collection, The Elisha Whittelsey Fund, 1949
1.4 Virgil Solis/public domain
1.5 Dmitry Bogdanov/CC BY
1.6 drawing from Pierre Pomet's 1737 *A Compleat History of drugs* page 284
1.7 Kim Traynor/CC BY-SA
1.8 WSA
1.9 © The Trustees of the British Museum
1.10 Hans Burgkmair the Elder/public domain

Principal Displays of the Society's Arms

2.1, 2.6, 2.8a, 2.9, 2.13, 2.15, 2.19 Brian Ellis
2.2 © The Trustees of the British Museum
2.3 Wellcome Collection/CC BY
2.4 Heritage Image Partnership Ltd/Alamy Stock Photo
2.7 © The Trustees of the British Museum
2.5, 2.8b, 2.10–2.12, 2.14, 2.16–2.18 WSA
2.20 sketches by C.R.B. Barrett in his 1905 *History of the Society of Apothecaries of London* pages xxxix & 287

Other Uses of the Society's Arms

3.1–3.3, 3.6, 3.8, 3.13, 3.15, 3.20, 3.25–3.26, 3.31–3.33 WSA
3.4–3.5, 3.9, 3.12, 3.14, 3.16–3.17, 3.29, 3.40 Ian Lomas
3.7 sketch by C.R.B. Barrett in his 1905 *History of the Society of Apothecaries of London* page 292
3.10 Richard Goddard
3.11 Michael Farthing
3.18–3.19, 3.21–3.24, 3.27–3.28, 3.30, 3.34–3.39 Brian Ellis

Armorial Glass in the Great Hall

4.1–4.2 Ian Lomas
4.3–4.7, 4.14–4.15, 4.18–4.19, 4.22–4.24 Brian Ellis
4.8–4.9 V&A, Archive of Art and Design, AAD/1977/1, James Powell & Sons (Whitefriars Ltd)
4.10, 4.12–4.13, 4.16, 4.20–4.21 WSA
4.11 *The Builder* 7 Dec 1917
4.17 by kind permission of Country Life Picture Library

The Great Staircase Windows

5.1, 5.4, 5.6 WSA
5.3, 5.5 sketches by C.R.B. Barrett in his 1905 *History of the Society of Apothecaries of London* pages 85 & 273
5.7 *The Builder* 7 Dec 1917
5.8–5.9, 5.13–5.17, 5.19 Brian Ellis
5.10–5.11 Ian Lomas
5.12 © The Society of Antiquaries of London
5.20 by kind permission of Country Life Picture Library

'The Apothecary' Window in the Great Hall

Spear, 6.3–6.4, 6.9 by kind permission of Alan Brooks
6.1–6.2, 6.5–6.7 William Shand
6.8 WSA

Whitefriars in Black Friars: Carl Edwards and his legacy at Apothecaries' Hall

Edwards, 7.1–7.3, 7.5 by kind permission of Caroline Benyon
7.4, 7.16 WSA
7.6–7.11, 7.14–7.15, 7.17 Brian Ellis
7.12–7.13 Ian Lomas

Royal Heraldry at the Hall

8.1 Kaihsu/public domain
8.2 Sodacan/CC BY-SA
8.3–8.4, 8.6 Brian Ellis
8.5 WSA
8.7 Ian Lomas
8.8 Photo: Dreamstime; & by kind permission of the Vicar of St Dunstan's, Rev Ann Pollington
8.9 Sodacan/CC BY-SA

The Bristow Panel in the Great Hall

9.1 Brian Ellis
9.2 sketch from William Page's 1912 *A History of the County of Hertford*: Volume 3 page 63
9.3 William Shand
9.4 The Bodleian Libraries, the University of Oxford: MS. Gough Herts. 4, fol. 1 66v
9.5–9.8 William Shand: by kind permission of the Priest-in-charge, St Peter & St Paul, Kimpton with St Lawrence, Ayot St Lawrence, the Rev Linda Williams

The Landing and Library Windows and the Missing Panel

10.1, 10.4–10.5 Brian Ellis
10.2–10.3, 10.6–10.7 WSA

Heraldic Strays

11.1–11.2 Brian Ellis
11.3 WSA
11.4–11.11 Ian Lomas
11.12 Ian @ Cornish churches
11.13 frontispiece to Philip Miller's 1730 *Catalogus Plantarum Officialium quae in Horto Botanico Chelseyano aluntur*
11.14–11.15 WSA
11.16 Philip Beddows
11.17 Art Directors & TRIP/Alamy Stock Photo
11.18 by kind permission of Bradford Museums & Galleries
11.19 by kind permission of Christ's Hospital School

Description and Explanation of the Stained Glass Panels in the Great Hall

Pages 165, 167–208, 210–212, 214–217, 219–235, 237–242 Brian Ellis
Pages 166, 209, 213, 236 Ian Lomas
Page 218 WSA

Index

A

B

C

D

E

F

G

H

I

J

K

L

M

N

O

P

T

U

V

W

Y

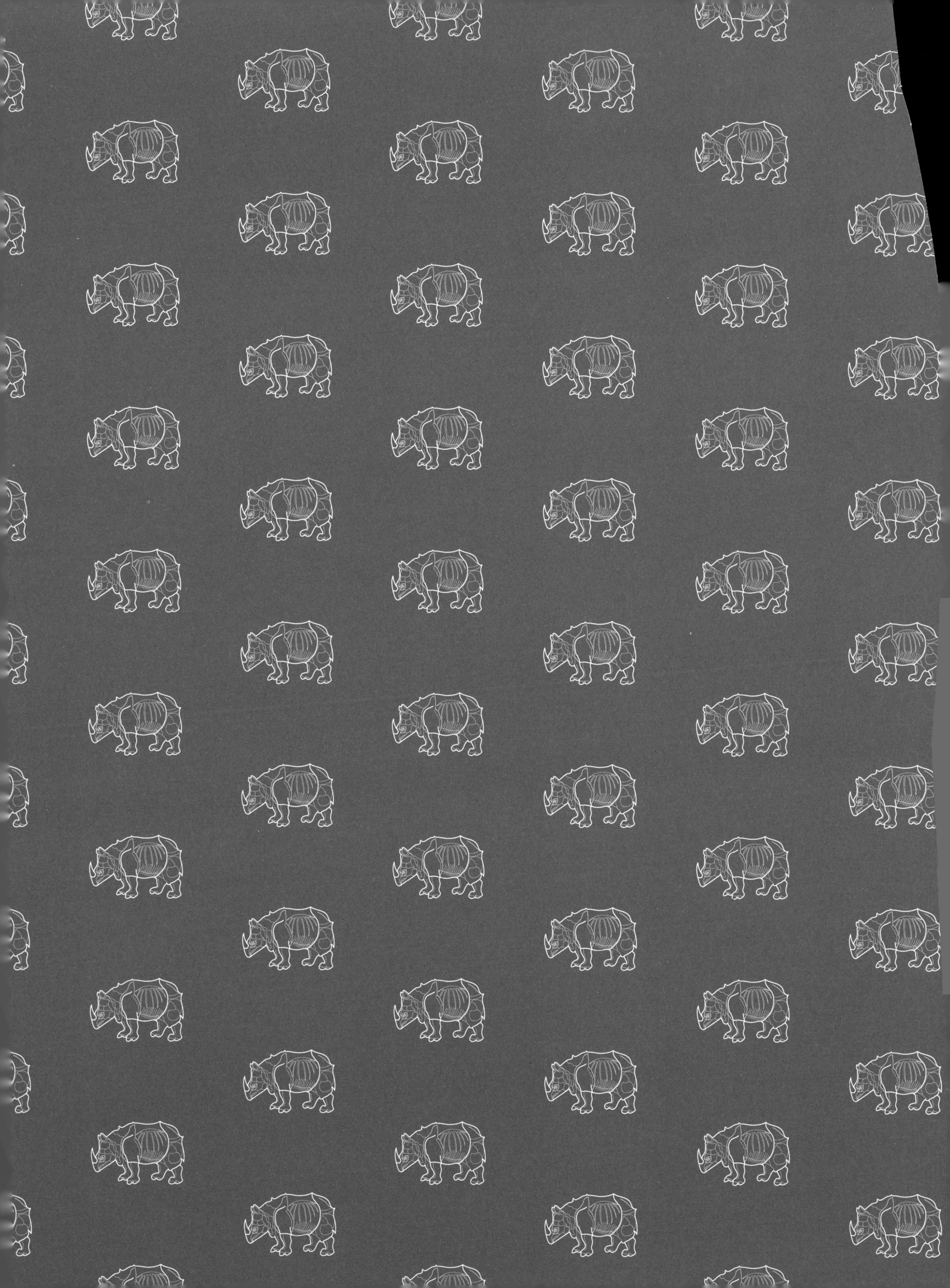